GW01279146

PLACENTAL FUNCTION AND FETAL NUTRITION

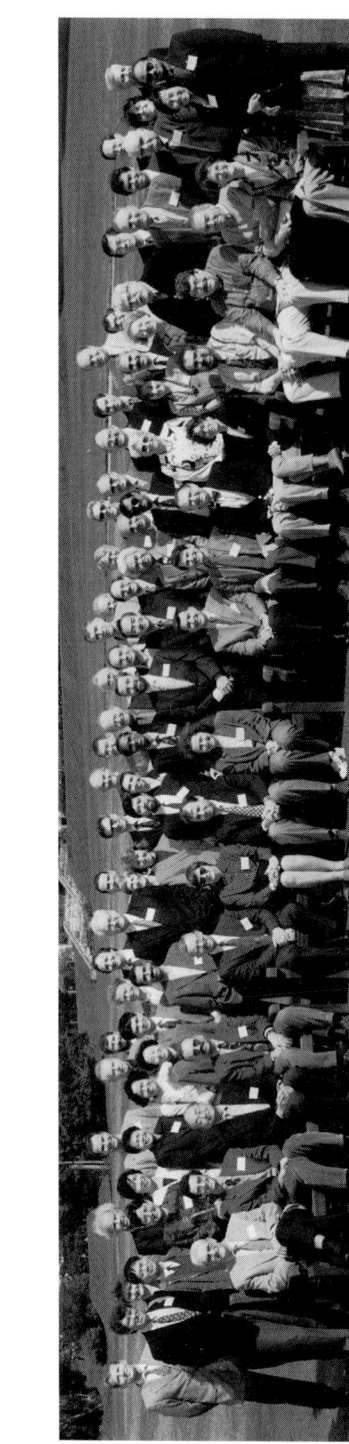

The 39th Nestlé Nutrition Workshop, Placental Function and Fetal Nutrition, was held in Ashdown Park, Sussex, England, in the spring of 1996.

Behind: M. Kohler, D. Briggs, A. Staudach, T. Schwenzer, E. Friedrich, K. Nicolaides, P. Finne, P. Soothill, M. Maganaris, N. Lashneva (+ in front), C. Costalos, K. Page (+ in front), N.M. Shilina, A. Fournie, J. Dobbing, P. Aggett, J. Girard, J. Milliez, D. Candy, M. Mikati, U. Preysch, S.K. Nassar, C. Sibley, H. Schneider, T. Chard, K. Godfrey, A. Jensen, A.A. Pourvaghar, G. Csakany, M.S.W. Lum, A.A. Yahava, G.S.H. Yeo, A. Varvarigou, R. Claydon.
1st Row: S. Devane, Qi Pei Liu, Y. Ma, A. Shen, G. Dimaano, Z. Wang, S. Liu, P. Lumbiganon, M. El-Essa, J. Gadzinowski, L. Grahnquist, H.Z. Abidin, S. Nalliah, P. Steenhout, B. Hadibroto, Z.T. Tjaniago, K. Taher, L. Cedard, C. Williams, P. Duc-Goiran, A. Marini, G. Meschia, N. Mumjiev, S. Achanna, S. Sethavanich.
Seated: E. Herrera, H. Valensise, E.S. Ogata, M.J. Soares, R.V. Anthony, D.M. Campbell, M.T. Clandinin, J.A. Owens, F. Haschke, R.D.H. Boyd, F.C. Battaglia, A.M. Marconi, F. Talamantes, M.J. Rennie, G. Pardi, R. Huch.

Nestlé Nutrition Workshop Series
Volume 39

PLACENTAL FUNCTION AND FETAL NUTRITION

Editor

Frederick C. Battaglia
University of Colorado
Health Sciences Center
Department of Pediatrics
Denver, Colorado, U.S.A.

NESTLÉ NUTRITION SERVICES

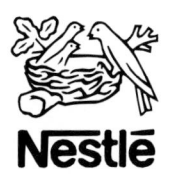

LIPPINCOTT–RAVEN ■ PHILADELPHIA–NEW YORK

Acquisitions Editor: Joyce-Rachel John
Manufacturing Manager: Dennis Teston
Production Manager: Lawrence Bernstein
Production Editor: Jeffrey Gruenglas
Indexer: Victoria Boyle
Compositor: Maryland Composition
Printer: Quebecor-Kingsport

Nestec Ltd., 55 Avenue Nestlé, CH-1800 Vevey, Switzerland
Lippincott-Raven Publishers, 227 East Washington Square,
Philadelphia, Pennsylvania 19106

© 1997, by Nestec Ltd. and Lippincott-Raven Publishers. All rights reserved. This book is protected by copyright. No part of it may be reproduced, stored in a retrieval system, or transmitted, in any form or by any means—electronic, mechanical, photocopy, recording, or otherwise—without the prior written consent of the publisher, except for brief quotations embodied in critical articles and reviews. For information write **Lippincott-Raven Publishers, 227 East Washington Square, Philadelphia, PA 19106-3780.**

Materials appearing in this book prepared by individuals as part of their official duties as U.S. Government employees are not covered by the above-mentioned copyright.

Printed in the United States of America

9 8 7 6 5 4 3 2 1

Library of Congress Cataloging-in-Publication Data

Placental function and fetal nutrition / editor, Frederick C. Battaglia; Nestlé Nutrition Services.
 p. cm.—(Nestlé Nutrition workshop series ; v. 39)
 "39th Nestlé Nutrition Workshop which was held at Ashdown Park Hotel in East Sussex, England in the spring of 1996"—Pref.
 Includes bibliographical references and index.
 ISBN 0-7817-1406-0
 1. Fetus—Nutrition—Congresses. 2. Placenta—Physiology—Congresses. 3. Maternal-fetal exchange—Congresses. I. Battaglia, Frederick C., 1932- . II. Nestlé Nutrition Services. III. Nestlé Nutrition Workshop (39th : 1996 : East Sussex, England) IV. Series.
 [DNLM: 1. Placenta—physiology—congresses. 2. Fetus—embryology—congresses. 3. Nutrition—in pregnancy—congresses. 4. Fetal Transport—physiology—congresses. W1 NE228 v.39 1997 / WQ 212 P698 1997]
RG615.P53 1997
612.6'3—dc21
DNLM/DLC
for Library of Congress

Care has been taken to confirm the accuracy of the information presented and to describe generally accepted practices. However, the authors, editors, and publisher are not responsible for errors or omissions or for any consequences from application of the information in this book and make no warranty, express or implied, with respect to the contents of the publication.

The authors, editors, and publisher have exerted every effort to ensure that drug selection and dosage set forth in this text are in accordance with current recommendations and practice at the time of publication. However, in view of ongoing research, changes in government regulations, and the constant flow of information relating to drug therapy and drug reactions, the reader is urged to check the package insert for each drug for any change in indications and dosage and for added warnings and precautions. This is particularly important when the recommended agent is a new or infrequently employed drug.

Some drugs and medical devices presented in this publication have Food and Drug Administration (FDA) clearance for limited use in restricted research settings. It is the responsibility of the health care provider to ascertain the FDA status of each drug or device planned for use in their clinical practice.

Preface

This book is the result of the 39th Nestlé Nutrition Workshop which was held at Ashdown Park Hotel in East Sussex, United Kingdom, in the spring of 1996. International experts in placental function and fetal nutrition were invited to discuss their work. The experts included basic scientists and clinical scientists. Ashdown Park provided a magnificent setting for a conference, one which encouraged informal discussion apart from the formal program.

The topic of placental function and fetal nutrition is an extremely important and timely one. The development and growth of a child is determined to a great extent by its *in utero* development. Fetal growth restriction, or intrauterine growth retardation, is a striking example of clinical pathology associated with placental dysfunction and fetal malnutrition. It is now clear that such effects can have long-term implications. The timeliness of this Workshop comes from the availability of new imaging and research techniques, which permit studies in human pregnancy as well as in basic research.

The conference had five sessions, in each of which a mixture of basic and clinical research topics was presented. This format led to lively exchange and discussion among basic scientists and clinicians. It was quickly apparent that a great deal of progress had been made towards understanding placental transport and metabolism and that some of the concepts which have emerged from basic research are now addressable in human pregnancies.

While many questions remain unanswered, it was clear that a far more precise description of normal fetal growth and metabolism is emerging, with the possibility of exploring how specific maternal diseases affect fetal and placental nutrition. Within the lively discussion that followed all presentations, there were suggestions with potential therapeutic application to human pregnancies.

FREDERICK C. BATTAGLIA, M.D.
Division of Perinatal Medicine
Department of Pediatrics
University of Colorado School of Medicine
Denver, Colorado, U.S.A.

Foreword

The placenta plays a central role in the nutrition of the fetus. It provides nutrients and removes waste products. Placental size and structure, developmental and pathological processes, as well as metabolic interactions with the fetus, cooperate with placental transport and metabolic mechanisms to affect placental-fetal nutrient exchange both quantitatively and qualitatively. It is generally accepted that small placental size is the major determinant of intrauterine growth retardation (IUGR) in infants. Even though placental glucose transfer appears to be unchanged in IUGR it remains unclear whether the efficiency of placental amino acids transport is altered. Lipid transport, placental hormone production, polypeptide growth factors, and signals originating from the fetus can also limit fetal growth.

The 39th Nestlé Nutrition Workshop, held in Ashdown Park, Sussex, United Kingdom and chaired by Professor F. Battaglia, allowed an interactive discussion between basic and clinically applied research in this field. It provided an opportunity not only to digest the progress made in our understanding of placental function and fetal nutrition, but also to outline the important questions for the future; among them, the prevention of IUGR and the nutritional requirements of the newborn with IUGR.

Professor F. Haschke, M.D.
Vice-President
Nestec Ltd.
Vevey, Switzerland

Contents

Techniques for the Study of Placental Transport—Transfer of
  Chloride as an Example 1
*R.D.H. Boyd, I.M. Doughty, J. Glazier, S. Greenwood,
  and C.P. Sibley*

Placental Delivery of Amino Acids. Utilization and Production
  vs. Transport 21
Giacomo Meschia

Molecular Mechanisms of Placental Development 31
Michael J. Soares

Fetal Liver and the Placenta: An Interactive System 47
Frederick C. Battaglia

The Endocrine Function of the Placenta: Interactions Between
  Trophic Peptides and Hormones 59
Lise Cedard

The Endocrine Function of the Placenta: Human Placental Growth
  Hormone Variant 75
Frank Talamantes

Development of Hormone Receptors Within the Fetus 85
Russell V. Anthony, M.D. Fanning, and L.C. Richter

Regulation of Gene Expression by Nutrients During the
  Perinatal Period 103
*Jean Girard, S. Hauguel-de Mouzon, F. Chatelain, P. Boileau,
  S. Thumelin, and J-P Pégorier*

Oxygenation *In Utero*: Placental Determinants and
  Fetal Requirements 123
Julie A. Owens, K.L. Kind, and J.S. Robinson

Placental Transport in Fetal Growth Retardation 143
Edward S. Ogata, R.H. Lane, R.A. Simmons, and G.J. Reid

Fetal Lipid Requirements: Implications in Fetal
   Growth Retardation 157
Jacqueline Jumpsen, J. Van Aerde, and M. Thomas Clandinin

Maternal Lipid Metabolism and Its Implications for Fetal Growth .. 169
Emilio Herrera and M.A. Munilla

Oxygen Consumption and Protein Metabolism in the Human Fetus   183
Michael J. Rennie

Nutrient Supply in Human Fetal Growth Retardation 191
Anna Maria Marconi

Maternal Vascular Disease and Fetal Growth 199
Carlo Romanini and H. Valensise

Fetal Growth and Long-Term Consequences in Animal Models of
   Growth Retardation 215
Kathleen Holemans, L. Aerts and F.A. Van Assche

Drug Abuse 231
Doris M. Campbell

Effects of Maternal Smoking on Placental Structure and Function .. 247
*K.R. Page, P. Bush D.R. Abramovich, P.J. Aggett, M.D. Burke,
   and T.M. Mayhew*

Concluding Remarks 251

Subject Index 253

Contributors

Speakers

Russell V. Anthony
Animal Reproduction and Biotechnology
  Laboratory
Department of Physiology
Colorado State University
Fort Collins, Colorado 80523-1683,
  U.S.A.

Federick C. Battaglia
Department of Pediatrics
University of Colorado Health
  Sciences Center
4200 E. Ninth Avenue, B-199
Denver, Colorado 80262, U.S.A.

R.D.H. Boyd
St. George's Hospital Medical School
Cranmer Terrace
London SW17 ORE, United Kingdom

Doris M. Campbell
Department of Obstetrics & Gynaecology
University of Aberdeen
Aberdeen Maternity Hospital
Foresterhill
Aberdeen AB9 2ZD, United Kingdom

Lise Cedard
INSERM U 361
Maternité Baudelocque
Reprod. et Physiopathologie Obstétricale
123 Bld de Port-Royal
75014 Paris, France

M.Thomas Clandinin
Department of Agricultural, Food &
  Nutritional Science and
Department of Medicine
University of Alberta
4-10 Agriculture/Forestry Centre
Edmonton, Alberta T6G 2P5, Canada

Jean Girard
Centre de Recherche sur l'Endocrinologie
  Moléculaire et le Développement
Centre National de la Recherche
  Scientifique
9 Rue Jules Hetzel
92190 Meudon, France

Emilio Herrera
Universidad San Pablo-CEU
Urbanización Montepríncipe
Ctra. Boadilla del Monte, km 5,300
E-28668 Madrid, Spain

Anna Maria Marconi
Department of Obstetrics & Gynaecology
University of Milan-IBMS San Paolo
Via Antonio di Rudiní 8
20144 Milan, Italy

Giacomo Meschia
Department of Physiology
University of Colorado School
  of Medicine
4200 E. Ninth Avenue C240
Denver, Colorado 80262, U.S.A.

Edward S. Ogata
The Children's Memorial Hospital
2300 Children's Plaza, #45
Chicago, Illinois 60614, U.S.A.

Julie A. Owens
Department of Physiology
University of Adelaide
Adelaide, South Australia, 5005, Australia

Michael J. Rennie
Department of Anatomy & Physiology
University of Dundee
Dundee DD1 4HN, United Kingdom

Carlo Romanini
Department of Obstetrics & Gynaecology
Università di Roma-Tor Vergata
Piazza dell'Umanesimo 10
I-00144 Roma, Italy

Michael J. Soares
Department of Physiology
University of Kansas Medical Center
3901 Rainbow Blvd.
Kansas City, Kansas 66160, U.S.A.

Frank Talamantes
Department of Biology
University of California
Sinsheimer Laboratories
Santa Cruz, California 95064, U.S.A.

F.A. Van Assche
Department of Obstetrics and Gynecology
Uz Gasthuisberg
Herestraat 49
B-3000 Leuven, Belgium

Speakers
(no manuscript provided)

Giorgio Pardi
Department of Obstetrics & Gynaecology
University of Milan-IBMS San Paolo
Via Antonia di Rudiní 8
20144 Milan, Italy

Alfred Staudach
Landeskrankenanstalten
Frauenklinik
Mullner Hauptstraße 48
A-5020 Salzburg, Austria

Session Chairmen

Frederick C. Battaglia / *Denver, USA*
Stuart Campbell / *London, United Kingdom*
Tim Chard / *London, United Kingdom*
Kypros Nicolaides / *London, United Kingdom*
Peter Soothill / *Bristol, United Kingdom*

Invited Attendees

Siva Achanna / *Malaysia*
Peter J. Aggett / *United Kingdom*
Stuart Campbell / *United Kingdom*
David C.A. Candy / *United Kingdom*
Tim Chard / *United Kingdom*
Christos Costalos / *Greece*
G.M. Csakany / *Hungary*
Sean Devane / *United Kingdom*
John Dobbing / *United Kingdom*
P. Duc-Goiran / *France*
Mazen El-Essa / *Kuwait*
Per Finne / *Norway*
Alain Fournie / *France*
Ernst Friedrich / *Germany*
Janusz Gadzinowski / *Poland*
Keith Godfrey / *United Kingdom*
Lena Grahnquist / *Sweden*
Budi R. Hadibroto / *Indonesia*
Renate Huch / *Switzerland*
Arne Jensen / *Germany*
Abu Taher Khan / *Bangladesh*
Nina V. Lashneva / *Russia*
Qi Pei Liu / *P.R. China*
Shunyun Liu / *P.R. China*
Milton Stew Wah Lum / *Malaysia*

CONTRIBUTORS

Pisake Lumbiganon / *Thailand*
Yanyan Ma / *P.R. China*
Antonio Marini / *Italy*
Mohamad Mikati / *Lebanon*
Jacques Milliez / *France*
Nikola Mumjiev / *Bulgaria*
S. Nalliah / *West Malaysia*
Salah Kamel Nassar / *Egypt*
Kypros Nicolaides / *United Kingdom*
K.R. Page / *United Kingdom*
A-A Pourvaghar / *Iran*
Tom Sanders / *United Kingdom*
Henning Schneider / *Switzerland*
Thomas Schwenzer / *Germany*
Soisaang Sethavanich / *Thailand*
Natalia M. Shilina / *Russia*
Colin Sibley / *United Kingdom*
Peter Soothill / *United Kingdom*
G.S.H. Yeo / *Singapore*
Z.T. Tjaniago / *Indonesia*
Herbert Valensise / *Italy*
Anastasia Varvarigou-Frima / *Greece*
Zhi-qiong Wang / *P.R. China*

Christine Williams / *United Kingdom*
Abd. Aziz Yahava / *Malaysia*
Hakimi Zainal Abidin / *Malaysia*

Nestlé Representatives

Denise Briggs / *Croydon, United Kingdom*
Ralph Claydon / *Croydon, United Kingdom*
Gemma Dimaano / *Manila, Philippines*
Bianca-Maria Exl / *Munich, Germany*
Ferdinand Haschke / *Vevey, Switzerland*
Manfred Kohler / *Munich, Germany*
Michalis Maganaris / *Athens, Greece*
Ulrich Preysch / *Vevey, Switzerland*
Anna Shen / *Beijing, P.R. China*
Philippe Steenhout / *Vevey, Switzerland*
Pat Wright / *Croydon, United Kingdom*

Nestlé Nutrition Workshop Series

Volume 39: Placental Function and Fetal Nutrition
Frederick C. Battaglia, Editor; 288 pp., 1997.
Volume 38: Diarrheal Disease
Michael Gracey and John A. Walker-Smith, Editors; 368 pp., 1997.
Volume 37: Feeding from Toddlers to Adolescence
Angel Ballabriga, Editor; 320 pp., 1996.
Volume 36: Long-Term Consequences of Early Feeding
John Boulton, Zvi Laron, and Jean Rey, Editors; 256 pp., 1996.
Volume 35: Diabetes
Richard M. Cowett, Editor; 320 pp., 1995.
Volume 34: Intestinal Immunology and Food Allergy
Alain L. de Weck and Hugh A. Sampson, Editors; 320 pp., 1995.
Volume 33: Protein Metabolism During Infancy
Niels C. R. Räihä, Editor; 264 p., 1994.
Volume 32: Nutrition of the Low Birthweight Infant
Bernard L. Salle and Paul R. Swyer, Editors; 240 pp., 1993.
Volume 31: Birth Risks
J. David Baum, Editor; 256 pp., 1993.
Volume 30: Nutritional Anemias
Samuel J. Fomon and Stanley Zlotkin, Editors; 232 pp., 1992.
Volume 29: Nutrition of the Elderly
Hamish N. Munro and Günter Schlierf, Editors; 248 pp., 1992.
Volume 28: Polyunsaturated Fatty Acids in Human Nutrition
Umberto Bracco and Richard J. Deckelbaum, Editors; 256 pp., 1992.
Volume 27: For a Better Nutrition in the 21st Century
Peter Leathwood, Marc Horisberger, and W. Philip T. James, Editors; 272 pp., 1993.
Volume 26: Perinatology
Erich Saling, Editor, 208 pp., 1992.
Volume 25: Sugars in Nutrition
Michael Gracey, Norman Kretchmer, and Ettore Ross, Editors; 304 pp., 1991.
Volume 24: Inborn Errors of Metabolism
Jürgen Schaub, François Van Hoof, and Henri L. Vis, Editors; 320 pp., 1991.
Volume 23: Trace Elements in Nutrition of Children—II
Ranjit Kumar Chandra, Editor, 248 pp., 1991.

Volume 22: History of Pediatrics 1850–1950
Buford L. Nichols, Jr., Angel Ballabriga, and Norman Kretchmer, Editors; 320 pp., 1991.
Volume 21: Rickets
Francis H. Glorieux, Editor; 304 pp., 1991.

PLACENTAL FUNCTION AND FETAL NUTRITION

Techniques for the Study of Placental Transport—Transfer of Chloride as an Example

R. D. H. Boyd, I. M. Doughty, J. Glazier, S. Greenwood, C. P. Sibley

Department of Child Health and School of Biological Sciences, University of Manchester, Manchester, United Kingdom

"It is therefore quite futile to inject some substance . . . into the maternal circulation of the rat at the end of pregnancy, and then, if it goes through into the foetal circulation, to report that 'the placenta is permeable to' whatever it was that was injected. Yet such wide conclusions have only too often been drawn although the only right conclusion would have been that, in the animal in question and at the time in question, placental permeability to the substance in question showed itself." J. Needham, *Chemical Embryology*, p. 1486 (1).

In what was the first systematic review of placental transfer mechanisms, Needham (1) grappled with three key issues: first, placental transfer has to be considered quantitatively—it is not an all-or-none phenomenon; second, it varies between species; and third, it will change over the course of gestation. A further central concept was established 10 years later with the introduction of radioisotopes. Flexner's series of articles (for example, ref. 2) made clear the vast quantitative difference there might be between unidirectional and net maternofetal fluxes; placental transfer is a two-way process, so that fetal accumulation depends on the quantitative difference between two unidirectional fluxes. Note the use of *maternofetal* rather than transplacental. Here we will consider exclusively transplacental transfer, but the two should not be considered synonymous, because for some solutes in some species, immunoglobulins, for example (3), nonplacental routes predominate, and such routes may make some contribution to the transport of other solutes—an underinvestigated issue.

A full analysis of transplacental transfer of a given cell, organism, molecular complex, or molecule (and we concentrate on molecules here) requires at least the following knowledge: (a) the species and its gestational age; (b) the flux rate of the molecule in each direction across placenta; (c) the route taken in crossing the placenta (paracellular, or alternatively crossing placental cell membranes by lipophilic diffusion, endocytosis, or through membrane transporters or channels) and its rate-limiting step, which may be different for different permeants; (d) interactions of the molecule within the placenta, including equilibration with similar molecules within the placenta and metabolic interconversions; (e) the external driving forces for movement between the maternal and fetal microcirculations at the placental exchange

TABLE 1A. *Methods of placental transfer study that maintain orientation*

Method	Variable measured	Details	Comment
Carcass analysis	Net flux	Analysis of conceptus content of different gestational ages	Reliable only for nonmetabolized solutes, e.g., calcium. Includes all maternofetal routes. Poor time resolution.
Accumulation or loss of exogenous tracer	Unidirectional flux	Fetal tracer content estimated directly or indirectly	If plasma concentrations are not low on the side away from tracer injection, hybrid of net and unidirectional flux is measured.
Umbilical and/or uterine arteriovenous differences *in situ*	Unidirectional or net flux	Cordocentesis, chronic preparation or at delivery	Unsteady state artifact is likely if measured at delivery.
Cotyledonary perfusion	Unidirectional or net flux	Steady-state transfer	Perfusion might alter passive permeability and thus wrongly estimate proportion of specific transport.
	Kinetics of uptake and back flux from maternal and fetal circulation	Single pass, indicator dilution	Can demonstrate transport asymmetry. May not reflect rate-limiting element of transfer unless combined with steady-state studies.
Intact villus	Kinetics of uptake or release Electrophysiologic study		May not reflect rate-limiting element of transplacental transport. May be "housekeeping," not transport functions.
Ussing technique	Ion fluxes and short circuit current		Pig only.

Modified from Sibley and Boyd (12), in which fuller references are provided.

area, that is, concentration differences, electrical potential differences, or solvent flow between them, bearing in mind that these may not be uniform over the entire surface of the placental exchange area because of flow limitation[1] and that exchange areas for different molecules may be diverse; (f) any internal driving forces that allow transport to be "uphill" through local release of chemically stored energy or in the form of cotransport; and finally (g) a detailed knowledge of the molecular mechanisms involved and of the control mechanisms for transfer.

Information from all these perspectives is not available for any molecule, for any species, or at any gestational age, perhaps reflecting the relative paucity of placental transport research. However, for any placental transport study, the choice of technique clearly needs to depend on the question to which an answer is being sought.

---

[1] Flow limitation is a term used to describe the situation in which the rate-limiting element of maternol-fetal exchange is the rate of delivery or removal of the molecule in question to the placental exchange area by either the maternal or fetal circulation or both. It is a concept central to the exchange of highly permeable molecules, such as respiratory gases and lipid-soluble drugs. It is not considered in this chapter, but it is well covered in Meschia *et al.* (4) and Faber and Thornburg (5).

Here we have chosen to use studies of chloride to indicate the range of techniques available and to indicate some of the conclusions that can be drawn from them. Chloride is an important extracellular ion accumulated in large amounts by the fetus. It may also play a role in fetal and placental pH control and in homeostasis of placental intracellular volume. There has recently been a considerable increase of understanding of its role and transport mechanism within placenta. Its transfer is not importantly flow-limited.

Before considering chloride studies in some detail, we should note that there are two broad approaches to transport investigations: (a) those in which the orientation of placenta is maintained. Transport mechanisms inferred from most such studies can often be shown to contribute to maternofetal exchange (Table 1A); (b) studies in which orientation is not maintained or in which transport across only part of the thickness of the exchange barrier is analyzed. These transport mechanisms may contribute to maternofetal exchange but may also reflect aspects of placental homeostasis or "housekeeping" (Table 1B).

There is also a hierarchy of scale, from the complex to the simple, large to small, from the intact placenta *in situ* in the free-ranging animal (or woman) through anesthesia, singly or dually perfused placenta or cotyledon, individual villus, placental cell to membrane preparations, transport protein, its messenger RNA, or gene. In general, experimental control increases as simplicity increases. Sadly, certainty as to the qualitative or quantitative role of any function does the reverse.

Each technique involves its own assumptions and potential sources of error, some of which are touched on below. Measurement of external driving forces across the exchange area, such as concentration differences between maternal and fetal plasma

TABLE 1B. *Methods of placental transfer study in which orientation is not maintained*

Method	Variable measured	Details	Comment
Slices; fragments	Kinetics of individual systems	Uptake or efflux studies	May be "housekeeping" rather than transplacental transport systems.
Membrane vesicles	Kinetics of individual systems	Microvillous (maternal facing) Basal (fetal facing)	May be "housekeeping" rather than transplacental transport systems.
Cultured cytotrophoblast	Uptake/efflux Transmembrane potential difference and ion channel characteristics		Care needs to be taken that placental cells rather than other lineages are being studied. Cells may never terminally differentiate into transporting syncytium. May be "housekeeping."
Molecular study of transport proteins and their expression	Biochemical and functional characterization	Location, comparability, function in transport systems	Essential elements in all transport other than paracellular or lipophilic routes.
Receptor binding studies	Affinity/number	Over 25 described	May have "housekeeping," endocrine transport, or other function.

Modified from Sibley and Boyd (12), in which fuller references are provided.

(see Table II in Morriss et al., ref. 6) and electrical potential differences (7,8), if any, is required for interpretation of transport studies. Thus, if fetal plasma concentration is higher than maternal, maternofetal active transport is more likely, but other explanations are also possible. Indirect inferences about control mechanisms and transport mechanisms may also be drawn from study of the endocrine or genetic manipulation of transport or following alteration of the energy supply within the placenta.

CHLORIDE

All the techniques in Table 1A and 1B except single-pass analysis and slice studies have been applied to the investigation of chloride in the placenta.

Carcass Analysis

By term, the human fetus has accumulated a net content of some 160 mM of chloride (9) from a maternal plasma whose chloride concentration is probably lower than fetal (Hellmuth, quoted in ref. 1; 5,10); the reverse is the case in sheep (11). It seems likely that if the extrafetal fluids whose electrolytes do not definitely reach them transplacentally (uncertainty on this point is a weakness of the methodology) are excluded, the proportionate content of chloride is likely to be broadly similar in different mammals, although it probably changes during gestation (Fig. 1). Transplacental net chloride fluxes in different species thus reflect relative fractional daily

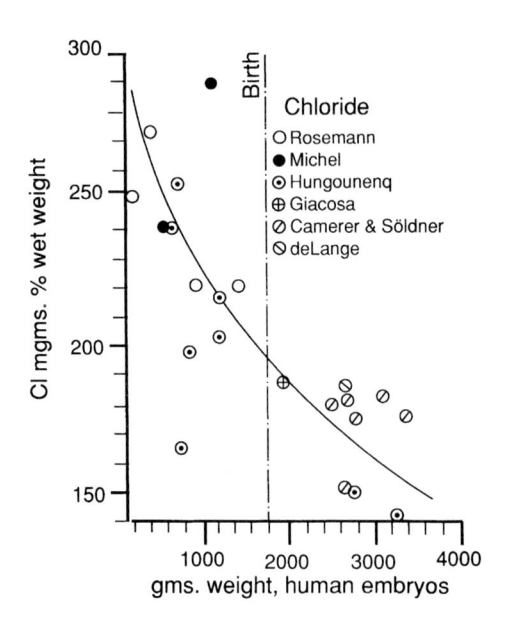

FIG. 1. Gestational fall in proportional fetal chloride content—human. From Needham (1).

TABLE 2. *"External" driving forces for chloride movement between maternal and fetal plasma across the placental exchange area*

Force		Reference
Concentration difference (*in vivo*)		
Human 5–6 mM	fetus higher	Bissonnette et al. 1994 (10)
Sheep 5.47 ± 1.31 mM	fetus lower	Armentrout et al. 1977 (46)
Electrical		
Human villous core (mature intermediate *in vitro*)	3 mV (median) negative to intervillous space	Greenwood et al. 1993 (8)
Solvent drag		
Rabbit midgestation	14 nl/s/g placenta	Faber 1995 (19)

increases in fetal weight; these are high for rat or rabbit, intermediate for sheep, and low for human. Such differences in growth rate are likely to be reflected in the proportionate importance of the different routes for chloride transport across the placenta. The net flux (nM/min/g placenta) averaged over the length of gestation is about 0.79 for a 3.5-kg newborn human, perhaps 1.74 for a 4-kg sheep, and 10.6 for a 5-g rat. Because of the changing fetal growth rate and body composition over gestation, such averaging is obviously problematic.

The estimated transplacental driving forces for chloride are given in Table 2.

In Vivo Unidirectional Fluxes

Unidirectional fluxes for chloride have been measured by all the methods listed in Table 1A, although not in a single species and sometimes in only one direction.

The sheep has the advantage of allowing fetomaternal flux or clearance measurements (for a distinction between them, see, for example, Sibley and Boyd, ref. 12) under chronic conditions with little fetal disturbance—the special power of this preparation. However, assumptions have to be made in calculating the flux. Thornburg et al. (13) estimated its value from fetal plasma disappearance curves by assuming a volume of distribution for chloride in the fetus. Boyd et al. (14) did so by measurement of uterine arteriovenous differences after isotope injection to the fetus. This approach involves the assumption that the uterine blood flow measured by a diffusion technique is appropriate to the uterine venous sampling site used. Reassuringly, the results are rather similar and substantially higher than the net flux (Table 3). Faber and Anderson (11) have recently calculated the reflection coefficient for chloride across the placenta of the same species to be 0.68 ± 0.04 when flux is modified by rendering the mother hypertonic. They suggest that this low value for the reflection coefficient contributes to explaining the paradox that the fetal lamb can accumulate water in the presence of a higher maternal plasma osmolality than fetal, chloride being an important contributor to the higher maternal concentration. Unidirectional maternofetal chloride flux has not been measured in the sheep. Furthermore, studies of flux across the perfused sheep placenta of chloride or of most

TABLE 3. *Chloride flux (nM/min/g placenta)*

	Net	Unidirectional	Reference
Sheep	—	320 ± 40	Boyd et al. 1981 (fetomaternal) (14)
	1.74	—	This chapter
Rat	—	7400 ± 800	Štulc et al. 1996 (maternofetal) (17)
	10.6	—	This chapter
Human	—	3800 ± 200	Doughty et al. 1996 (maternofetal) (40)
	0.79	—	McCance and Widdowson 1961 (9)

other solutes have not been made—perhaps a pity in view of the extensive *in vivo* data available for this species.

In the rat, unlike the sheep, no measurements of unidirectional chloride flux have been reported across the placenta of the unanesthetized pregnant animal. Unidirectional fluxes in the unanesthetized state have, however, been measured for other solutes, including calcium (15). The measurements for calcium flux across the placenta of the unanesthetized rat are rather close in value to those measured across the placenta of the anesthetized animal or across the perfused rat placenta, not true of the guinea pig. This allows some confidence to be placed in the data for chloride fluxes across the latter two rat preparations, although there are some quantitative differences in value between them (16,17). Maternofetal clearance across the intact placenta of anesthetized rats (37.3 ± 12.9 mL/min) is about 20 times greater than that of the presumed extracellular marker chromium EDTA (ethylenediamine-tetraacetic acid), whereas its diffusion coefficient in water is only four times higher (Fig. 2A). This raises the possibility that most transplacental chloride movement in this species is transcellular, and other evidence in the perfused placenta amply supports this. For example, the inhibitor DIDS (4,4'-diiosothiocyanostilbene-2,2'-disulfonate), which inhibits anion exchange in other systems, reduces chloride flux to about 25% of its control value but does not affect chromium EDTA (Fig. 2A). The transfer mechanism is fully saturated at physiologic concentrations of chloride. It does not heavily depend on energy supply within the placenta, in keeping with the notion that exchange rather than active transport is involved; neither cyanide nor cooling has very much effect on the process. The transport mechanism has a high affinity for nitrate and bromide, less for lactate, and little for gluconate, as can be inferred from the effect of replacing chloride with other anions (Fig. 2 B,C). Maternofetal flux is highly dependent on fetal bicarbonate.

It is not clear how far the results from rats, with their short gestation period and high net fluxes per gram of placenta, can be applied to other species (18). In the rabbit, in which clearances have been measured in midgestation (19), the maternofetal flux appears to be considerably lower per gram of placenta. In the nonhuman primate, although unidirectional clearances are fairly high when compared per gram with those of the sheep, there is rather little restriction compared with that of urea (20). We will return to the human data below.

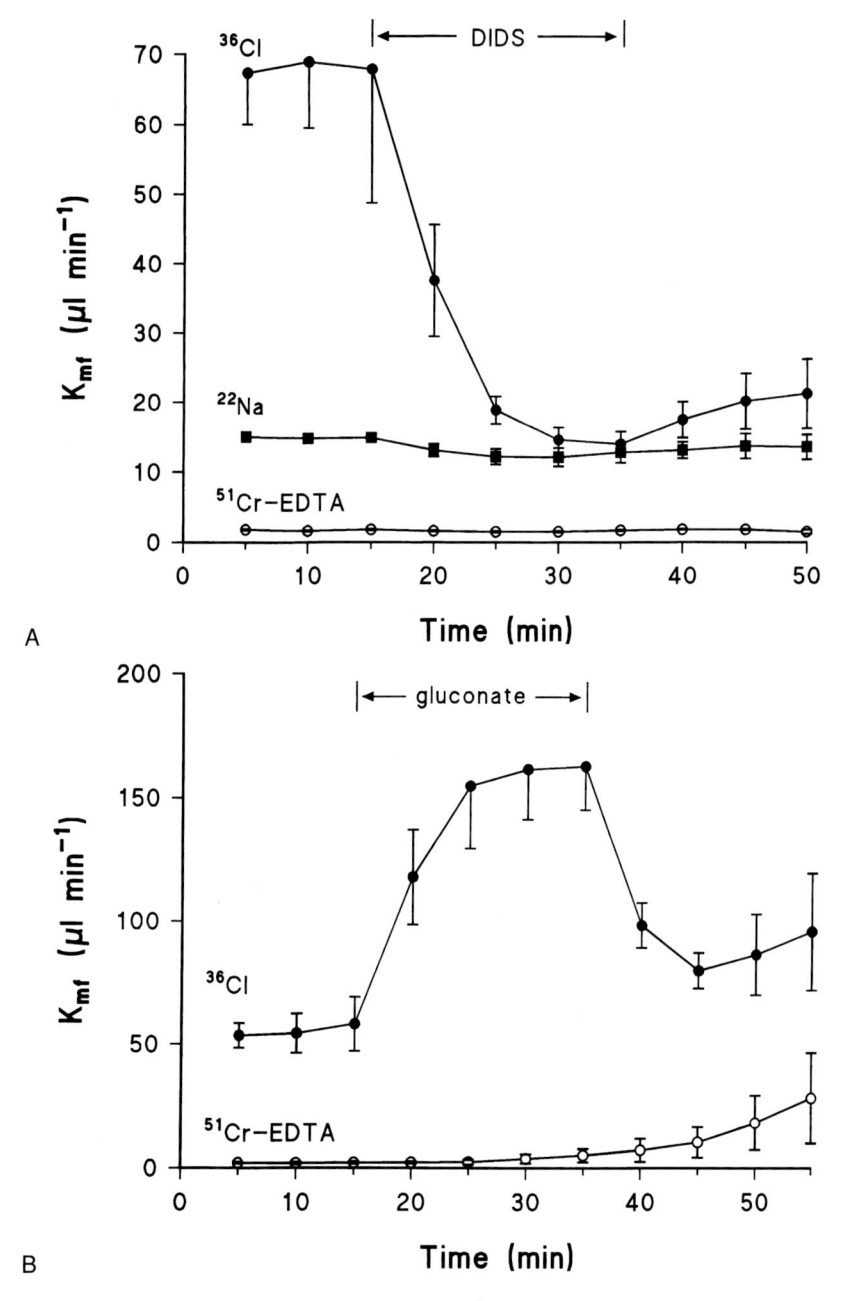

FIG. 2. Maternofetal chloride clearance (K_{mf} μl·min^{-1}) across perfused rat placenta. **A:** Effect of 0.1 mM DIDS in umbilical perfusate on the maternofetal transfer of individual solutes: n = 3 ± SEM. Umbilical perfusion. **B:** Effect of lowering chloride concentrations in maternal perfusate to 50 mM by replacement of sodium chloride with sodium gluconate. Dual perfusion.

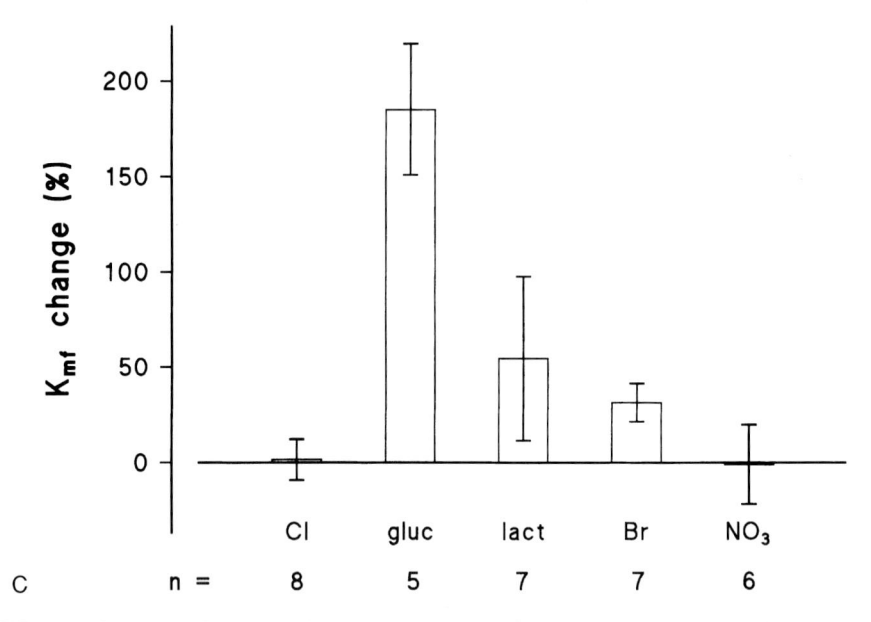

FIG. 2. *(Continued)* **C:** Anion selectively assessed by effect on K_{mf} of substitution with a range of anions as in 2B. From Štulc et al. (17), with kind permission of the *American Journal of Physiology*.

Other Techniques

Vesicle Studies

Numerous investigations have been made of chloride movements into or out of vesicles reconstituted from the microvillous (maternal facing) membrane of the syncytiotrophoblast. The membrane is isolated by homogenization, precipitation with divalent cations, and differential centrifugation to produce a fraction high in the microvillous membrane enzyme alkaline phosphatase. The membrane is then encouraged to form vesicles by shear stress. The great majority of studies are on human material. It is also possible to study the rat placenta in this way (for example, Glazier et al., ref. 21), but chloride transport has not yet been investigated in vesicles from this species. Although not all studies are concordant in their results, the following broad conclusions (see Table 4 and Fig. 4A) can be drawn about mechanisms allowing chloride transfer across the microvillous membrane. Various assays have been used to measure chloride movement into the vesicles and to determine its kinetics.

1. The presence of an anion exchanger responsible for perhaps 30% of the chloride flux into vesicles, for example, measured using ^{36}Cl (22);
2. A DPC (diphenylamine-2-carboxylate)-inhibitable conductance imposing voltage dependence on chloride flux, for example, measured by fluorescence quenching (23);

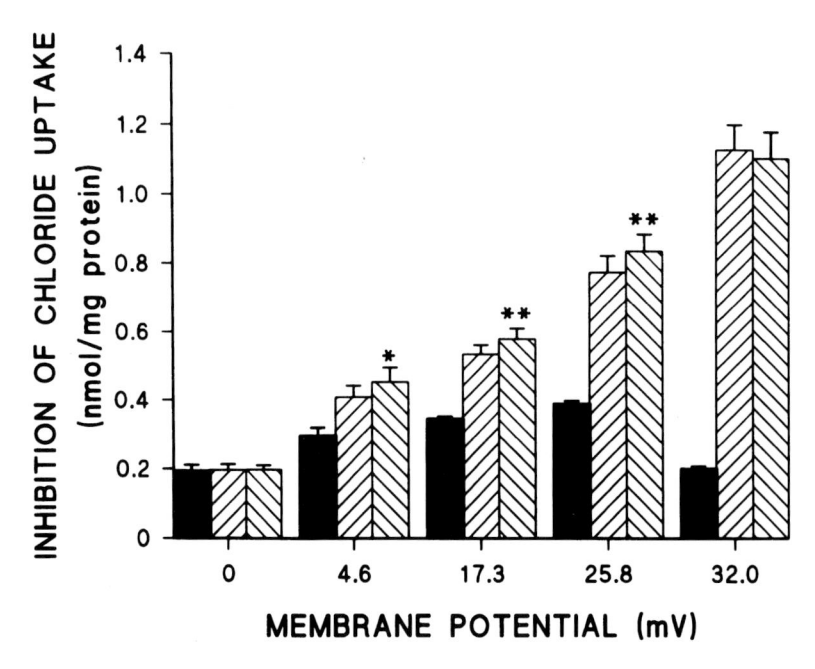

FIG. 3. Inhibitable chloride uptake into human microvillous membrane vesicles as a function of imposed potential differences. From Byrne et al. (24), with kind permission of Elsevier Science Publishers, Amsterdam, The Netherlands.

3. Another conductance pathway, DIDS-inhibitable, maximally active at a vesicle inside positive potential of approximately +25 mV (24), measured using ^{36}Cl uptake (Fig. 3).

Interestingly, a study by Placchi et al. (25) showed that chloride conductance may be controlled by protein kinase A-dependent phosphorylation.

Basal membrane from the fetal face of syncytiotrophoblast is harder to isolate than microvillous and, in the case of chloride, has been little studied. Illsley and Sellers (26) did note a lower ratio of chloride to potassium permeability in membranes from the basal rather than the microvillous surface.

The great power of the vesicle technique is its relative simplicity at the bench coupled with the ability to manipulate and dissect the kinetics of transport systems. Possible contamination with transporting membranes other than those desired may be a source of error. Assessment of this depends on the availability of biochemical markers for the membrane whose ultrastructural localization is known; this is clearer for the human than other species. Normal cofactors and driving gradients may be absent. Use of vesicle results to compare different gestational ages or clinical groups also requires demonstration that vesicle purity and geometry are not grossly different (for example, Mahendran et al., ref. 27; Kuruvilla et al., ref. 28). Comparison of flux into vesicles to that across the whole organ is very speculative.

Intact Individual Villi

These have been used to a limited extent in the investigation of chloride transport. A chloride conductance has been demonstrated at the microvillous membrane using microelectrode techniques (8). The maxi chloride channel identified using single-channel patch clamp methods (29) might contribute to this chloride conductance. The channel was inhibited by DIDS but was inactivated at potentials more extreme than approximately ±20 mV. Patch clamp methods give rapid information about channels and their manipulation, just as vesicles do for conductance, but deriving their activity *in vivo* requires further information, such as knowledge of the membrane potential difference. For example, the maxi chloride channel is open at a potential difference close to the median microvillous membrane potential difference of −22 mV, but this latter measurement has been made only *in vitro* in the absence of a fetal circulation (8). An early study of the sodium dependence of rubidium efflux from villous clumps (30) suggested the possible presence on the microvillous membrane of a sodium-chloride-potassium cotransporter, but no confirmatory evidence for this has been found. A successful single villous perfusion technique would be a major advance that we have so far failed to achieve.

Cytotrophoblast Cells

About 30% of such cells isolated *in vitro* have been shown to express a channel with electrophysiologic properties similar to those of CFTR (cystic fibrosis transmembrane conductance regulator), a maxi chloride channel, and a channel of intermediate conductance (20 pS) (31). Using whole-cell patch clamp recordings, Kibble *et al.* (32) have demonstrated the presence of two different chloride currents, one activated by increased cytosolic calcium ion and inhibited by DIDS and the other similar to volume regulatory chloride currents showing the outward rectification seen in other cell types (Table 4 and Fig. 4B). It is not known whether these currents are present in syncytiotrophoblast after differentiation. Cytotrophoblast cells do not form part of the exchange barrier at term, so the information they give on transport is by inference, as they do evolve into syncytiotrophoblast, which does form part of the exchange barrier.

Molecular Studies

Limited molecular studies have been made of potential chloride transport molecules or of their gene expression. Vanderpuye *et al.* (33) showed some years ago that the band 3 isoform of erythrocyte membrane proteins, a candidate anion transporter, was present on the basal but not the maternal microvillous membrane. Powell *et al.* (34), in a preliminary report, found by contrast that it was present in higher concentration in microvillous than basal membranes. Faller *et al.* (35) report the presence of CFTR protein by immunoblotting, and its messenger RNA has been

TABLE 4. *Chloride transporters and channels in human placenta*

	Site	Inhibitor/activator	Selected references[a]	Technique
Transporters				
Na:2Cl:K	Syncytiotrophoblast—Microvillous membrane		Boyd (30)	Intact villi; inferred
Cl:HCO$_3$	Syncytiotrophoblast—Microvillous membrane		Shennan, Illsley, Byrne, Grassl (22,23,24,47)	Vesicle kinetics[b]
Cl:HCO$_3$	Syncytiotrophoblast—Basal membrane		Vanderpuye (33)	Immunoblotting
Channels				
Maxi chloride (300 pS)	Syncytiotrophoblast—Microvillous membrane	DIDS	Brown (29)	Single-channel recording Intact villi
Maxi chloride (300 pS)	Cell membrane	DIDS	Byrne (31)	Single-channel recording Cytotrophoblast cells
Intermediate chloride (25 pS)		DPC	Greenwood (48)	
Small chloride (9 pS) CFTR		Activated by PKA/ATP	Byrne (49)	
Outward rectifying conductance (Ca^{2+}-dependent)	Whole cell	DIDS	Kibble (32)	Whole-cell recording Cytotrophoblast cells
Swelling-activated conductance		DIDS	Kibble, Bissonnette (32,50)	
Linear conductance		Activated by cAMP, HCG	Cronier (51)	Whole-cell recording
CFTR MDR			Mylona, Dechecchi (36, 52)	RTPCR

DIDS, 4,4'-diiosothiocyanostilbene-2,2'-disulfonate; DPC, diphenylamine-2-carboxylate; HCG, human chorionic gonadotrophin; CFTR, cystic fibrosis transmembrane conductance regulator; MDR, multidrug resistance gene; RTPCR, reverse transcriptase polymerase chain reaction.
[a] Full references can be found in Kibble *et al.* (32).
[b] Vesicle studies have also shown chloride conductances, but the responsible channels are not yet certain.

reported to be present on the basis of reverse transcriptase polymerase chain reaction (RTPCR) studies (36) (Table 4). Interestingly, Western blotting of a microvillous membrane preparation indicates the presence of the anion exchanger band 3 at a concentration in equally loaded gels similar to that found in blood cells (I. M. Doughty, *unpublished observations*), suggesting that chloride-bicarbonate exchange might be as important at the maternofetal boundary as it is in the red cell chloride shift.

Perfused Human Placenta

Dancis *et al.* (37) noted in an early study of the perfused human placental cotyledon at term, as Battaglia *et al.* (20) had in the *in situ* monkey placenta, that chloride

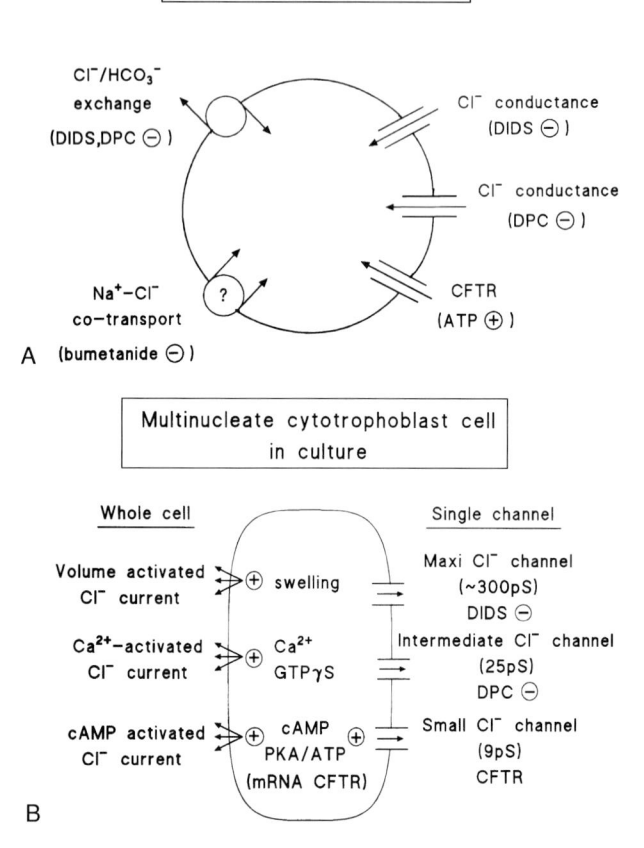

FIG. 4. Chloride transport mechanisms: human placental trophoblast (for sources, see text and reference list). **A:** Mechanisms demonstrable in microvillous syncytiotrophoblast membrane reconstituted into vesicles. **B:** Mechanisms demonstrable by electrophysiologic techniques in syncytialized cultured cytotrophoblast.

clearance was much closer to that of the small, highly permeable molecule urea in primate than in sheep. This led to the assumption for a number of years that transcellular movement as opposed to paracellular diffusional flux of chloride was unlikely to be present in either primate. In support of this simple view is the finding in the human of a relatively high permeability to presumed extracellular markers (38,39), suggesting a major, rather open, transcellular route.

Whether all transplacental chloride movement in the human is paracellular has recently been reinvestigated using the perfused human placental cotyledon by Doughty et al. (40). Like Dancis et al. (37), we noted a high chloride permeability.

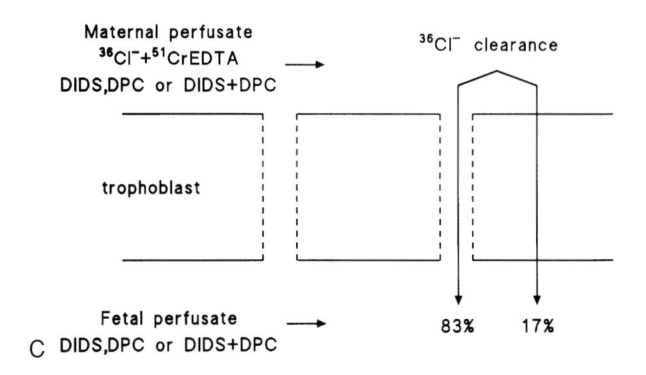

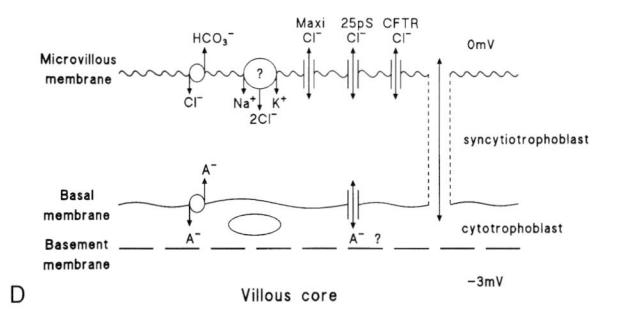

TRANSFER OF CHLORIDE IN PLACENTAL TRANSPORT

Perfused human placental cotyledon

FIG. 4. *(Continued)* **C:** Mechanisms demonstrable in the perfused placental lobule (40). **D:** Mechanisms of placental chloride transport for which there is direct or indirect evidence.

The quantitative value was not identifiably different from that predicted from simultaneous measurement of creatinine or chromium EDTA fluxes, assuming that all three pass through unrestricted water channels across placenta. However, careful analysis of the relative effects on these three permeants of the addition of DIDS or DPC singly or jointly to the perfusate suggests that approximately 7% of transfer appears to be by a DIDS-inhibitable route and perhaps 15% by a route inhibitable by DPC or DPC plus DIDS (Fig. 4C). As mentioned, this may be important in generating the observed higher fetal than maternal concentration for chloride in women found at cordocentesis.

The strengths and weaknesses of the perfused human cotyledon have been reviewed elsewhere (41). The technique has not yet been reliably applied to preterm or midgestational material, at which stage control of placental transfer might be more important than at term.

Implications

Because of the broad relationship between the diffusion coefficient in water and the placental permeability of small extracellular solutes, there has been a general consensus (for example, Faber and Thornburg, ref. 5) that there is a paracellular pathway across the rate-limiting barrier of the placental exchange area. This paracellular route must be accessible to small ions, such as chloride. Indeed, it has sometimes been assumed that this is the only important route of maternofetal chloride exchange. The experiments discussed above indicate the importance of the following questions: first, what is the proportionate quantitative importance of the transcellular to paracellular routes? The most likely answer is very high in the rat and probably the pig (42), and low but not zero in the human. Second, where is biologic control of fetal chloride accretion exerted? The answer is not yet apparent.

According to Stulc (43), calculation of the importance of the paracellular path in sheep may have been an overestimate, as the partial lipid solubility of the extracellular permeants used was ignored in earlier studies. His recalculation of data from the sheep solves the earlier paradox that chloride (and sodium) permeability was too low for the estimated paracellular pore dimensions and density in that species.

It seems unlikely that the several chloride channels and chloride exchangers mentioned above (summarized in Table 4 and Fig. 4D) are solely concerned with maternofetal exchange of that ion. There may be direct or more complex interactions with the transfer of a range of other anions, such as bicarbonate (17) or iodide (22), an interesting ion actively accumulated in several species (for example, see Canning *et al.*, ref. 44). Indirect interaction with amino acid transport might also be important through the effect of intracellular hypertonicity induced by amino acids controlling basal side chloride channel opening (10). Such volume-sensitive chloride channels are, as mentioned, present in cytotrophoblast cells during syncytialization. At first sight, it might appear redundant for an "epithelium" such as the placenta, bathed on both faces by plasma of relatively constant composition, to require a volume regulatory mechanism within its cells or syncytium. However, pregnant animals and humans will have evolved under conditions of environmental stress more significant than those present during most placental studies. We might therefore predict that volume regulatory mechanisms will be more prominent in the placenta of those species subject to diurnal or seasonal changes in maternal plasma composition. There are also further reasons why trophoblast might need a responsive volume regulatory capacity even in the presence of constant plasma isotonicity—for example, to balance any phasic secretion of placental hormones and the associated solute uptake necessary to sustain their synthesis. Nothing is known of the validity of this notion for the trophoblast.

UTILIZATION OF TECHNIQUES

This review of chloride transport studies indicates, as would review of the transport of any other solute, the major weakness of placental research. The hallmark of placenta is, as emphasized by Needham (1), species diversity in function as in structure. Nevertheless, we fail repeatedly to deploy the available techniques across species. Thus, the sheep is a gold standard for physiologic studies of fetoplacental metabolism, for some endocrine investigations, and for cardiovascular and salt and water balance studies, but there has been little or no investigation of molecular transport mechanisms or electrophysiology below the level of maternofetal electrical potentials in sheep placenta. Conversely, in the rat, transport across the intact placenta has been extensively studied both *in vivo* and *in vitro*, but there has again been no detailed electrophysiology and little work on its transport proteins. The same could be said with greater emphasis for rabbit and guinea pig despite important studies at the intact placental level. Systematic transport study across mouse placenta has yet to begin, despite its extensive use in immunology and the opportunities for transgenic manipulation of placental function that it offers. Even within the limited field of transport studies, some solutes have been predominantly studied in one species, some in another.

The human provides an exciting field for transport studies through the emerging ability to correlate *in vitro* work on the tissue using a wide range of techniques with *in vivo* stable isotope studies (for example, Chien *et al.*, ref. 45), and the greatest bulk of placental research is conducted in this species. Nevertheless, the amount of information is still extremely patchy and interpretation must remain speculative.

REFERENCES

1. Needham J. *Chemical Embryology*. Cambridge: Cambridge University Press; 1931.
2. Flexner LB, Cowie DB, Hellman LM, Wilde WS, Vosburgh GS. The permeability of the human placenta to sodium in normal and abnormal pregnancies. *Am J Obstet Gynecol* 1948;55:469–480.
3. Brambell FWR. The passive immunity of the young animal. *Biol Rev* 1958;33:488–531.
4. Meschia G, Battaglia FC, Bruns PD. Theoretical and experimental study of transplacental diffusion. *J Appl Physiol* 1967;22:1171–1178.
5. Faber JJ, Thornburg KL. *Placental Physiology*. New York: Raven Press; 1983.
6. Morriss FM, Boyd RDH, Mahendran D. Placental transport. In: Knobil E, Neill JD, eds. *Physiology of Reproduction*. 2nd ed. New York: Raven Press; 1994:814–861 (vol 2).
7. McNaughton TG, Power GG. Current topic: The maternal-fetal electrical potential difference: new findings and a perspective. *Placenta* 1991;12:185–197.
8. Greenwood SL, Boyd RDH, Sibley CP. Transtrophoblast and microvillus membrane potential difference in mature intermediate human placental villi. *Am J Physiol* 1993;265:C460–C466.
9. McCance RA, Widdowson EM. Mineral metabolism of the foetus and new-born. *Br Med Bull* 1961; 17:132–136.
10. Bissonnette JM, Weiner CP, Power GG. Amino acid uptake and chloride conductances in human placenta. *Placenta* 1994;15:445–446.
11. Faber JJ, Anderson DF. Concentrations of Na^+ and Cl^- in transplacental ultrafiltrate in sheep. *J Physiol (Lond)* 1995; 487: 159–167.
12. Sibley CP, Boyd RDH. Mechanisms of transfer across the human placenta. In: Polin RA, Fox WW, eds. *Fetal and Neonatal Physiology*. 1st ed. Philadelphia: WB Saunders; 1992.
13. Thornburg KL, Binder ND, Faber JJ. Diffusion permeability and ultrafiltration-reflection-coefficients of Na^+ and Cl^- in the near term placenta of the sheep. *J Dev Physiol* 1979;1:47–60.
14. Boyd RDH, Canning JF, Stacey TE, Ward RHT. Steady-state ion distribution and feto-maternal ion fluxes across the sheep placenta. *Placenta* 1981; (Suppl 2):229–234.
15. Štulc J, Štulcová B. Transport of calcium by the placenta of the rat. *J Physiol (Lond)* 1986;371: 1–16.

16. Štulc J, Husain S, Boyd RDH, Sibley CP. Mechanisms of chloride transport across the *in situ* perfused placenta of the anaesthetized rat. *J Physiol (Lond)* 1992;452:94P(abst).
17. Štulc J, Štuclová B, Husain S, Sibley CP. Transfer of Cl⁻ across the placenta of the anesthetized rat. *Am J Physiol* 1996;271:1107–1114.
18. Sibley CP. Mechanisms of ion transfer by the rat placenta: a model for the human placenta? *Placenta* 1994;15:675–691.
19. Faber JJ. Transplacental clearances of inert hydrophilic tracers in rabbits of 18 days' gestation. *Placenta* 1995;16:403–412.
20. Battaglia FC, Behrman RE, Meschia G, Seeds AE, Bruns PD. Clearance of inert molecules, Na, and Cl ions across the primate placenta. *Am J Obstet Gynecol* 1968;102:1135–1143.
21. Glazier JD, Sibley CP, Carter AM. Effect of fetal growth restriction on system A amino acid transporter activity in the maternal facing plasma membrane of rat syncytiotrophoblast. *Pediatr Res* 1996; 40:325–329.
22. Shennan DB, Davis B, Boyd CAR. Chloride transport in human placental microvillus membrane vesicles. *Pflügers Arch* 1986;406:60–64.
23. Illsley NP, Glaubensklee C, Davis B, Verkman AS. Chloride transport across placental microvillous membranes measured by fluorescence. *Am J Physiol* 1988;255:C789–C797.
24. Byrne S, Glazier JD, Greenwood SL, Mahendran D, Sibley CP. Chloride transport by human placental microvillous membrane vesicles. *Biochim Biophys Acta* 1993;1153:122–126.
25. Placchi P, Lombardo R, Tamanini A, Brusa P, Berton G, Cabrini G. cAMP-dependent protein kinase inhibits the chloride conductance in apical membrane vesicles of human placenta. *J Membr Biol* 1991;119:25–32.
26. Illsley NP, Sellers MC. Ion conductances in the microvillous and basal membrane vesicles isolated from human placental syncytiotrophoblast. *Placenta* 1992;13:25–34.
27. Mahendran D, Byrne S, Donnai P, D'Souza SW, Glazier JD, Jones CJP, et al. Na⁺ transport, H⁺ concentration gradient dissipation and system A amino acid transporter activity in purified microvillous plasma membrane isolated from first trimester human placenta: comparison to the term microvillous membrane. *Am J Obstet Gynecol* 1994;171:1534–1440.
28. Kuruvilla AG, D'Souza SW, Glazier JD, Mahendran D, Maresh MJ, Sibley CP. Altered activity of the system A amino acid transporter in microvillous membrane vesicles from placentas of macrosomic babies born to diabetic women. *J Clin Invest* 1994;94:689–695.
29. Brown PD, Greenwood SL, Robinson J, Boyd RDH. Chloride channels of high conductance in the microvillous membrane of term human placenta. *Placenta* 1993;14:103–115.
30. Boyd CAR. Cotransport systems in the brush border membrane of the human placenta. *Ciba Found Symp* 1983;95:300–314.
31. Byrne S, Greenwood SL, Sibley CP. Chloride channels in trophoblast cells cultured from human placenta. In: Escobar H, Baquero F, Suarez L, eds. *Clinical Ecology of Cystic Fibrosis.* Amsterdam: Elsevier; 1993:3–8.
32. Kibble JD, Greenwood SL, Clarson LH, Sibley CP. A Ca^{2+}-activated whole-cell Cl⁻ conductance in human placental cytotrophoblast cells activated via a G protein. *J Membr Biol* 1996;151:131–138.
33. Vanderpuye OA, Kelley LK, Morrison MM, Smith CH. The apical and basal plasma membranes of the human placental syncytiotrophoblast contain different erythrocyte membrane protein isoforms. Evidence for placental forms of band 3 and spectrin. *Biochim Biophys Acta* 1988;943:277–287.
34. Powell TL, Dehlin M, Westergren DO, Ingcarsson K, Jansson T. Identification of ion transporter isoforms in human placenta. *Placenta* 1995;16:A58(abst).
35. Faller DP, Egan DA, Ryan MP. Evidence for location of the CFTR in human placental apical membrane vesicles. *Am J Physiol* 1995;269:C148–C155.
36. Mylona P, Glazier JD, Greenwood SL, Sides MK, Sibley CP. Expression of the cystic fibrosis transmembrane conductance regulator and multidrug resistance genes during development and differentiation in the human placenta. *Placenta* 1995;16:A50(abst).
37. Dancis J, Kammerman S, Jansen V, Schneider H, Levitz M. Transfer of urea, sodium, and chloride across the perfused human placenta. *Am J Obstet Gynecol* 1981;141:677–681.
38. Thornburg KL, Burry KJ, Adams AK, Kirk EP, Faber JJ. Permeability of placenta to insulin. *Am J Obstet Gynecol* 1988;158:1165–1169.
39. Bain MD, Copas DK, Taylor A, Landon MJ, Stacey TE. Permeability of the human placenta *in vivo* to four non-metabolised hydrophilic molecules. *J Physiol (Lond)* 1990;431:505–513.
40. Doughty IM, Glazier JD, Greenwood SL, Boyd RDH, Sibley CP. Mechanisms of materno-fetal chloride transfer across the *in vitro* perfused human placental cotyledon. *Am J Physiol (in press).*

41. Schneider H, Panigel M, Dancis J. Transfer across the perfused human placenta of antipyrine, sodium and leucine. *Am J Obstet Gynecol* 1972;114:822–828.
42. Boyd RDH, Glazier JD, Moore WMO, Sibley CP, Ward BS. Effect of chloride replacement on the electrical activity of the pig placenta *in vitro*. *J Physiol (Lond)* 1985;371:270P(abst).
43. Štulc J. Transfer pathways across the sheep placenta. *Placenta* 1996;17:377–379.
44. Canning JF, Stacey TE, Ward RHT, Boyd RDH. Radioiodide transfer across sheep placenta. *Am J Physiol* 1986;250:R112–R119.
45. Chien PFW, Smith K, Watt P, Scrimgeour CM, Taylor DJ, Rennie MJ. Protein turnover in the human fetus studied at term using stable isotope tracer amino acids. *Am J Physiol* 1993;265:E31–E35.
46. Armentrout T, Katz S, Thornburg KL, Faber JJ. Osmotic flow through the placental barrier of chronically prepared sheep. *Am J Physiol* 1977;233:H466–H474.
47. Grassl SM. G/HCO$_3$ exchange in human placental vesicles. *J Biol Chem* 1989;264:11103–11106.
48. Greenwood SL, Byrne S, Sibley CP. A chloride channel of 25 pS conductance in choriocarcinoma cells and cytotrophoblasts in culture. *Placenta* 1993;14:A26(abst).
49. Byrne S, Greenwood SL, Sibley CP. A chloride channel of small conductance in cytotrophoblast cells isolated from human term placenta. *Placenta* 1995;16:A10(abst).
50. Bissonnette J, Maylie B, Fiorillo C, Maylie J. Volume regulated chloride channels in human cytotrophoblast. *Placenta* 1995;16:A7(abst).
51. Cronier L, Bois P, Herve JC, Malassine A. Effect of human chorionic gonadotrophin on chloride current in human syncytiotrophoblasts in culture. *Placenta* 1995;17:599–609.
52. Dechecchi MC, Cabrini G. Chloride conductance in membrane vesicles from human placenta measured using a fluorescent probe. Implications for cystic fibrosis. *Biochim Biophys Acta* 1988;945:113–120.

DISCUSSION

Dr. Battaglia: Do we know yet how specific these transporter proteins are? In enzymology we often gave different names to the same protein depending on which pathway of metabolism it was regulating. This made us think of biology in far too complex a manner. In fact, one protein can have multiple functions. So I wonder how thoroughly that question has been investigated for these chloride transporters.

Dr. Boyd: Evidence is emerging that what you say may be completely right. Dave Shennan has done interesting work on volume regulatory release of amino acids, particularly aspartate and taurine (1). I believe the channel is DIDS-inhibitable, and it looks as though it may be a nonspecific anion channel, so that amino acid loss through intact villi may be via the same channel as chloride. There are even more interesting data showing that the protein of one of the amino acid transporters is probably also a viral receptor, and so the virus may be making use of an amino acid transporter protein to latch on. Thus, there is an interface between microbiology and transport (2). A general point is that I think we are particularly bad at crosstalk in placentology because we come from so many different disciplines. I don't understand endocrinology, and it may be that my colleagues in endocrinology don't understand transport. Immunologists study all these proteins and call them different things. There must be a lot of overlap.

Dr. Soothill: Coming from the human field, when one observes the techniques you describe, one is always concerned that the amount of destruction involved in creating the microspheres or in the separation of the placenta from the maternal surface during delivery may make it very difficult to extrapolate to *in vivo* systems. How can we test whether the extensive research that has gone on in these models does apply to the human *in vivo*?

Dr. Boyd: There are increasing possibilities of doing ethical studies *in vivo*. It looks as though stable isotopes provide a tremendous field for studying the undisturbed human, and of course you can make inferences in other ways—for example, Ken Thornburg and Terry

Stacey et al. have studied inert substances like vitamin B_{12} or certain sugars given to the mother before delivery and then looked at their presence in fetal urine and have drawn conclusions about placental permeability from that. There is also the possibility of doing electrophysiologic studies through catheters being used for antenatal diagnoses. So you begin to piece together what goes on *in vivo*.

Dr. Marconi: Biopsies of the placenta may be taken during pregnancy in selected cases. How far are we from applying the methodology you have described to that tiny piece of placenta so that we can tell how it is working?

Dr. Boyd: The only constraint is the ethical one. You can study individual villi, so if you can provide enough tissue, you could do it tomorrow.

Dr. Marconi: But how much is enough? Chorionic villous sampling is already used within 12 weeks for prenatal diagnosis, so it is certainly feasible.

Dr. Boyd: If you came here with three villi tomorrow, we could do electrophysiologic studies on them. However, we don't have a direct question to ask yet in the clinical setting, and in a sense, we are all casting around for that.

Dr. Sibley: As Dr. Boyd says, we can do electrophysiologic studies on one villus. Thus, if we get one villus, we can measure electrical potentials. The difficulty is translating that into something useful in terms of the whole placenta *in vivo*, but I think it is possible. What you need to do to view it as a whole—as we have tried to do with chloride—is to do electrophysiologic measurements at the single membrane level and then build them up into a model using whole perfused placentas, so you can get some idea of what the single molecule measurements mean in terms of the whole placenta. Once we begin to know more about what these transporter proteins are—and I agree that many of them may be more than just transporters—and once we know what their molecular structure is, then we can apply molecular biology techniques to isolate messenger RNA and determine how much of those proteins are there and what they do. Once we have done that we can start to make inferences from that single measurement on one villus.

Dr. Talamantes: In clinical disorders like cystic fibrosis, in which there are chloride transport abnormalities and other types of disorder, has there been an examination of what goes on in the placenta?

Dr. Boyd: Yes there has, but the findings have been disappointing. I think I am right in saying that nobody has currently shown a convincing, reproducible transport defect in placental tissues in cystic fibrosis. Is that a correct statement, Colin?

Dr. Sibley: This is true. CFTR is present in the placenta, but we don't know if babies with cystic fibrosis have a placental transport defect. The kidney also expresses CFTR at high levels, but it does not seem to be particularly affected in cystic fibrosis. There is still a lot of argument about whether the CFTR protein just transports chloride or whether it transports ATP, for example, so we might be looking at the wrong thing at the moment.

Dr. Page: You raised the intriguing possibility of various changes that can occur in gestation that we can't get at very easily in the human but that we know must occur from animal models. Do we have patterns from either culture or microvillus preparations from earlier stages in gestation that show changes in transporters that might reflect changes that we know are going on in animal models?

Dr. Boyd: We certainly do, from comparing first-trimester material (obtained at termination, not at biopsy) with term material, and Dr. Sibley will tell us precisely what those differences are, because he was involved in a study of amino acid transporters.

Dr. Sibley: We have done quite a lot of work comparing first-trimester (psychosocial) termination placenta material with term placenta material, and we found a variety of changes.

Some transport activities increase between the first trimester and term. For example, the system A amino acid transporter activity goes up between first trimester and term; other transporters—for example, sodium-proton exchanger and chloride-bicarbonate exchanger—don't change at all, and we suspect that sodium-potassium ATPase activity actually goes down from the first trimester to term. So we do see differences between first trimester and term, and the fact that they do not all go in the same direction shows that they are controlled changes that reflect changes in fetal growth patterns, and are not simply global changes caused by the placenta maturing or dying. In the rat, we have shown that there are marked increases in passive permeability and in a variety of transport proteins in late pregnancy, but these don't exactly reflect the changes we see in the human. One of the important things you have to remember in species comparison is the vastly different growth rates, placental weights, and blood flow geometries, all of which determine how that particular species transports solids. That is why it is very difficult to make those species comparisons.

Dr. Rennie: Do you think there are membrane-mediated transport events that modulate metabolism of the placenta *per se*? Within the mother there are substantial variations in concentration of various important solutes—amino acids, for example, and possibly others—and it is not clear to me to what extent the placenta or the fetus responds to these. But it is very clear that in adult animals the metabolism of the liver, for example, is markedly regulated by the state of hydration of the cell. Thus, if you stretch the liver cell, it becomes anabolic and accumulates protein, glycogen, and fat; if you shrink it, it becomes catabolic. You can mimic most of the endocrinologic effects that modulate liver metabolism by making the cell bigger or smaller. In other words, it appears that membrane-associated stretch is very important in the liver. So I wonder whether volume regulatory effects in the placenta might not be associated with a well-regulated mechanism for modulating placental metabolism. That is something we haven't really thought about up to now.

Dr. Boyd: That is an extremely interesting idea and exactly the sort of remark I hope to get out of this conference. I think it is exactly the sort of way in which one might integrate the available data.

Dr. Soothill: I wonder whether you would like to comment on research that might be going on in these models for interventions to improve or alter placental transfer. Are people currently investigating those?

Dr. Boyd: I think the answer perhaps is not very much so far. I think we are beginning to edge toward a period in which there are various kinds of interventions to improve transport, or prevent transport when there are unwanted solutes in the maternal circulation, whether they be viruses, proteins, or drugs that require blocking.

Dr. Sibley: Strauss in Philadelphia recently showed exciting data suggesting that there is a possibility of gene therapy at the placenta using viral particles to transfect different tissues. He showed that using the right sort of virus you can actually get the right gene into a mouse placenta. I think this is an exciting intervention, but we are a long way from being sure of the outcome at present.

Dr. Soothill: Do you think that the placental perfusion technique would help us with that?

Dr. Schneider: You have to bear in mind that until now in most laboratories the time available for working with perfusion systems has been quite limited—usually not more than 1 to 2 hours. Richard Miller in Rochester has recently extended perfusion work to 12 to 24 hours, and we have lately also extended the duration of our experiments to up to 8 hours and have actually started to do intervention work with insulin-like growth factor-1 (IGF-1), although this is very preliminary. The question is whether these effects, like those of IGF-1, can really be successfully studied over these limited time periods in culture.

Dr. Soothill: Can you test both the maternal and the fetal side in your system?

Dr. Schneider: Definitely, that is one of the strong aspects.

Dr. Battaglia: As I understood it, you described all chloride transport that was not DIDS-inhibitable as paracellular. I very much doubt this is the case. It seems to me you could still be left with quite a lot that is being transported by specific transporters, just not DIDS-inhibitable. I see nothing in the perfused human placenta data that says it is that leaky and nondiscriminating.

Dr. Schneider: It is true, the placenta is not as leaky as this might suggest. The work that Dr. Boyd briefly mentioned by Kent Thornburg on the transfer of urea and various sugars, in which he measured the permeability figure *in vivo* and compared it with the *in vitro* data, shows that placental integrity *in vitro* is quite well preserved. What we and others have done is to look at the effect of an increase in hydrostatic pressure in the fetal villous circulation on transfer integrity, and we have shown that there is a big difference between the guinea pig and the human placenta. The human placenta *in vitro* is much more resistant to these hydrostatic pressure changes than the guinea pig placenta. Minor changes in pressure in the *in vitro* guinea pig placenta will increase permeability enormously; fortunately for us, the human placenta is quite a bit more resilient.

Dr. Boyd: I would like to come back on that point. I think the evidence is moving a bit in your direction that most substances are transported through the cell, but there is a big experimental block to overcome first, and that is the way that both *in vivo* and *in vitro* the primate placenta lets through a string of apparently untransported molecules—chromium EDTA, erythritol, vitamin B_{12} when the transport is saturated, lactulose, and one or two others—and the simplest explanation for this is that there is a substantial paracellular pathway that is about the same in the perfused model as *in vivo* near term. My way of getting around is to say that earlier on the placenta might be tighter, but there isn't really a lot of evidence for that.

Dr. Battaglia: If you block with only one inhibitor, you can't necessarily ascribe any remaining transport to a paracellular pathway.

Dr. Sibley: If you take our permeability data and you normalize them for diffusion coefficient, then the chloride permeability coefficient is very similar to the two extracellular tracers we use. We showed chromium EDTA and mannitol, but we have also used L-glucose, and those three, together with chloride, showed very similar normalized permeabilities, which suggests that most of the chloride really is paracellular. So our evidence isn't just based on DIDS inhibition.

REFERENCES

1. Shennan DB, McNeillie SA. Volume-activated amino acid efflux from term human placental tissue: stimulation of efflux via a pathway sensitive to anion transport inhibitors. *Placenta* 1995;16:297–308.
2. Wang H, Kavanaugh MP, North RA, *et al.* Cell-surface receptor for ecotropic murine retroviruses is a basic amino-acid transporter. *Nature* 1991;352:729–731.

Placental Delivery of Amino Acids. Utilization and Production vs. Transport

Giacomo Meschia

Department of Physiology, University of Colorado Health Sciences Center, Campus Box C-240, 4200 East Ninth Avenue, Denver, Colorado 80262, USA

Early studies of amino acid transport across the ovine placenta suggested that amino acids taken up by the placenta from the maternal circulation are delivered to the fetus with no major loss (placental amino acid utilization) or addition (placental amino acid production) (1). Recent data indicate that for some amino acids, this suggestion is not valid, and that amino acid metabolism is an important aspect of placental function. The new information is based on several lines of evidence.

COMPARISON OF UTERINE AND UMBILICAL UPTAKE OF AMINO ACIDS

In sheep, the net flux of metabolic substrates between maternal circulation and pregnant uterus (uterine uptake) and the net flux of metabolic substrates between placenta and fetus (umbilical uptake) have been estimated using an application of the Fick principle (2). In this application, uterine uptake of any given substrate is estimated by measuring uterine blood flow (ml/min) and the concentration difference of the substrate between maternal arterial and uterine venous blood (μmol/ml). The uterine uptake (μmol/min) is then calculated as the product of uterine blood flow and concentration difference. Umbilical uptake is similarly estimated by measuring umbilical blood flow and the concentration difference of the substrate between umbilical venous and umbilical arterial blood. When uterine and umbilical uptakes are estimated in the same animal preparation, they provide information about placental metabolism. A uterine uptake that is greater than umbilical uptake indicates utilization by the uteroplacental tissues, whereas an umbilical uptake that is greater than uterine uptake indicates placental production.

The application of the Fick principle to the study of placental amino acid metabolism *in vivo* has been difficult to implement for the following reasons: (a) with few exceptions, the concentration differences of each amino acid across the uterine and umbilical circulations are a relatively small percentage of the arterial concentration,

Thus, a large number of measurements are required to compensate for the noise introduced by random analytic error, (b) in the chromatographic measurements of amino acid concentrations, incomplete peak separation may provide unreliable information about certain amino acids. Early attempts to measure serine uptakes were biased by this error (3), and (c) free amino acid concentrations can be measured in either whole blood or plasma. The choice of which concentration is measured affects the accuracy of the uptake estimate. For example, plasma carries glutamate at a much lower concentration than red cells and is the only blood compartment that exchanges glutamate with the placenta and other organs (4). As a result, glutamate uptake is best estimated as the product of so-called plasma flow [blood flow x (1—fractional hematocrit)] and the plasma glutamate concentration difference. Plasma concentration differences of amino acids for which plasma is not the only blood compartment of exchange must be converted to whole blood differences and then multiplied by blood flow. For leucine, conversion factors have been estimated by measuring the volume of distribution of tracer amino acid added to maternal and fetal blood incubated *in vitro* (5).

The interpretation of the results of uptake calculations raises theoretical concerns in addition to the practical concerns listed above. For example, the uptake calculations assume that in passing through the placenta, maternal and fetal blood do not produce free amino acids. This would not be the case if blood proteins and peptides were rapidly hydrolyzed by the placenta and became a significant source of free amino acids at the site of transplacental exchange. However, there has been no evidence thus far to suggest that processes other than placental uptake and release of amino acids play a significant role in determining the concentration differences of amino acids across the uterine and umbilical circulations.

In the last 2 years, we have begun a long-term project in which simultaneously measured uterine and umbilical blood flows and plasma concentration differences of amino acids across the uterine and umbilical circulations are used to explore placental amino acid metabolism *in vivo* through the application of the Fick principle. Thus far, this project has provided information about uptakes of most of the neutral and acidic amino acids in 15 pregnant sheep, studied under normal physiologic conditions and at approximately 130 days' gestation (about 2 weeks before term). There are three notable results: (a) the branched-chain amino acids leucine, valine, and isoleucine show uterine uptakes that are significantly greater than umbilical uptakes, (b) there is a fairly large serine uptake by the pregnant uterus with no significant umbilical serine uptake. The opposite occurs with glycine: no significant uterine uptake and a large umbilical uptake, and (c) glutamate shows a large uptake by the placenta from the umbilical circulation (negative uptake). These results are confirmed and explained by other lines of evidence, including tracer studies. As placental uptake of glutamate is discussed in another chapter in this volume (**Fetal Liver and the Placenta: An Interactive System**), the remainder of the discussion focuses primarily on the branched-chain amino acids glycine and serine.

PLACENTAL UTILIZATION OF BRANCHED-CHAIN AMINO ACIDS

In addition to the data already mentioned, uterine uptakes of branched-chain amino acids that are significantly greater than umbilical uptakes have been observed in two previous studies (5,6). The placenta releases into the fetal and maternal circulations the keto acids formed in the deamination of leucine (ketoisocaproic acid) (5,7,8), valine (ketoisovaleric acid) (8), and isoleucine (α-keto-β-methylvaleric acid) (8). When tracer leucine is infused into the fetus, approximately 10% is deaminted in the placenta (7). We conclude from this evidence that branched-chain amino acids entering the placenta are rapidly deaminated, and that this catabolic process reduces the flux of branched-chain amino acids from placenta to fetus.

In exploring the functional meaning of branched-chain amino acid deamination within the placenta, we note that it results in the formation of glutamate through transamination with α-ketoglutarate. Therefore, the placenta has an endogenous source of glutamate from branched-chain amino acid transamination as well as an exogenous source from the uptake of fetal glutamate. The oxidation of glutamate by placental mitochondria generates NADPH (reduced nicotinamide adenine dinucleotide phosphate), which can then be used for steroid synthesis (9). This information suggests that placental branched-chain amino acid deamination may be linked to steroidogenesis.

Through glutamate oxidation, the deamination of branched-chain amino acids ultimately results in the formation of ammonia. The uteroplacental tissues take up branched-chain amino acids at a combined rate of approximately 20 μmol/min/kg fetus and release them into the fetal circulation at the combined rate of approximately 13 μmol/min/kg fetus. This indicates a net uteroplacental branched-chain amino acid utilization rate of approximately 7 μmol/min/kg fetus. The ovine uteroplacental tissues excrete ammonia in both the maternal and fetal circulations at an estimated rate of 10 μmol/min/kg fetus (10). Therefore, the comparison of uteroplacental branched-chain amino acid utilization and ammonia excretion (7 *vs.* 10 μmol/min/kg fetus) suggests that deamination of branched-chain amino acids is one of the main contributors to placental ammonia production.

Recently, ovine placental transport and fetal utilization of leucine at 130 days' gestation have been compared between control ewes and ewes in which severe intrauterine growth retardation (IUGR) had been induced by exposure to heat stress in early and midpregnancy (5). Leucine fluxes were measured by means of leucine tracers simultaneously infused into the maternal and fetal circulations. Several fluxes were reduced in the IUGR group, even when expressed per kilogram of fetus. There were significant reductions in uteroplacental utilization, fetal disposal rate, transport from mother to fetus, back flux from fetus to placenta, and decarboxylation of fetal leucine. Uteroplacental utilization and transport from mother to fetus were also significantly reduced per gram placenta. These data indicate that maternal leucine flux into the IUGR placenta was markedly reduced and that most of the reduced flux was routed into fetal utilization through a decrease in placental leucine catabolism and a decrease in the leucine flux from fetus to placenta. It is apparent, therefore, that placental branched-chain amino acid metabolism may be altered in IUGR pregnancies and that the amount of branched-chain amino acids available for fetal consumption depends on the interplay between placental transport and placental metabolism of these amino acids.

PLACENTAL GLYCINE PRODUCTION

Several studies have shown a relatively large fetal uptake of glycine at the approximate rate of 5 μmol/min/kg fetus (11). As there is no demonstrable uptake of glycine by the pregnant uterus, the data suggest that most of the glycine delivered by the placenta to the fetus is produced within the placenta. Glycine can be formed from serine by the following reaction:

Serine + Tetrahydrofolate $\rightarrow$ Glycine + Methylenetetrahydrofolate + H_2O

Therefore, the glycine data focus attention on placental serine metabolism. There are three possible sources of serine for the placenta: the fetal circulation, the maternal circulation, and serine synthesized within the placenta.

Several attempts have been made to establish whether there is a net flux of serine into the placenta from the fetal circulation. This flux has been difficult to detect, because the concentration of serine in fetal blood and plasma is very high (approximately 700 μM). In three studies of the sheep fetus in late gestation, the estimated net flux ranged from statistically insignificant to approximately 2 μmol/min/kg fetus (12). For the unpublished observations in the 15 late-gestation fetuses, the mean net flux was 1.23 ± 0.84 μmol/min/kg fetus and not significantly different from zero. However, two studies of amino acid uptake in the midgestational fetus were able to demonstrate a significant net flux of serine into the placenta from the fetus (12). Furthermore, the infusion of L-[1-^{13}C] serine into the fetal circulation has shown placental uptake of the tracer serine and significant placental output of [1-^{13}C] glycine, both in late and midgestation (12). The combined tracee and tracer evidence indicates that fetal serine is one of the sources for the production of glycine by the placenta, although not a major source in late gestation.

The unpublished data in 15 late-gestation fetuses show a relatively large uptake of maternal serine by the pregnant uterus, equal to about 80% of placental glycine output into the umbilical circulation. This comparison suggests that in late gestation the placenta uses primarily maternal serine for the production of fetal glycine. To test the hypothesis that maternal serine is converted to fetal glycine by the placenta, we infused L-[1-^{13}C] serine intravenously into the mother and sampled maternal and fetal plasma for tracer serine and glycine enrichments. These experiments showed no enrichment of fetal serine and a significant enrichment of fetal glycine. However, the interpretation of the data was made somewhat difficult by the fact that the maternal infusion of tracer serine labeled maternal glycine, raising the question of whether the tracer glycine transported into the fetus by the placenta had been formed in the mother rather than in the placenta. In separate experiments designed to answer this question, tracer glycine was infused into the mother. The tracer glycine infusion showed mother-to-fetus glycine transport, but at a rate that could explain only a small fraction of the fetal glycine labeling in the tracer serine experiments. Therefore, the combined results of maternal tracer serine and glycine infusion supported the hypothesis that maternal serine is used by the placenta to form fetal glycine. For a more direct proof of placental conversion of serine to glycine, we performed a different experiment, using a twin preparation (13). In this preparation, we used the local infusion of tracer serine into one uterine artery to expose the placenta of one twin (experimental placenta) to a higher concentration of tracer serine than the placenta of the other twin (control placenta). No tracer serine could be detected in either fetus. Glycine enrichments in uterine venous and umbilical arterial and venous plasma were significantly higher for the experimental placenta, thus demonstrating placental conversion of maternal serine into glycine.

The question of whether serine synthesized within the placenta is a significant source for the formation of fetal glycine remains unanswered. During the constant infusion of tracer serine into the maternal circulation, umbilical venous glycine enrichment is about 5% of maternal serine enrichment. This indicates that maternal serine entering the placenta is diluted by placental serine and that the glycine formed from the maternal serine is further diluted by placental glycine. Because the ovine placenta has a high protein turnover rate (5,14), it is unclear whether this dilution results from the release of serine and glycine by placental proteins or includes *de novo* synthesis of placental serine.

In the conversion of serine to glycine, each β carbon of serine becomes an "activated one-carbon unit" through the formation of methylenetetrahydrofolate. These carbon units are used in a large number of biosynthetic processes (e.g., purine synthesis). Therefore, the conversion of serine to glycine within the placenta may have the main function of synthesizing metabolic substrates that are important for fetal growth and depend on the availability of activated one-carbon units for their synthesis. Further studies focused on the placental utilization of β serine carbon are needed to explore the validity of this hypothesis.

SUMMARY

Studies of placental amino acid metabolism, by means of *in vivo* tracer methodology, have shown that the ovine placenta deaminates leucine and converts both maternal and fetal serine into fetal glycine. There is evidence that in addition to leucine, the placenta deaminates the other two branched-chain amino acids—isoleucine and valine. The comparison of branched-chain amino acid uptake by the pregnant uterus and by the umbilical circulation (20 *vs.* 13 μmol/min/kg fetus) suggests that the branched-chain amino acid deamination rate by the placenta could be as high as

7 μmol/min/kg fetus. The transamination of branched-chain amino acid with α-ketoglutarate produces glutamate, which is an oxidative substrate for placental mitochondria. In addition, the placenta oxidizes glutamate derived from fetal plasma. Glutamate oxidation by placental mitochondria has been linked to NADPH production and steroidogenesis. In the heat stress model of ovine fetal growth retardation, both placental transport and placental utilization of leucine are reduced.

Although maternal serine enters the placenta, there is no placental transport of maternal serine into the fetus. The comparison of uterine serine uptake with umbilical glycine intake indicates that in late gestation, maternal serine contributes about 80% of the glycine delivered to the fetus by the placenta. One important function of serine-to-glycine conversion is the generation of methylenetetrahydrofolate, which is a substrate for a variety of essential biosynthetic processes. It is not clear, however, what functional advantage, if any, is provided by localization of the entire conversion of maternal serine to fetal glycine in the placenta rather than the fetus.

ACKNOWLEDGMENT

This work was supported by NIH Grant HD-01866, "Physiological Study of the Placenta," and NIH Grant HD-29188, "Fetal and Placental Metabolism of Threonine and Alanine."

REFERENCES

1. Holzman IR, Lemons JA, Meschia G, Battaglia FC. Uterine uptake of amino acids and glutamine-glutamate balance across the placenta of the pregnant ewe. *J Dev Physiol* 1979;1:137–149.
2. Meschia G, Battaglia FC, Hay WW, Sparks JW. Utilization of substrates by the ovine placenta *in vivo*. *Fed Proc* 1980;39:245–249.
3. Bell AW, Kennaugh JM, Battaglia FC, Meschia G. Uptake of amino acids and ammonia at mid-gestation by the fetal lamb. *Q J Exp Physiol* 1989;74:635–643.
4. Moores RR, Vaughn PR, Battaglia FC, Fennessey PV, Wilkening RB, Meschia G. Glutamate metabolism in the fetus and placenta of late gestation sheep. *Am J Physiol* 1994;267(*Regul Integr Comp Physiol* 36):R89–R96.
5. Ross JC, Fennessey PV, Wilkening RB, Battaglia FC, Meschia G. Placental transport and fetal utilization of leucine in a model of fetal growth retardation. *Am J Physiol* 1996;270(*Endocrinol Metab* 33):E491–E503.
6. Liechty EA, Kelley J, Lemons JA. Effect of fasting on uteroplacental amino acid metabolism in the pregnant sheep. *Biol Neonate* 1991;60:207–214.
7. Loy GL, Quick AN, Hay WW, Meschia G, Battaglia FC, Fennessey PV. Fetoplacental deamination and decarboxylation of leucine. *Am J Physiol* 1990;259(*Endocrinol Metab* 22):E492–E497.
8. Smeaton TC, Owens JA, Kind KL, Robinson JS. The placenta releases branched-chain keto acids into the umbilical and uterine circulations in the pregnant sheep. *J Dev Physiol* 1989;12:95–99.
9. Klimek J, Makarewicz W, Swierczynski J, Bossy-Bukato G, Zelewski L. Mitochondrial glutamine and glutamate metabolism in human placenta and its possible link with progesterone biosynthesis. *Trophoblast Res* 1993;7:77–86.
10. Holzman IR, Lemons JA, Meschia G, Battaglia FC. Ammonia production by the pregnant uterus. *Proc Soc Exp Biol Med* 1977;156:27–30.
11. Cetin I, Sparks JW, Quick AN, Marconi AM, Meschia G, Battaglia FC, *et al.* Glycine turnover and oxidation and hepatic serine synthesis from glycine in fetal lambs. *Am J Physiol* 1991;260(*Endocrinol Metab* 23):E371–E378.

12. Moores RR, Carter BS, Meschia G, Fennessey PV, Battaglia FC. Placental and fetal serine fluxes at midgestation in the fetal lamb. *Am J Physiol* 1994;267(*Endocrinol Metab* 30):E150–E155.
13. Moores RR, Rietberg CC, Battaglia FC, Fennessey PV, Meschia G. Metabolism and transport of maternal serine by the ovine placenta: glycine production and absence of serine transport into the fetus. *Pediatr Res* 1993;33:590–594.
14. Carrol MJ, Young M. The relationship between placental protein synthesis and transfer of amino acids. *Biochem J* 1983;210:99–105.

DISCUSSION

Dr. Rennie: It looks as though the maternal tracer enrichment of your leucine was quite different in the IUGR and control animals—one was about 6 mol% excess and the other was about 4. Was that a reflection of the maternal turnover, or did you put different amounts of tracer in?

Dr. Meschia: You are quite right, there was a lower turnover of leucine in the growth-retarded than in the IUGR mother, and that correlated with nutrition. When we exposed the sheep to heat stress in a 40°C chamber for several hours, our first concern was whether we were producing growth retardation because of effects on maternal nutrition. But in fact maternal nutrition was not much affected by heat stress in early and midgestation. However, when the sheep were taken out of the chamber, there was a reduced food intake, and we attributed this to the fact that they were carrying a much smaller fetus and placenta, and the mammary glands were not so well developed.

Dr. Soothill: But you said in your talk that you believed this was caused by reduced transfer. But the other hypothesis is that there is reduced protein turnover and protein uptake within the fetus. How did you separate those two?

Dr. Meschia: First of all, there is reduced uptake of leucine by the mother, but when one looks at the concentration of leucine in maternal blood, it is not altered. The fetal leucine concentration is reduced compared with control. There is a decreased disposal rate of leucine in the fetus that is almost exclusively caused by the fact that there is less entry of leucine into the fetus and less back flux of leucine into the placenta. So it is the dysfunction of the placenta that explains the decreased disposal rate of fetal leucine.

Dr. Jensen: Is there any relation between oxygen delivery to the placenta/fetus and the reduced leucine disposal rate?

Dr. Meschia: As I have already indicated, these fetuses tend to be hypoxic, and that is because of an increased PO_2 gradient between maternal blood and fetal blood. It is not caused by decreased uterine perfusion. Although in absolute terms there is less blood flow in the growth-retarded conceptus, when one looks at uterine blood flow per kilogram of fetus or per kilogram of conceptus, then there is no difference. The fetus is hypoxic because there is a larger gradient of PO_2 between mother and fetus. In other words, the diffusing capacity of the placenta for oxygen is reduced. Oxygen consumption by the uteroplacental mass is not reduced, so this reduction of leucine utilization seems rather specific.

Dr. Jensen: Would that lead us to the conclusion that the transporter system for leucine and the reduced disposal rate are regulated on the fetal side rather than on the maternal side?

Dr. Meschia: It is extremely difficult to establish cause and effect from *in vivo* data. There is definitely decreased transport of leucine into the placenta. I indicated that this is probably a primary event compared with other things, such as a decrease in leucine concentration in the fetus. But I would not go so far as to claim a cause-and-effect relationship—that is really difficult to establish.

Dr. Marini: In your model, did you have any chance of measuring heat shock proteins in the maternal myocardium?

Dr. Meschia: We haven't done that yet. But we have in mind to measure heat shock proteins in the placenta to see if they appear under these conditions. We really have not yet understood the pathogenesis. What we can exclude is that this defect in transport of amino acid has anything to do with decreased blood flow. It is definitely a problem of transport.

Dr. Godfrey: One of the very important things to bear in mind is the likelihood that these amino acid relationships are very different in early and late pregnancy. For example, we have indirect data suggesting that indices of glycine insufficiency are telling us very different things in human early and late pregnancy. Do you have any data that might bear on that in your models?

Dr. Meschia: We have no data yet in early pregnancy.

Dr. Herrera: Is there any relationship between decreased protein synthesis and the rate of leucine transfer in the growth-retarded fetuses?

Dr. Meschia: We do not see significant changes in protein synthesis. I have to be very careful here. What we study, of course, is the turnover of plasma leucine, and we can estimate how much of the flux of leucine is into protein rather than oxidation. We find that the flux into protein is no different per kilogram of fetus than in the normal, although it could be 10% or 20% less, in which case it would be very difficult to establish a statistically significant difference. I want to point out that from ultrasonographic scans one can see that this growth retardation begins rather early in gestation; one can therefore assume that this severe growth retardation that one sees at the end of pregnancy is the accumulated effect of a relatively small difference in growth rates over a long time, and that is why it is not easy, in my opinion, to see changes in protein synthesis per kilogram of fetus.

Dr. Rennie: When we measure glycine transfer, as we can in the human situation, we do get a substantial glycine transfer from the mother to the fetus. Under IUGR conditions, although there is a substantial decrement of leucine transfer, we find there is no decrement of glycine transfer but an increased glycine back flux. So it appears that the two amino acids differ in that leucine does not get across as fast as glycine, but glycine appears not to be used so fast and therefore it comes back to the mother. I don't know whether this is a sheep difference or a model difference, because our model and yours are really very different. But I think it is fascinating that there are these differences. I wonder whether you found any differences in serine-to-glycine transfer in your growth-retarded animals. I don't think you have touched on that.

Dr. Meschia: We have not studied the serine-to-glycine conversion in the growth-retarded. You are quite right that we have to be very careful about the species differences. The paracellular pathway of transport seems to be absent in the sheep. So any transport of amino acid you see from mother to fetus definitely involves transporters. There is definitely a species difference here. The sheep placenta seems to act only via transporters; there is no evidence that amino acids are transported in any other way in the sheep.

Dr. Marconi: We have done human pregnancy studies that are quite similar to those done in the sheep by the group in Denver, infusing a bolus of leucine and glycine at the time of fetal blood sampling in normal fetuses, and we find exactly the same thing, that the transplacental passage of leucine and the fetal-maternal ratio is very close to 1, whereas the enrichment of glycine in the fetus is negligible.

Dr. Rennie: That is a very interesting difference, I think.

Dr. Sibley: We have shown that the activity of the system A transporter in the microvillous membrane of growth-retarded human placentas is about half that of normally grown fetuses.

The system A transporter will transport glycine, so we would predict a decrease in glycine transfer from those data, but there are a number of things we don't know in relating that to the *in vivo* situation, such as what the driving pulses are, what the intracellular concentrations are, and what the relative maternofetal concentrations are; but there is certainly a defect in the plasma membrane of the human placenta and in the main transporter that would transport glycine. Unfortunately, nobody has yet looked at the system L transport, which is the one that would transport leucine in the human placenta. I should also add that our system A data hold for both small-for-gestational-age (SGA) fetuses and those with severe growth retardation.

Dr. Soothill: So are you suggesting that these differences might relate to different transporter molecules?

Dr. Sibley: Yes, but this is not the whole story.

Dr. Meschia: I am aware of your results. There is no question that the literature shows more and more that in growth retardation there is a defect in transport of amino acids, such as the system A amino acids. One must bear in mind that the transport of amino acids from mother to fetus involves at least two steps—transport into the placenta and transport out of the placenta—and there could be also a problem in terms of transport out of the placenta. For instance, the sheep placenta has definitely got a system A transport, and yet we see virtually no serine and very little glycine transport into the fetus. So we have to think globally.

Dr. Marconi: I was very surprised when I saw that the reduction in umbilical uptake was mainly caused by a reduction in the direct flux of leucine from mother to fetus and not by a decreased contribution from the placental pool. How do you explain that? One would expect a similar reduction in both sources.

Dr. Meschia: The protein turnover in the placenta was expressed per kilogram of fetus, so one would have to express it per gram of placenta, but in whatever units you express it, it does not look as though the protein turnover in the placenta is really much affected, and this is consistent with the fact that the oxygen consumption of the placenta (per gram of placenta) is not really much different. I don't see a problem in combining this information with the fact that there is less leucine transported into the placenta. At this age the placenta is not growing, and there is no accretion of proteins in the placenta, so protein turnover could still go on with virtually no input of exogenous leucine.

Dr. Marconi: Yes, but as a clinician I would expect the placenta not to be working very well as an organ, but instead you tell us that the transport systems from mother to the placenta are not working, while placental metabolism reflected by protein turnover is working somehow! Is there some kind of compensation?

Dr. Meschia: I wish I knew. When you look at these placentae, you cannot see changes in oxygen consumption and yet you can see changes in leucine utilization. Perhaps this is because with leucine utilization we are looking at a single substrate.

Dr. Boyd: You have touched on a question that always worries me, and that is the matter of the denominator—whether one should be dividing by placental weight, placental surface area, fetal weight, fetal lean body mass, and so on. I haven't got any answers, but I just wonder if you could reflect for a moment on that difficulty, which really runs right across the field.

Dr. Meschia: This is very important. First of all, why did I divide the transport fluxes by kilogram of fetus? The reason for this is that if you look at a normal and a growth-retarded individual, of course the growth-retarded will have a reduction in anything you measure because it is smaller. It would be very difficult to imagine that the growth-retarded individual would consume the same amount of oxygen in absolute terms as the normal. So you have to normalize the data. Consider oxygen consumption. If you take oxygen consumption in absolute terms, of course the growth-retarded individual has a much lower oxygen consumption than the normal, but per kilogram of fetus the oxygen consumption appears to be about the same. So I could have used oxygen consumption of the fetus as the normalizing variable and I would have exactly the same results. So the idea of doing fluxes per kilogram of fetus or per rate of fetal oxygen consumption is to exclude trivial data because of the fact that we are dealing with two different masses.

Dr. Soothill: I think that is a very important point in terms of the human observational data, because we have nearly always compared it with the normal cases at that gestational age, and there are important differences there.

Dr. Owens: When we produce experimental intrauterine growth retardation in sheep, we produce it in a different way, by restricting implantation and producing a placenta that is small because it has fewer cotyledons. In a recent study, when we looked at protein synthesis rates within that restricted placenta in late gestation, we actually found, along with reduced oxygen consumption per kilogram of placenta, a reduced rate of protein synthesis within the placenta in the most restricted placentae. So this differs a little from what you were finding, and my guess would be that the restricted placenta produced by heat stress as opposed to restricted implantation is quite different in terms of structure, although it may be exposed to a similar metabolic and endocrine milieu late in gestation. Coming back to this question of the cause of reduced leucine entry in your growth retardation model in late gestation, I wonder to what extent you have looked at structural changes within the placenta as being partly if not solely responsible for that. What I am thinking of is reductions in surface area per gram of that placenta, changes in diffusion distance perhaps, and so on. I can see clearly that people are very interested in changes in the relative abundance of relevant transporters, but I think it is also important to know what is happening structurally within the placenta.

Dr. Meschia: We looked years ago for histologic changes and could not establish any definite changes, but we are planning to do this again, now that we have more experience. This is a very important question. Is a gram of placenta in the growth-retarded individual the same as a gram of placenta in the normal?

Dr. Marini: From a clinical point of view, as neonatologists we know that the composition of an IUGR neonate is completely different from that of an appropriate gestational age preterm baby.

Molecular Mechanisms of Placental Development

Michael J. Soares

Department of Physiology, University of Kansas Medical Center, Kansas City, Kansas 66160, USA

The placenta possesses features allowing it to modify the maternal reproductive tract into a hospitable and nutritive environment for the developing embryo and fetus. These fundamental tasks are accomplished through the differentiation of the trophoblast cell lineage. Mature trophoblast cell phenotypes are characterized by their acquisition of functions that contribute to the modification of the maternal environment and the development of the embryo/fetus. These adaptive functions include (a) invasion, (b) nutrient and waste transport, (c) metabolism, (d) evasion of the maternal immune system, and (e) production of hormones and cytokines. Identification of a particular trophoblast cell phenotype can be achieved through analysis of the activities of batteries of genes associated with each function. The orchestration of molecular events responsible for directing trophoblast cell differentiation is largely unknown.

The purpose of this chapter is to review our present understanding of the molecular mechanisms involved in controlling the development of the trophoblast cell lineage. Our analysis is primarily directed to rodent and primate models. The reader is also referred to other recent reviews on related aspects of placental development (1-5).

TROPHOBLAST CELL LINEAGE: RODENT AND HUMAN

Trophoblast cells represent the first lineage arising from the embryo and progress along a multilineage pathway. Differentiation is probably influenced by an inherent genetic program and environmental signals emanating from embryonic and maternal compartments. It is well established that there are important interactions of the inner cell mass (ICM) and its derivatives with trophectoderm (1). This early bidirectional signaling system is believed to govern initial phases of trophoblast growth and differentiation. Developmental pathways leading from the trophoblast progenitor (trophectoderm) to one of several differentiated trophoblast end points are yet to be

TABLE 1. *Rodent and human trophoblast cell lineages*

Rodent
  Trophoblast giant cells
  Spongiotrophoblast cells
  Glycogen cells
  Syncytial trophoblast cells
Human
  Cytotrophoblast cells (villous or extravillous)
  Syncytial trophoblast cells (villous or extravillous)
  Villous intermediate trophoblast cells
  Extravillous mononuclear trophoblast cells

clarified. Both rodent and human trophoblast cells organize into a hemochorial type of placenta, with maternal blood directly bathing trophoblast cells.

The rodent trophoblast cell lineage consists of at least four distinct differentiated phenotypes (2,6) (Table 1): (a) trophoblast giant cell, (b) spongiotrophoblast cell, (c) glycogen cell, and (d) syncytial trophoblast cell. These cell types can be distinguished on the basis of their morphology, intraplacental location, and pattern of gene expression. Trophoblast giant cells arise through endoreduplication, are located at the placental-uterine interface, and have a prominent endocrine role. Spongiotrophoblast and glycogen cells are embedded within the chorioallantoic placenta and participate in endocrine and metabolic functions, respectively. Syncytial trophoblast cells are believed to arise from the fusion of trophoblast precursors, are located at the placental-fetal interface, and have a prominent role in nutrient and waste transport.

The following description of the human trophoblast cell lineage (Table 1) is derived from discussions by Ringler and Strauss (7), Aplin (8), and Kaufmann and Burton (9). Human trophoblast cells can be located inside or outside villous structures.

Intravillous Trophoblast

Intravillous trophoblast cells are generally classified in two categories: *cytotrophoblast* cells and *syncytial trophoblast* cells. The number of nuclei in a cell largely provides the criterion for trophoblast cell classification: mononuclear cells are cytotrophoblast cells, and multinuclear cells are syncytial trophoblast cells. Unfortunately, the cytotrophoblast category is inherently confusing, describing both stem and differentiated cell types. The term cytotrophoblast should be restricted to proliferative mononuclear trophoblast cells that are progenitors for differentiated trophoblast cell types. Nonproliferative mononuclear trophoblast cells progressing along the differentiation pathway should be referred to as *villous intermediate trophoblast* cells (7). Syntial formation through fusion of mononuclear trophoblast cells is clearly a hallmark of end-stage human intravillous trophoblast cell differentiation. Syncytial trophoblast cells are key parenchymal cell types of the placenta, possessing important endocrine and transport properties. Various human choriocarcinoma cell lines may represent intermediate mononuclear stages progressing along the differentiated pathway (10).

Extravillous Trophoblast

The extravillous trophoblast lineage consists of mononuclear trophoblast and syncytial trophoblast cells. These cells develop outside the villous structure, contribute to the formation of the smooth chorion, chorionic plate, basal plate, and cell columns, and have previously been assigned an array of different names (9). Again, three cell populations can be identified: a proliferative population, referred to as *extravillous cytotrophoblast* cells; nonproliferative differentiated mononuclear trophoblast cells, referred to as *extravillous mononuclear trophoblast* cells; and a multinucleated differentiated population, referred to as *extravillous syncytial trophoblast* cells. The term *intermediate* has been avoided because it implies a transitory population between cytotrophoblast and syncytial trophoblast cell populations and not an endstage differentiated phenotype. Functionally, the extravillous cell populations behave differently from villous trophoblast. In addition to some endocrine activities, extravillous trophoblast cells also contribute to the establishment of the uteroplacental interface. Environmental factors probably contribute to differences in the phenotypes shown by villous and extravillous trophoblast.

GENOMIC IMPRINTING AND TROPHOBLAST CELL DEVELOPMENT

Genomic imprinting represents a process of allele-specific control of gene expression and is paramount to the development of the trophoblast lineage (11–13). Through a series of elegant zygotic nuclear transfer experiments, the paternal genetic contribution was shown to be essential for placental development (14,15). Androgenetic zygotes (exclusively paternally derived) show extensive development of extraembryonic tissues, including trophoblast, but limited development of the embryo proper, whereas gynogenetic zygotes (exclusively maternally derived) show limited development of extraembryonic tissues but more extensive development of the embryo proper. Additional support for the involvement of paternally imprinted genes in trophoblast development was derived from the genesis of hydatidiform moles, benign types of gestational trophoblast disease characterized by an excessive formation of trophoblast structures. The genetic makeup of the majority of complete hydatidiform moles is exclusively paternal, whereas partial hydatidiform moles are generally triploid, with two paternal contributions and a single maternal contribution (11). Approximately 20 genes have been shown to have a paternal or maternal allele-specific pattern of expression (13,16). Two of these genes, insulin-like growth factor-2 (IGF-2) and *Mash-2*, have been implicated in the development of trophoblast cells (see below).

Some imprinted genes are located in clusters on chromosomes that have previously been connected with the control of trophoblast development (2,17). Although regulatory mechanisms responsible for genomic imprinting have not been determined, allele-specific DNA methylation has received considerable attention (13,18). Identification of additional genes involved in the regulation of the trophoblast cell lineage may be forthcoming from studies on genomic imprinting.

STRATEGIES FOR THE DISCOVERY OF GENES PIVOTAL TO DEVELOPMENT OF THE TROPHOBLAST CELL LINEAGE

Two principal tactics have been used to dissect cell differentiation: (a) *in vitro* approaches using cell culture and (b) *in vivo* approaches involving gene targeting and the generation of transgenic mice.

In Vitro Strategies

Significant progress in understanding molecular mechanisms associated with the differentiation of any cell lineage is greatly facilitated by the establishment of *in vitro* models (2,6). Several *in vitro* strategies have been used in the study of trophoblast cell biology.

Primary Cultures

As a rule, trophoblast cell primary cultures have been problematic. They are difficult to isolate to homogeneity, they do not proliferate, and they do not readily assimilate or express transgenes. On a positive side, the cells spontaneously differentiate in culture and can provide a window into various aspects of trophoblast cell differentiation (7,19,20).

Spontaneous Placenta-Derived Cell Lines

Trophoblast cell lines can be established from normal placentae (21,22). The cells proliferate well; however, they do not readily show characteristics unique to differentiated trophoblast cells, and consequently precise determinations of their *in vivo* counterparts have been difficult.

Virally Transformed Cell Lines

Another strategy yielding some success involves the immortalization of trophoblast cells with recombinant viruses containing Simian virus 40 (23). These cell lines (HP-A1, HP-A2, HP-W1) express at least some genes characteristic of the trophoblast cell lineage and are responsive to some known modulators of trophoblast cell function (23).

Trophoblast Tumor-Derived Cell Lines

The derivation of cell lines from spontaneous trophoblast tumors (choriocarcinoma) has proved to be an effective approach for the development of *in vitro* models. Human choriocarcinoma cell lines (BeWo, JEG, Jar, HM, HCCM-5, NUC-1, HT-H) have been available for the past two decades (reviewed in ref. 7). These cells retain the ability to show aspects of differentiated function, especially the expression of chorionic gonadotrophin (CG) subunit genes, and have effectively been used to characterize trophoblast cell-specific gene expression. Human choriocarcinoma cell lines tend to have a mixed phenotype, possessing ability to proliferate and express differentiated function simultaneously. Some sublines may be more useful than the original parent cell lines (24,25). The specific part of the trophoblast lineage represented in the human choriocarcinoma cell lines is not entirely apparent.

Cell lines have also been generated from a rat choriocarcinoma (26–28). One of the rat choriocarcinoma cell lines, Rcho-1, has proved to be very useful. Rcho-1 trophoblast cells can be experimentally manipulated to proliferate or differentiate (28–30). Differentiation is restricted to the trophoblast giant-cell lineage and includes the expression of members of the placental prolactin gene family and two hydroxylases involved in steroid hormone biosynthesis (28,29,31–33). These cells have also been shown to be useful for studying transcriptional control of trophoblast giant-cell-specific genes (31–37).

Overview

An ideal culture system would permit the experimental manipulation of a population of stem cells to proliferate or differentiate in specific directions along a multilineage pathway. Although perfection has not been achieved, several different *in vitro* models are available that allow dissection of elements of trophoblast cell differentiation and the control of trophoblast cell-specific gene expression. Collectively, the immortalized cell populations can be considered caricatures of normal development and represent valuable resources for dissecting regulatory mechanisms (38). An important key is in determining which regulatory mechanisms correspond to normal *vs.* transformed phenotypes.

Gene Targeting and Transgenic Strategies

These approaches take advantage of our expanding abilities to manipulate the genetic constitution of the mouse. Embryonic stem cell and homologous recombination strategies are effective means for disrupting specific gene activities during development (39,40). Introduction of transgenes by pronuclear injection has also proved to be a useful *in vivo* approach for mapping trophoblast cell-specific gene promoter activities (41–44). Human and rodent promoters for trophoblast cell-specific genes have been used to direct transgene expression to the mouse placenta (42–44). These trophoblast cell-specific promoters may prove to be essential components of targeting vectors used for the delivery of perturbing agents that will aid in the dissection of the trophoblast cell lineage regulatory network. Gene targeting and transgenic strategies are most effective when coupled with *in vitro* trophoblast cell culture systems. The recent derivation of a rhesus monkey embryonic stem cell line may provide new opportunities for studying trophoblast cell differentiation in a primate model (45).

PUTATIVE TROPHOBLAST REGULATORY GENES

An assortment of genes has been implicated in the control of trophoblast cell differentiation (Table 2). These genes have been identified through both *in vitro* and *in vivo* experimental approaches. Some regulatory genes may be specific only to the trophoblast cell lineage, whereas others may have a broader spectrum of involvement in the regulation of trophoblast and nontrophoblast developmental processes.

Extracellular Regulatory Signal/Receptor Systems

Several cell signaling systems have been implicated in trophoblast-specific processes fundamental to differentiation. *E-cadherin* is a homotypic cell-cell adhesion molecule critical for the establishment of the tight trophectoderm epithelium of the blastocyst (46). Targeted disruption of E-cadherin leads to preimplantation lethality (46). Another recently identified cell-cell adhesion molecule, termed *trophinin*, has been implicated in the initial trophoblast-endometrial interactions involved in implantation (47). As gestation progresses, a heterotypic cell-cell adhesion system

TABLE 2. *Putative trophoblast regulatory genes*

Extracellular regulatory signal receptor systems
  E-cadherin
  Trophinin
  Vascular cell adhesion molecule-1 (VCAM-1)/α4-integrin
  Hepatocyte growth factor (HGF)/*c-met*
  Epidermal growth factor (EGF) family of ligands/EGF receptor
  Insulin-like growth factor-2 (IGF-2)
Cytoplasmic signaling components
  Src family tyrosine protein kinases
  vav
Nuclear signaling factors
  Thing-1/*Hxt*/e-Hand
  Mash-2
  GATA factors

has been shown to be pivotal for placental morphogenesis. *Vascular cell adhesion molecule-1* (VCAM-1) is expressed at the tip of the invading allantoic mesenchyme, and its receptor, *α4-integrin*, is expressed on the surface of trophoblast cells (48–50). *Hepatocyte growth factor/scatter factor* (HGF/SF) and its receptor, the transmembrane tyrosine kinase *c-met*, have a similar pattern of expression (51). Collectively, VCAM-1/α4-integrin and HGF/SF/*c-met* represent two important signaling systems responsible for determining the surface area available for maternal-fetal exchange. Murine null mutations in any one of these genes results in a disruption of placental development and prenatal lethality (51–54). The actions of these signaling systems would appear to be targeted to the progenitor population for syncytial trophoblast cells. Possible involvement of either the VCAM-1/α4-integrin or HGF/SF/*c-met* pathways in the regulation of placental development in primates is yet to be demonstrated.

Two other growth factor receptor systems have been implicated in the control of placental development. The *epidermal growth factor* (EGF) *receptor* signaling pathway appears to participate in the control of implantation and placental morphogenesis in rodents (55,56), and in some aspects of syncytial trophoblast differentiation in the human (57). The identity of the EGF receptor ligand(s) involved in these important developmental processes has not been specified. Most interestingly, the EGF receptor null mutation shows a different phenotype depending on the genetic background of the mouse, suggesting the existence of additional modifier genes (55,56). Targeted disruption of the EGF receptor gene can lead to a defect in blastocyst-uterine interactions and peri-implantation lethality or to a defect in spongiotrophoblast cell differentiation and midgestation lethality (55,56). *Insulin-like growth factor-2* (IGF-2) is expressed in both rodent and primate placentae (58) and has been implicated in the control of placental growth (59). Murine fetuses with an IGF-2 null mutation are growth-retarded, as are their placentae (59). The placental defect appears to be associated with an aberration in glycogen cell development (60). The receptor signaling pathway mediating placental IGF-2 actions has not been identified.

Cytoplasmic Signaling Components

Thus far, only a few cytoplasmic components of signal transduction cascades have been implicated in trophoblast cell development. Two of the components are part of protein tyrosine kinase signaling pathways. Src family protein tyrosine kinases (*src*, *yes*, *lyn*) have been investigated in trophoblast cells committed to the trophoblast giant-cell lineage (T. Kamei, G. P. Hamlin, B. M. Chapman, and M. J. Soares, University of Kansas Medical Center, Kansas City, KS, *unpublished data*). *Src* is constitutively active, *yes* shows a biphasic pattern of activation associated with proliferation and differentiation, and *lyn* activation is differentiation-dependent. Disruption of tyrosine kinase activities results in an attenuation of differentiation-dependent trophoblast giant-cell gene activation. *Src* has also been postulated to participate in the differentiation of human syncytial trophoblast cells (61). A second cytoplasmic component implicated in trophoblast cell development is *vav* (62). Trophoblast cells are prominent sites for *vav* expression early during embryogenesis (62). Development of *vav* null mutant embryos arrests around the time of implantation, at least in part because of disrupted trophoblast differentiation (62). The *vav* protein possesses multiple functional domains relevant to signal transduction networks; however, a specific function for *vav* is yet to be determined. At this juncture, we can only speculate that *vav* participates in a tyrosine kinase signaling pathway regulating trophoblast cell growth, differentiation, or both. Finally, elements of the cyclic AMP-protein kinase A cascade have prominent modulatory effects on the phenotype of differentiated human trophoblast cells (63).

Nuclear Signaling Factors

This category of trophoblast regulatory genes is dominated by genes that encode for DNA binding proteins. Several *trans*-acting factors have been shown to control trophoblast cell-specific gene expression, trophoblast cell differentiation, or both.

Two members of the basic helix-loop-helix (bHLH) transcription factor family have been implicated in regulating the trophoblast cell lineage. First of all, in a search of developmentally important regulatory factors, three research groups independently identified the same bHLH transcription factor, referring to it as *Thing-1* (64), *Hxt* (37), or *e-HAND* (65). Thing-1/*Hxt*/e-HAND was shown to have a pattern of tissue-specific expression consistent with a trophoblast regulatory factor. Furthermore, Cross et al. (37) showed that overexpression of Thing-1/*Hxt*/e-HAND promoted various aspects of trophoblast differentiation, including stimulation of the placental lactogen-I (PL-I) gene promoter in cells committed to the trophoblast giant-cell lineage. Current data are compatible with Thing-1/*Hxt*/e-HAND serving as a regulator of the trophoblast giant-cell lineage. Another trophoblast-regulatory gene, *Mash-2*, encodes for a mammalian member of the achaete-scute family of bHLH transcription factors, is maternally imprinted, and possesses a trophoblast cell restricted pattern of expression (66–68). Targeted disruption of the murine *Mash-2* gene leads to failures in spongiotrophoblast and glycogen cell development and lethality by midgestation (66). Other trophoblast lineages do not appear to be directly affected. Trophoblast cell target genes for *Mash-2* action have yet to be determined. bHLH transcription factors interact with consensus nucleotide sequences termed *E-Boxes* (64), which are prevalent in the 5'-flanking region of several genes known to be specifically activated in trophoblast cells (31–37). It is important to appreciate that the activities of bHLH transcription factors are directly regulated through associations with Id and E-protein families (69). The involvement of Thing-1/*Hxt*/e-HAND and *Mash-2* in the control of primate placental development has not been reported.

GATA factors have been shown to participate in the transcriptional control of the PL-I gene in rodent trophoblast giant cells (36) and the CG α- and β-subunit genes in differentiated human trophoblast cells (70). Development of either GATA-2 or

GATA-3 null mutant embryos arrests at midgestation with a number of defects, including several in extraembryonic structures (71,72).

An assortment of other *cis*-elements and *trans*-acting factors has been connected with trophoblast cell-specific gene expression. AP-1 elements and their binding factors (including members of the *fos* and *jun* families) contribute to the regulation of both rodent and human trophoblast cell-specific genes (34,73). Cyclic AMP response elements (CREs) and their binding factors (including CRE binding proteins) have a fundamental role in the transcriptional regulation of the CG α- and β-subunit genes in human trophoblast cells (73,74). C/EBPb, a member of the bZIP class of transcription factors, has been postulated to regulate a pregnancy-specific glycoprotein expressed in the rat placenta, referred to as *RnCGM-3* (75). Several other *cis*-elements in trophoblast cell-specific genes have been identified; however, the proteins that interact with the DNA regulatory sequences have not been completely characterized (31,42,75–79). Additionally, other putative *trans*-acting factors (*Pem*, Rex-1) have been shown to have a trophoblast pattern of expression, which may implicate them as participants in the development of the placenta (80,81).

The regulation of trophoblast cell-specific gene expression is clearly multifactorial, involving the participation of several DNA regulatory elements and DNA binding proteins. Specificity is probably achieved through the precise combination of factors interacting with particular regions of regulatory DNA, Nilson's "combinatorial code" (82). Some regulatory factors may have pivotal roles in controlling the expression of batteries of genes directing the differentiated phenotype, whereas the participation of other regulatory factors may be more restricted. Analysis of trophoblast differentiation-specific gene activation represents an effective strategy for deciphering regulatory networks involved in the derivation of the trophoblast lineage.

Other Putative Regulatory Genes

Various other genes have been implicated in trophoblast cell development in the mouse. These genes have been identified by the characterization of several spontaneous and induced mutations that are associated with impaired placental development. Each mutation is linked to abnormalities in either trophoblast giant-cell or spongiotrophoblast cell development, and has been localized to chromosomes 2, 7, 9, 15, 17, or the X chromosome (see refs. 2 and 82). The product or products encoded by the disrupted genes have not been reported.

FINAL COMMENTS

It is imperative that future research be directed toward improving our understanding of both rodent and primate placental development. Research must progress toward elucidation of the molecular mechanisms underlying the derivation of the trophoblast cell lineage. The ability to manipulate the rodent genome provides a powerful tool in uncovering roles for putative primate placental regulatory factors.

However, to interpret experimentation with rodents, we need to identify cross-species commonalities in placental development. On the basis of our current knowledge, it is apparent that some aspects of primate placental development will be unique. Thus, progress in the establishment of nonhuman primate models is also required.

ACKNOWLEDGMENTS

I would like to thank past and present members of my laboratory and my collaborators. Research from the author's laboratory was supported by Grants HD-20676, HD-29036, and HD-29797 from the National Institute of Child Health and Human Development.

REFERENCES

1. Rossant J. Development of the extraembryonic lineages. *Semin Dev Biol* 1995;6:237–247.
2. Soares MJ, Chapman BM, Kamei T, Yamamoto T. Control of trophoblast cell differentiation: lessons from the genetics of early pregnancy loss and trophoblast neoplasia. *Dev Growth Differ* 1995;37: 355–364.
3. Cross JC, Werb Z, Fisher SJ. Implantation and the placenta: key pieces of the development puzzle. *Science* 1994;266:1508–1518.
4. Roberts RM, Xie S, Mathialagan N. Maternal recognition of pregnancy. *Biol Reprod* 1996;54: 294–302.
5. Desoye G, Shafrir E. Placental metabolism and its regulation in health and diabetes. *Mol Aspects Med* 1994;15:505–682.
6. Soares MJ, Faria TN, Hamlin GP, Lu X-J, Deb S. Trophoblast cell differentiation: expression of the placental prolactin family. In: Soares MJ, Handwerger S, Talamantes F, eds. *Trophoblast Cells: Pathways for Maternal-Embryonic Communication.* New York: Springer-Verlag; 1993:45–67.
7. Ringler GE, Strauss JF. *In vitro* system for the study of human placental endocrine function. *Endocr Rev* 1990;11:105–123.
8. Aplin J. Implantation, trophoblast differentiation, and haemochorial placentation: mechanistic evidence *in vivo* and *in vitro. J Cell Sci* 1991;99:681–692.
9. Kaufmann P, Burton G. Anatomy and genesis of the placenta. In: Knobil E, Neill JD, eds. *The Physiology of Reproduction.* 2nd ed. New York: Raven Press; 1994:441–484.
10. Sibley CP, Hochberg A, Boime I. Bromo-adenosine stimulates choriogonadotropin production in JAr and cytotrophoblast cells: evidence for effects on two stages of differentiation. *Mol Endocrinol* 1991;5:582–586.
11. Lawler SD, Fisher RA. The contribution of the paternal genome: hydatidiform mole and choriocarcinoma. In: Redman CWG, Sargent IL, Starkey PM, eds. *The Human Placenta. A Guide for Clinicians and Scientists.* Oxford: Blackwell Scientific Publications; 1993:82–112.
12. Varmuza S, Mann M. Genomic imprinting—defusing the ovarian time bomb. *Trends Genet* 1994; 10:118–123.
13. Franklin GC, Adam GIR, Ohlsson R. Genomic imprinting and mammalian development. *Placenta* 1996;17:3–14.
14. McGrath J, Solter D. Completion of mouse embryogenesis requires both the maternal and paternal genomes. *Cell* 1984;37:179–183.
15. Surani MAH, Barton SC, Norris ML. Nuclear transplantation in the mouse: heritable differences between parental genomes after activation of the embryonic genome. *Cell* 1986;45:127–136.
16. Leighton PA, Saam JR, Ingram RS, Tilghman SM. Genomic imprinting in mice: its function and mechanism. *Biol Reprod* 1996;54:273–278.
17. McLaren A. Genetics of the early mouse embryo. *Annu Rev Genet* 1976;10:361–388.
18. Latham KE, McGrath J, Solter D. Mechanistic and developmental aspects of genetic imprinting in mammals. *Int Rev Cytol* 1995;160:53–98.

19. Contractor SF, Sooranna SR. Trophoblast cell culture as a model for studying placental function. In: Redman CWG, Sargent IL, Starkey PM, eds. *The Human Placenta. A Guide for Clinicians and Scientists*. Oxford: Blackwell Scientific Publications; 1993:504–526.
20. Lu X-J, Deb S, Soares MJ. Spontaneous differentiation of trophoblast cells along the spongiotrophoblast pathway: expression of the placental prolactin gene family and modulation by retinoic acid. *Dev Biol* 1994;163:86–97.
21. Soares MJ, Schaber KD, Pinal CS, De SK, Bhatia P, Andrews GK. Establishment of a rat placental cell line expressing characteristics of extraembryonic membranes. *Dev Biol* 1987;124:134–144.
22. Yagel S, Casper RF, Powell W, Parhar RS, Lala PK. Characterization of pure human first-trimester cytotrophoblast cells in long-term culture: growth pattern, markers, and hormone production. *Am J Obstet Gynecol* 1989;160:938–945.
23. Lei K-J, Gluzman Y, Pan C-J, Chou JY. Immortalization of virus-free human placental cells that express tissue-specific functions. *Mol Endocrinol* 1992;6:703–712.
24. Kohler PO, Bridson WE. Isolation of hormone-producing clonal lines of human choriocarcinoma. *J Clin Endocrinol Metab* 1971;32:683–687.
25. Wice B, Menton D, Geuze H, Schwartz AL. Modulators of cyclic AMP metabolism induce syncytiotrophoblast formation *in vitro*. *Exp Cell Res* 1990;186:306–316.
26. Teshima S, Shimosato Y, Koide T, Kuroki M, Kikuchi Y, Aizawa M. Transplantable choriocarcinoma of rats induced by fetectomy and its biological activities. *Gann* 1983;74:205–212.
27. Verstuyf A, Sobis H, Goebels J, Fonteyn E, Cassiman J, Vandeputte M. Establishment and characterization of a continuous *in vitro* line from a rat choriocarcinoma. *Int J Cancer* 1990;45:752–756.
28. Faria TN, Soares MJ. Trophoblast cell differentiation: establishment, characterization, and modulation of a rat trophoblast cell line expressing members of the placental prolactin family. *Endocrinology* 1991;129:2895–2906.
29. Hamlin GP, Lu X-J, Roby KF, Soares MJ. Recapitulation of the pathway for trophoblast giant cell differentiation *in vitro*: stage-specific expression of members of the prolactin gene family. *Endocrinology* 1994;134:2390–2396.
30. Hamlin GP, Soares MJ. Regulation of DNA synthesis in proliferating and differentiating trophoblast cells: involvement of transferrin, transforming growth factor-β, and tyrosine kinases. *Endocrinology* 1995;136:322–331.
31. Yamamoto T, Chapman BM, Clemens JW, Richards JS, Soares MJ. Analysis of cytochrome P-450 side-chain cleavage gene promoter activation during trophoblast cell differentiation. *Mol Cell Endocrinol* 1995;113:183–194.
32. Yamamoto T, Roby KF, Kwok SCM, Soares MJ. Transcriptional activation of cytochrome P450 side chain cleavage enzyme expression during trophoblast cell differentiation. *J Biol Chem* 1994;269:6517–6523.
33. Yamamoto T, Chapman BM, Johnson DC, Givens CR, Mellon SH, Soares MJ. Cytochrome P450 17α-hydroxylase gene expression in rat differentiating trophoblast cells. *J Endocrinol* 1996;150:161–168.
34. Shida MM, Ng Y-K, Soares MJ, Linzer DIH. Trophoblast-specific transcription from the mouse placental lactogen-I gene promoter. *Mol Endocrinol* 1993;7:181–188.
35. Vuille J-C, Cattini PA, Bock ME, Verstuyf A, Schroedter IC, Duckworth ML, et al. Rat prolactin-like protein A partial gene and promoter structure: promoter activity in placental and pituitary cells. *Mol Cell Endocrinol* 1993;96:91–98.
36. Ng YK, George KM, Engel JD, Linzer DIH. GATA factor activity is required for the trophoblast-specific transcriptional regulation of the mouse placental lactogen I gene. *Development* 1994;120:3257–3266.
37. Cross JC, Flannery ML, Blanar MA, Steingrimsson E, Jenkins NA, Copeland NG, et al. Hxt encodes a basic helix-loop-helix transcription factor that regulates trophoblast cell development. *Development* 1995;121:2513—2523.
38. Pierce GB. Carcinoma is to embryology as mutation is to genetics. *Am Zool* 1985;25:707–712.
39. Hogan B, Beddington R, Costantini F, Lacy E. *Manipulating the Mouse Embryo. A Laboratory Manual*. 2nd ed. New York: Cold Spring Harbor Laboratory Press; 1994.
40. Sedivy JM, Joyner AL. *Gene Targeting*. New York: Freeman; 1992.
41. Winston JH, Hanten GR, Overbeek PA, Kellems RE. 5' Flanking sequences of the murine adenosine deaminase gene direct expression of a reporter gene to specific prenatal and postnatal tissues in transgenic mice. *J Biol Chem* 1992;267:13472–13479.

42. Calzonetti T, Stevenson L, Rossant J. A novel regulatory region is required for trophoblast-specific transcription in transgenic mice. *Dev Biol* 1995;171:615–626.
43. Bokar JA, Keri RA, Farmerie TA, Fenstermaker RA, Andersen B, Hamernik DL, *et al*. Expression of glycoprotein hormone α-subunit gene in the placenta requires a functional cyclic AMP response element whereas a different *cis*-acting element mediates pituitary-specific expression. *Mol Cell Biol* 1989;9:5113–5122.
44. Strauss BL, Pittman R, Pixley MR, Nilson JH, Boime I. Expression of the β subunit of chorionic gonadotropin in transgenic mice. *J Biol Chem* 1994;269:4968–4973.
45. Thomson JA, Kalishman J, Golos TG, Durning M, Harris CP, Becker RA, *et al*. Isolation of a primate embryonic stem cell line. *Proc Natl Acad Sci U S A* 1995;92:7844–7848.
46. Larue L, Ohsugi M, Hirchenhain J, Kemler R. E-cadherin null mutant embryos fail to form trophectoderm epithelium. *Proc Natl Acad Sci U S A* 1994;91:8263–8267.
47. Fukuda MN, Sato T, Nakayama J, Klier G, Mikami M, Aoki D, *et al*. Trophinin and tastin, a novel cell adhesion molecule complex with potential involvement in embryo implantation. *Genes Dev* 1995;9:1199–1210.
48. Gurtner GC, Davis V, Li H, McCoy MJ, Sharpe A, Cybulsky MI. Targeted disruption of the murine VCAM-1 gene: essential role of VCAM-1 in chorioallantoic fusion and placentation. *Genes Dev* 1995;9:1–14.
49. Kwee L, Baldwin HS, Shen HM, Stewart CL, Buck C, Buck CA, et al. Defective development of the embryonic and extraembryonic circulatory systems in vascular cell adhesion molecule (VCAM-1) deficient mice. *Development* 1995;121:489–503.
50. Yang JT, Rayburn H, Hynes RO. Cell adhesion events mediated by α4 integrins are essential in placental and cardiac development. *Development* 1995;121:549–560.
51. Uehara Y, Kitamura N. Hepatocyte growth factor/scatter factor and the placenta. *Placenta* 1996;17:97–101.
52. Uehara Y, Minowa O, Mori C, Shiota K, Kuno J, Noda T, et al. Placental defect and embryonic lethality in mice lacking hepatocyte growth factor/scatter factor. *Nature* 1995;373:702–705.
53. Schmidt C, Bladt F, Goedecke S, Brinkmann V, Zschiesche W, Sharpe M, *et al*. Scatter factor/hepatocyte growth factor is essential for liver development. *Nature* 1995;373:699–702.
54. Bladt F, Riethmacher D, Isenmann S, Aguzzi A, Birchmeier C. Essential role for the c-met receptor in the migration of myogenic precursor cells into the limb bud. *Nature* 1995;376:768–771.
55. Sibilia M, Wagner EF. Strain-dependent epithelial defects in mice lacking the EGF receptor. *Science* 1995;269:234–238.
56. Threadgill DW, Dlugosz AA, Hansen LA, Tennenbaum T, Lichti U, Yee D, *et al*. Targeted disruption of mouse EGF receptor: effect of genetic background on mutant phenotype. *Science* 1995;269:230–234.
57. Morrish DW, Bhardwaj D, Dabbagh LK, Marusyk H, Siy O. Epidermal growth factor induces differentiation and secretion of human chorionic gonadotropin and placental lactogen in normal human placenta. *J Clin Endocrinol Metab* 1987;65:1282–1290.
58. Zhou J, Bondy C. Insulin-like growth factor-II and its binding proteins in placental development. *Endocrinology* 1992;131:1230–1240.
59. Baker J, Liu JP, Robertson EJ, Efstratiadis A. Role of insulin-like growth factors in embryonic and postnatal growth. *Cell* 1993;75:73–82.
60. Lopez MF, Dikkes P, Zurakowski D, Villa-Komaroff L. Insulin-like growth factor-II affects the appearance and glycogen content of glycogen cells in the murine placenta. *Endocrinology* 1996;137:2100—2108.
61. Rebut-Bonneton C, Boutemy-Roulier S, Evain-Brion D. Modulation of pp60c-src activity and cellular localization during differentiation of human trophoblast cells in culture. *J Cell Sci* 1993;105:629–636.
62. Zmuidzinas A, Fischer K-D, Lira SA, Forrester L, Bryant S, Bernstein A, et al. The *vav* proto-oncogene is required early in embryogenesis but not for hematopoietic development *in vitro*. *EMBO J* 1995;14:1–11.
63. Strauss JF, Kido S, Sayegh R, Sakuragi N, Gafvels ME. The cAMP signalling system and human trophoblast function. *Placenta* 1992;13:389–403.
64. Hollenberg SM, Sternglanz R, Cheng PF, Weintraub H. Identification of a new family of tissue-specific basic helix-loop-helix proteins with a two-hybrid system. *Mol Cell Biol* 1995;15:3813–3822.
65. Cserjesi P, Brown D, Lyons GE, Olson EN. Expression of the novel basic helix-loop-helix gene eHAND in neural crest derivatives and extraembryonic membranes during mouse development. *Dev Biol* 1995;170:664–678.

66. Guillemot F, Nagy A, Auerbach A, Rossant J, Joyner A. Essential role of Mash-2 in extraembryonic development. *Nature* 1994;371:333–336.
67. Guillemot F, Caspary T, Tilghman SM, Copeland NG, Gilbert DJ, Jenkins NA, et al. Genomic imprinting of Mash-2, a mouse gene required for trophoblast development. *Nat Genet* 1995;9: 235–241.
68. McLaughlin KJ, Szabo P, Haegel H, Mann JR. Mouse embryos with paternal duplication of an imprinted chromosome 7 region die at midgestation and lack placental spongiotrophoblast. *Development* 1996;122:265–270.
69. Weintraub H. MyoD family and myogenesis: redundancy, networks, and thresholds. *Cell* 1993;75: 1241–1244.
70. Steger DJ, Hecht JH, Mellon PM. GATA-binding proteins regulate the human gonadotropin α-subunit gene in the placenta and pituitary gland. *Mol Cell Biol* 1994;14:5592–5602.
71. Pandolfi PP, Roth ME, Karis A, Leonard MW, Dzierzak E, Grosveld FG, et al. Targeted disruption of the GATA3 gene causes severe abnormalities in the nervous system and in fetal liver hematopoiesis. *Nat Genet* 1995;11:40–44.
72. Tsai F-Y, Keller G, Kuo FC, Weiss M, Chen J, Rosenblatt M, et al. An early haematopoietic defect in mice lacking the transcription factor GATA-2. *Nature* 1994;371:221–226.
73. Jameson, JL, Hollenberg AN. Regulation of chorionic gonadotropin gene expression. *Endocr Rev* 1993;14:203–221.
74. Pittman RH, Nilson JH. The α-subunit of the glycoprotein hormones: evolution of a combinatorial code for placenta-specific expression. In: Soares MJ, Handwerger S, Talamantes F, eds. *Trophoblast Cells: Pathways for Maternal-Embryonic Communication.* New York: Springer-Verlag; 1993:45–67.
75. Chen H, Lin B, Chen C-L, Johnson PF, Chou JY. Role of the transcription factor C/EBPb in expression of a rat pregnancy-specific glycoprotein gene. *DNA Cell Biol* 1995;14:681–688.
76. Steger DJ, Buscher M, Hecht JH, Mellon PL. Coordinate control of the α- and β-subunit genes of human chorionic gonadotrophin by trophoblast-specific element-binding protein. *Mol Endocrinol* 1993;12:1579–1589.
77. Hum DW, Aza-Blanc P, Miller WL. Characterization of placental transcriptional activation of the human gene for P450scc. *DNA Cell Biol* 1995;14:451–463.
78. Jiang S-W, Eberhardt NL. Involvement of a protein distinct from transcription enhancer factor-1 (TEF-1) in mediating human chorionic somatomammotropin gene enhancer function through the GT-IIC enhanson in choriocarcinoma and COS cells. *J Biol Chem* 1995;270:13906–13915.
79. Fitzpatrick SL, Walker WH, Saunders GF. Genetic elements regulating human placental lactogen expression. In: Soares MJ, Handwerger S, Talamantes F, eds. *Trophoblast Cells: Pathways for Maternal-Embryonic Communication.* New York: Springer-Verlag; 1993:273–285.
80. Lin T-P, Labosky PA, Grabell LB, Kozak CA, Pitman JL, Kleeman J, et al. The *Pem* homeobox gene is X-linked and exclusively expressed in extraembryonic tissues during early murine development. *Dev Biol* 1994;166:170–179.
81. Rogers MB, Hosler BA, Gudas LJ. Specific expression of a retinoic acid-regulated, zinc-finger gene, Rex-1, in preimplantation embryos, trophoblast and spermatocytes. *Development* 1991;113:815–824.
82. Zechner U, Reule M, Orth A, Bonhomme F, Strack B, Guenet J-L, et al. An X-chromosome linked locus contributes to abnormal placental development in mouse interspecific hybrids. *Nat Genet* 1996; 12:398–403.

DISCUSSION

Dr. Milliez: How much do we know about the relation between genomic imprinting and the enzymes that are critical for implantation. In other words, are these genes paternally derived?

Dr. Soares: There are two imprinted genes that have been shown to be involved in placental development: *Mash-2* and IGF-2. *Mash-2* is a transcription factor. It is a member of a class of transcription factors called basic helix-loop-helix transcription factors, and these have been shown in other systems to be extremely important for development, for example, in muscle. If you mutate the *Mash-2* gene, you get a phenotype that is very similar to what I showed you for one of the phenotypes associated with mutation of the EGF receptor. Under these conditions, the spongiotrophoblast component of the placenta does not develop. The target genes for *Mash-2* have not been identified. The second gene is for IGF-2, which is a growth factor and is known to be produced in the placenta, with receptors also located in the placenta. The target for IGF-2, at least as far as I can see from the literature, appears to be the glycogen cell population. The size of the placenta in IGF-2 mutant mice is smaller, but the success of the pregnancy is not affected overall. There are a number of other imprinted genes that may very well be important for placental development. Overall, there may be 15 genes that have been shown to be clearly imprinted, either paternally or maternally. Whether some of those are also involved in placental development remains to be determined.

Dr. Ogata: With respect to signal transduction, I know that in the rat fetal liver there are some mechanisms in place that can modify the signal transduction cascade, and you can see this also in the mouse, and you can use a transgenic strategy to alter signal transduction pathways. Do you have any information in the placenta concerning this?

Dr. Soares: I don't believe so. I should like to emphasize the species diversity with regard to placental structure, and with regard to function in hormone production. Rodent placentae don't produce chorionic gonadotrophin, yet they appear to have the transcriptional machinery to activate the genes in a transgene situation.

Dr. Boyd: I am glad you made that comment, because I was about to ask you a general point about species diversity. The central enigma about the placenta is why on earth is there this extraordinary structural and functional diversity. I was wondering whether you molecular people could come at that from a different angle. The blastocyst doesn't look very different between species; could you map and then maybe interfere with the diverging species changes? Is that a train of thought that has any merit?

Dr. Soares: I think it has considerable merit. We are just now getting closer to developing the molecular tools to allow us to dissect some of those types of events. But there are really only a handful of genes that are somewhat trophoblast-specific and that are beginning to be understood now in terms of their regulation, which would enable us to manipulate them.

Dr. Wang: There is a high incidence of the trophoblast disease in women of low socioeconomic status. Do you think there is a relationship between nutrition and trophoblast cell development?

Dr. Soares: I don't know. I suspect that a key factor, as Professor Boyd was saying, is for us to gain insight into some of these key regulatory genes, which might be important for the development of trophoblast cells and the organization of the placenta. Then we might also have potential parameters to monitor the effects of nutritional abnormalities and maybe have a better idea of what specifically to look for and to see how the specific activation of a certain group of genes might be influenced.

Dr. Owens: I would like to comment on the question of nutrition and trophoblast cell development. Our work has been looking at the guinea pig and the impact of mild to moderate maternal nutritional restriction from before pregnancy and in early pregnancy on the developing blastocyst. A reduction in maternal nutritional intake to only 85% of *ad libitum* control has a very large impact on the number of cells present in the trophectoderm in the day 6 blastocyst, such that the ratio of cells in the inner cell mass, that will go on to be the fetus, to that in the trophectoderm is increased by up to 10-fold. This is in a very large number of animals now. We know that most of those animals would go on to be pregnant, but we don't know the longer-term fetal and placental outcomes.

Dr. Soares: So you see some type of compensation with nutritional deprivation and you are actually getting more trophoblast?

Dr. Owens: In the cases described we are getting less trophoblast. However, if we restrict nutritional intake to 70% of *ad libitum* intake, we do find a redistribution of cells to the trophectoderm, and that is reflected in a relatively large placenta later in midgestation and near term. Perhaps that reflects persistence of one form of compensation if you like, but I guess that here we have a mild to moderate perturbation of the environment of the developing blastocyst having a very large impact on cell number in the trophectoderm at that stage, in some cases with long-term effects, so that nutrition is clearly far more important than we might have suspected, given the relatively minor demands on the mother at that stage. In the light of what you have reviewed, I think it would be important to look at the extent to which genes are regulated by nutritional and hormonal factors within the oviduct and the uterus.

Dr. Huch: Coming back to species differences, the depth of invasion of the trophoblast into the maternal tissue is different in different species, and textbook information indicates that this is regulated on the maternal side. Is this still correct in the light of the new information?

Dr. Soares: In the species in which there is more prominent invasion, especially in rodents and in the human, there is certainly evidence that the differentiated uterine stromal cells are a source of various regulators that influence trophoblast invasion, such as inhibitors of metalloproteinases, which may be directly involved in the invasive process by trophoblast cells, and also various cytokines like transforming growth factor β, which is known to influence or modulate trophoblast cell behavior and differentiation. In the case of domestic species, in which you really don't get invasion at all, I am not as familiar with the regulatory signals that are involved.

Dr. Owens: This may not be so relevant to the question of invasion and its molecular modulation and the difference between species, but it is my understanding that in the rodent, in the mouse at least, IGF-2 is paternally imprinted and the IGF-2 (type 2) receptor maternally, but in the human, where the fetus is placing much less of a demand on the mother in terms of what it needs to acquire, only the IGF-2 gene is paternally imprinted and the receptor is not maternally imprinted. That is an example of a species difference in the relative impact of the paternal *vs.* maternal genome.

Dr. Sibley: You mentioned the point that we have learned a lot from transgenic mice. The end point was not that they were interested in the placenta but they had to go through the process to get the transgenic mouse that they really wanted at the end. I'm wondering if we are losing a lot of information from people who have made transgenic mice or have failed to make transgenic mice because there was a lethality in the gene they have knocked out on the way to making it. Should we set up a register or an international journal in which we ask people to write in and tell us of failed transgenic models?

Dr. Soares: I think this is particularly evident with regard to the hepatocyte growth factor. Hepatocyte growth factor is presumably involved in liver development and also in other processes as well. I am sure the laboratories that were involved in creating the mutation had no interest at all in placental development, but that's where the initial defect was.

Placental Function and Fetal Nutrition,
edited by Frederick C. Battaglia,
Nestlé Nutrition Workshop Series, Vol. 39.
Nestec Ltd., Vevey/Lippincott-Raven Publishers,
Philadelphia, © 1997.

Fetal Liver and the Placenta: An Interactive System

Frederick C. Battaglia

Division of Perinatal Medicine, Departments of Pediatrics and Obstetrics-Gynecology, University of Colorado School of Medicine, Denver, Colorado 80262, USA

Fetal physiologists have centered their attention on the endocrine system when considering the potential interaction of one fetal organ with another or one fetal organ with the placenta. Our own studies in pregnant sheep showed an impressive correlation between placental size and the size of the fetal liver (Fig. 1). This observation—which is not a characteristic of the fetal brain, for example—suggests that the growth of the two organs is interrelated. In our earlier studies of carbohydrate metabolism, it rapidly became clear that the function of the fetal liver and the placenta must be integrated, at least with respect to glucose metabolism. In a series of studies (1–3), we showed that the placental delivery of glucose to the fetus was a function of the transplacental glucose gradient. The fetal hepatic production of glucose was also a function of the placental delivery of glucose. Only when the latter fell to low levels did the rate of fetal gluconeogenesis become significant (3). This makes good sense, of course, because if the fetal liver constantly produced glucose, it would decrease the transplacental gradient by raising fetal glucose concentration. This would then lead to reduced umbilical uptake. Hence, fetal hepatic glucose production, under normal circumstances, would be counterproductive, as it would substitute fetal carbon sources for maternal glucose carbon. These studies made us curious as to whether a similar interaction between fetal hepatic metabolism and placental transport and metabolism also existed for amino acids.

AMINO ACID TRANSPORT AND METABOLISM

The more we have studied different groups of amino acids, the more it has become clear that fetal hepatic metabolism and placental metabolism must be viewed as an integrated system. There has been a considerable body of evidence attesting to the organ-specific aspects of amino acid metabolism during adult life. The presumption has been that such specificity would apply to early postnatal life. Our studies have shown that this is also true of fetal development. In this chapter, I shall review three

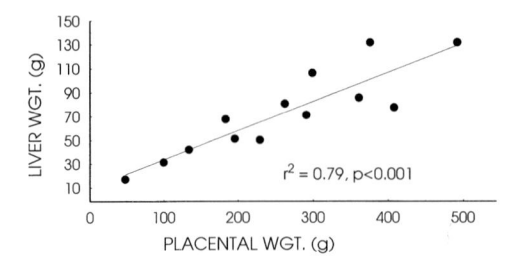

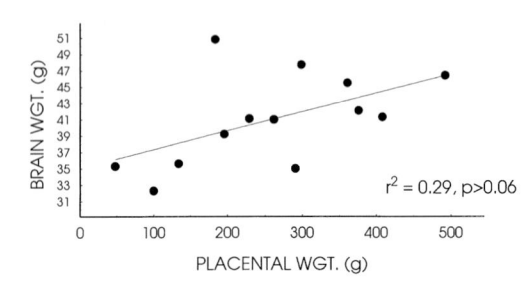

FIG. 1. Relationship of placental weight to fetal brain and liver weights. From Thureen et al. (12).

aspects of fetal hepatic and placental metabolism of amino acids: (a) their net uptake and/or release from both organs; (b) serine and glycine exchange; and (c) glutamine and glutamate exchange.

FETAL HEPATIC AND PLACENTAL AMINO ACID UPTAKE OR RELEASE

The uptake or release of amino acids from the placenta to the fetal circulation for the ovine fetus is reviewed in Meschia's chapter in this volume (**Placental Delivery of Amino Acids**). The estimate of net amino acid exchange has required updating as improvements in amino acid methodology have come along. The reasons for this rest with several facts peculiar to this stage of development, and these have been discussed in some detail by Meschia. The high rate of perfusion of the fetal liver and placenta is coupled with the fact that some amino acids are present at extremely high concentrations in the ovine fetus, further leading to a low extraction coefficient (e.g., threonine, with a fetal concentration of 366 μM and an umbilical extraction coefficient of 0.05). A specific analytic problem was posed by the particular pattern of umbilical arteriovenous differences for glutamine and glutamate, in that glutamine enters the umbilical circulation from the placenta in large amounts, resulting in a high umbilical venous concentration, whereas glutamate is almost totally cleared from the fetal plasma across the placenta, resulting in very low umbilical venous concentrations. By some modifications in the HPLC methodology, this difficulty can be overcome (4).

Some years ago, we measured the concentration differences of amino acids across

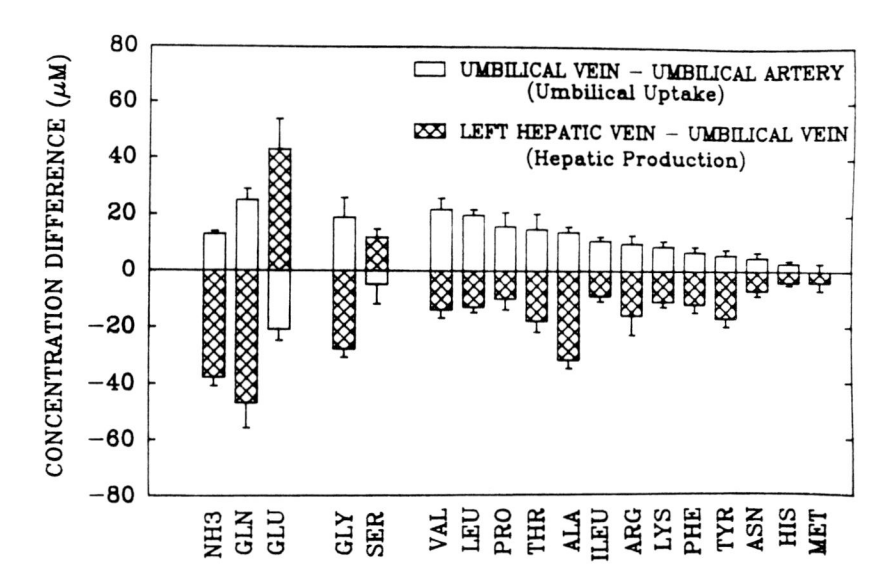

FIG. 2. Comparison of arteriovenous differences (μM) of individual amino acids and ammonia across fetal left hepatic lobe and umbilical circulation. From Marconi et al. (5), with permission.

the fetal hepatic circulation and the umbilical circulation. Figure 2 summarizes the data from that study (5). For most amino acids, there is a large uptake into the fetal liver from the placenta. However, some differences from postnatal life are striking. We have already commented on the absence of a net glucose release from the fetal liver, despite large hepatic uptakes of alanine, glutamine, and lactate. In postnatal life, a large uptake of these compounds would be associated with hepatic glucose production. In addition, glutamate and serine are produced in the fetal liver and taken up from the fetal circulation and delivered to the placenta and other fetal organs. In one sense, glutamate production by the fetal liver serves as an alternative to hepatic glucose production, although the combined uptake of lactate, alanine, and glutamine far exceeds net glutamate output. The uterine uptake of amino acids can be measured, although with considerably less precision, given the fact that uterine blood flow is almost twice umbilical flow (see **Placental Delivery of Amino Acids**). One of the striking comparisons is between uterine glycine uptake, which is not measurable, and umbilical glycine uptake, which is quite large. Taken together, these observations point to a high rate of placental glycine production.

FETAL HEPATIC AND PLACENTAL SERINE-GLYCINE EXCHANGE

We have studied serine (6,7) and glycine (8,9) exchange between the fetal liver and placenta, as well as their fetal plasma fluxes. These were the first studies that clearly demonstrated to us that the supply of amino acids to the fetus is not only a

FETAL LIVER   **PLACENTA**

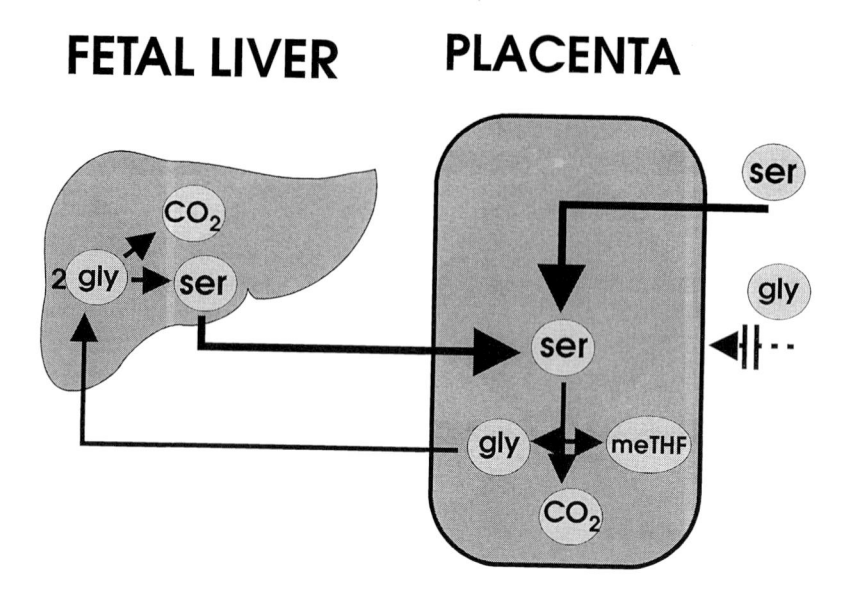

FIG. 3. Interorgan exchange of glycine and serine. Serine taken up from both circulations into the placenta can be used for glycine production. *MeTHF*, methylenetetrahydrofolate.

function of transplacental transport but also of placental production or fetal production. In fact, for serine and glycine, the ovine fetal requirements are almost solely met by production within the placenta or fetus. Figure 3 presents a summary in diagrammatic form of the conclusions from these studies, in which stable isotopic tracer methodology was used for *in vivo* investigation in the late-gestation fetal lamb. An impressive organ specificity is shown by these amino acids. Fetal serine oxidation represents 7.9 ± 0.5% of infused L-[U-^{14}C]serine and occurs primarily in the carcass (approximately 80% of the total fetal CO_2 production). By contrast, glycine oxidation represents 11.3 ± 0.5% of the L-[1-^{14}C]glycine infused, and approximately 70% of total fetal oxidation can be accounted for by the hepatic rate of oxidation (8). Stoichiometrically, the molar ratio of fetal hepatic serine production and CO_2 production from glycine is approximately 1:1, consistent with the combined actions of serine hydroxymethyltransferase and glycine cleavage system, both of which have high activity in the fetal liver (8). Thus, in the fetal liver, glycine uptake is utilized, in part, for serine production and for oxidation. Two pathways of fetal serine utilization have been established from these studies: (a) uptake and utilization by the placenta for glycine production, and (b) uptake and oxidation in the fetal skeletal tissues.

In the placenta, there is an uptake of serine from both the maternal circulation and the fetal circulation. Clearly, therefore, all the fetal requirements for serine must be met by fetal production. Within the placenta, some of the serine is utilized for glycine production as well as for CO_2 production. The consequence of this serine to glycine flux is the production of methylenetetrahydrofolate (MeTHF). This compound is also produced from glycine oxidation within the placenta. The fate of the MeTHF within the placenta is not known, although it may contribute not only to nucleic acid synthesis but also to homocysteine-methionine interconversion.

Figure 4 presents the relationships between fetal serine concentration, fetal plasma disposal rate, fetal serine oxidation, and fetal glycine derived from fetal plasma serine (6). Clearly, an increase in fetal serine concentration increases the disposal rate and the flux to CO_2 and glycine production.

To test if maternal plasma serine was also utilized for placental production of glycine, we carried out a series of studies in twin pregnancies (9). L-[1-^{13}C]serine was infused into the maternal artery supplying only one uterine horn. The fetus and placenta of that horn were the "experimental" horn, with the other uterine horn and its fetus and placenta serving as a "control." Despite almost 300 minutes of infusion that led to a maternal uterine venous enrichment of approximately 18%, there was no detectable serine enrichment in either fetal circulation. However, glycine enrichments were higher in the uterine and umbilical veins of the experimental horn compared with either the maternal and fetal arterial enrichments, or compared with the venous enrichments in the control horn. These results established that maternal plasma serine is also utilized for placental glycine production and that there is no detectable transplacental transport of serine for the ovine placenta.

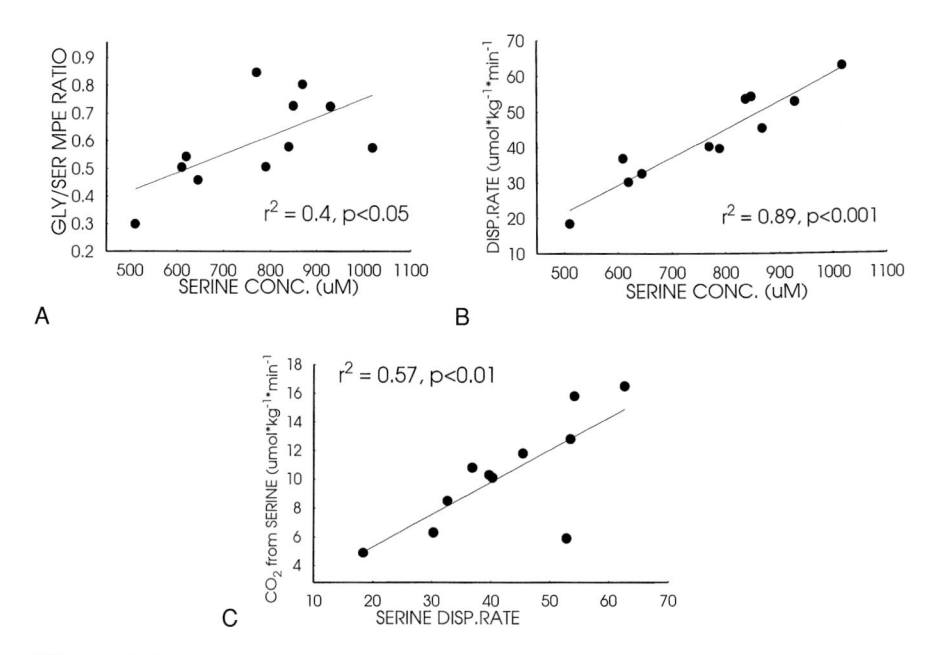

FIG. 4. A: Relates the fetal plasma glycine-serine enrichment ratio to fetal plasma serine concentration. **B:** Presents the fetal plasma serine disposal rate vs. fetal plasma serine concentration. **C:** Presents the serine flux to CO_2 per kilogram of fetal weight vs. the fetal plasma serine disposal rate (units as in B). Data from Cetin et al. (6), with permission.

The studies outlined above were carried out in late gestation, at approximately 120 days. However, we have studied fetal serine fluxes at midgestation as well (7). At this stage, one has a relatively large placenta (410 ± 20 g) and a relatively small fetus (145 ± 12 g). The fetal plasma serine disposal rate is enormous (61.8 ± 4.0 μmol/min/kg fetal weight), owing to a large uptake of serine from the fetal circulation into the placenta (approximately 80% of the total L-[1-^{13}C]serine infused). In none of the studies was it possible to demonstrate a significant transfer of fetal plasma serine or glycine into the maternal circulation. Thus, these amino acids are effectively trapped within the fetus or placenta, or both.

From these studies we can conclude that the fetal requirements for some nonessential amino acids are met primarily—if not entirely—by fetal or placental production rather than by transplacental transport, and that there is significant organ specificity to amino acid metabolism in fetal life, just as there is in postnatal life.

FETAL HEPATIC AND PLACENTAL EXCHANGE OF GLUTAMINE AND GLUTAMATE

Among amino acids, the most striking example of the fetal liver and placenta functioning as an integrated organ system is given by the interorgan fluxes of glutamine and glutamate. Even in the early studies, which did not utilize stable isotope tracer methodology but were simply directed at determining the net uptake or release of these amino acids across the fetal liver and placenta, certain striking features were observed (5). The glutamine taken up from the placenta into the fetal circulation was used by the fetal liver, and the glutamate produced by the fetal liver was used by the placenta. The fetal plasma glutamate was virtually cleared (60% extraction) across the fetal umbilical circulation. This striking interorgan exchange was then explored using stable isotope methodology (10).

L-[1,2-^{13}C$_2$]glutamine was infused into the fetal circulation. The entry of glutamine from the placenta accounted for approximately 60% of the fetal disposal rate. Approximately 45% of the glutamine taken up by the fetal liver was released from the fetal liver as glutamate, and the rate of fetal hepatic production accounted for almost the total fetal glutamate production. In adult humans, it has been estimated that on a daily protein diet containing one mole of amino acids, the molar ratio of hepatic glucose production to O$_2$ uptake would be about 0.15. Therefore, if the adult liver had to oxidize the glucose produced from amino acids completely, its O$_2$ consumption would increase by 90%. As 4.5 moles of O$_2$ are required to oxidize glutamate completely, the fetal liver would require an increase in O$_2$ consumption of 60% to 70% to oxidize the glutamate produced. Thus, the unique characteristic of the fetal liver—namely, a large net glutamate production—can be regarded as an excellent accommodation to the virtual absence of gluconeogenesis during fetal life.

In another study, L-[2,3,3,4,4-^{2}H$_5$]glutamate was infused into the fetal circulation (11). The fetal plasma disposal rate was 11.9 ± 1.3 μmol/min/kg fetal weight.

Given the low fetal arterial concentration of plasma glutamate (about 50 μM), this represents an extraordinary fetal plasma clearance of 200 ± 8 ml/min/kg fetus, which is greater than umbilical plasma flow. The placental extraction of fetal plasma glutamate was almost 90%. Most of the glutamate was oxidized, about 40% in the fetus and about 40% in the placenta. There was a small (6%) amount of the placental glutamate uptake returned to the fetus as glutamine, but the major disposal was placental oxidation.

The impact of the large placental uptake of fetal plasma glutamate can be seen when the fetal plasma clearances of six amino acids that have been studied using comparable methodology and over the same gestational age range are compared (11) (Table 1).

In summary, we have presented the following hypothesis: During fetal life, fetal hepatic gluconeogenesis is uncoupled from amino acid oxidation. By this view, the release of glutamate from the fetal liver is a consequence of such uncoupling. In addition, our data have shown that the rate of placental uptake and oxidation of glutamate is supply-limited. This led us to a second hypothesis: Fetal modulation of placental metabolic activity depends on glutamate oxidation. Glutamate oxidation generates NADPH (reduced nicotinamide adenine dinucleotide phosphate), a required cofactor for steroidogenesis. Thus, it is possible that endocrine effects on fetal hepatic amino acid metabolism might subsequently affect the placenta indirectly. Klimek *et al.* (13) have demonstrated a link between human placental mitochondrial oxidation of glutamate and synthesis.

From such hypotheses, we were led to question whether, associated with the profound endocrine changes during parturition, there were demonstrable changes in fetal hepatic glutamine and glutamate metabolism. The study we have recently concluded (4) used a fetal infusion of dexamethasone to induce parturition, which occurred at 47 ± 4 hours from the start of the fetal infusion. After 24 hours of dexamethasone infusion, there was a significant reduction in fetal hepatic glutamate output to one quarter of preparturition values. This led to a decrease in fetal glutamate concentration and in net placental glutamate uptake to one fifth of preparturition

TABLE 1. *Comparison of mean fetal arterial plasma concentrations, disposal rates, and clearances for five amino acids*

	Arterial plasma concentration, μM	Disposal rate, μmol/min/kg	Clearance, ml/min/kg	Reference
Glutamate	59	11.9	200	Present study
Tyrosine	87	1.8	21	20
Leucine	168	8.7	55	16
Alanine	295	15.5	52	8
Glycine	406	12.4	31	3
Serine	767	42.5	55	2

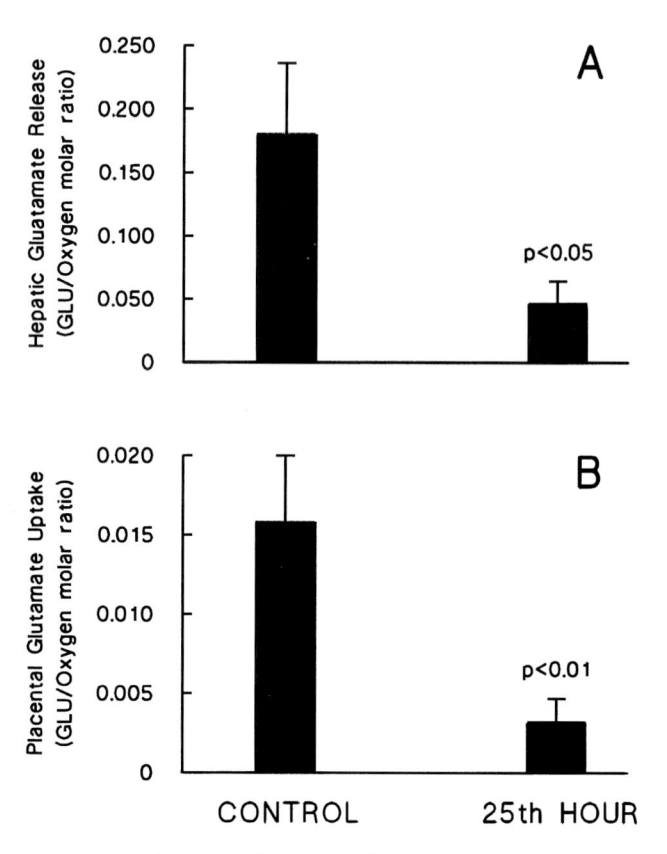

FIG. 5. Presents the arteriovenous differences of glutamate across the umbilical circulation and the differences in glutamate concentration between the fetal hepatic vein and umbilical vein. Both refer to plasma concentrations and are expressed as Glu (μmol)/O_2 content (μmol). Data from Moores et al. (11).

values. These changes are presented in Fig. 5. Thus, steroid-induced parturition is associated with profound changes in fetal hepatic glutamate metabolism. These changes may play a role in integrating changes in fetal hepatic and placental metabolism during parturition.

SUMMARY

The evidence we have accumulated for amino acid exchange and metabolism clearly demonstrates that the fetal liver and placenta function as an integrated system of organs. This is a striking characteristic with regard to serine-glycine interactions and glutamine-glutamate interactions. Their importance is at least in part a function of controlling one-carbon pools (serine-glycine) and NADPH supply (glutamine-glutamate). Functionally, the production of glutamate in the fetal liver serves as an alternative to glucose production for the release of carbon derived from amino acids.

ACKNOWLEDGMENT

This work was supported by NIH Grant HD-01866, "Physiological Study of the Placenta," and NIH Grant HD-29188, "Fetal and Placental Metabolism of Threonine and Alanine."

REFERENCES

1. Simmons MA, Battaglia FC, Meschia G. Placental transfer of glucose. *J Dev Physiol* 1979;1:227–243.
2. Hay WW, Sparks JW, Battaglia FC, Meschia G. Maternal-fetal glucose exchange: necessity of a 3 pool model. *Am J Physiol* 1984;246:E528–E534.
3. Hay WW, Sparks JW, Wilkening RB, Battaglia FC, Meschia G. Fetal glucose uptake and utilization as functions of maternal glucose concentration. *Am J Physiol* 1984;246:E237–E242.
4. Barbera A, Wilkening RW, Battaglia FC, Meschia G. Metabolic alterations in the fetal hepatic and umbilical circulations during glucocorticoid induced parturition in sheep. *Pediatr Res (in press)*.
5. Marconi AM, Battaglia FC, Meschia G, Sparks JW. A comparison of amino acid arteriovenous differences across the liver, hindlimb and placenta in the fetal lamb. *Am J Physiol* 1989;257: E909–E915.
6. Cetin I, Fennessey PV, Sparks JW, Meschia G, Battaglia FC. Fetal serine fluxes across the fetal liver, hindlimb and placenta in late gestation: the role of fetal serine in placental glycine production. *Am J Physiol* 1992;263:E786–E793.
7. Moores RR, Carter BS, Meschia G, Fennessey PV, Battaglia FC. Placental and fetal serine fluxes at mid-gestation in the fetal lamb. *Am J Physiol* 1994;267:E150–E155.
8. Cetin I, Sparks JW, Quick AN, Marconi AM, Meschia G, Battaglia FC, et al. Glycine turnover and oxidation and hepatic serine synthesis from glycine in fetal lambs. *Am J Physiol* 1991;260: E371–E378.
9. Moores RR, Rietberg CCT, Battaglia FC, Fennessey PV, Meschia G. Metabolism and transport of maternal serine by the ovine placenta: glycine production and absence of serine transport into the fetus. *Pediatr Res* 1993;33:590–594.
10. Vaughn PR, Lobo C, Battaglia FC, Fennessey PV, Wilkening RB, Meschia G. Glutamine-glutamate exchange between placenta and fetal liver. *Am J Physiol* 1995;268:E705–E711.
11. Moores RR, Vaughn PR, Battaglia FC, Fennessey PV, Wilkening RB, Meschia G. Glutamate metabolism in the fetus and placenta of late gestation sheep. *Am J Physiol* 1994;267:R89–R96.
12. Thureen PJ, Trembler KA, Meschia G, Makowski EL, Wilkening RB. Placental glucose transport in heat-induced fetal growth retardation. *Am J Physiol* 1992;263(*Regul Integr Comp Physiol* 32): R578–R585.
13. Klimek J, Makarewicz W, Swierczynski J, Bossy-Bukato G, Zelewski L. Mitochondrial glutamine and glutamate metabolism in human placenta and its possible link with progesterone biosynthesis. *Trophoblast Res* 1993;7:77–86.

DISCUSSION

Dr. Chard: To what extent can some of these things be extrapolated to the human? For example, it is not my understanding that in the human the most oxygenated blood goes to the liver.

Dr. Battaglia: There is a ductus venosus in the human as well, and a large fraction of umbilical venous blood is shunted through it. The question for the liver is what kind of blood perfuses it. It is perfused by that fraction of umbilical venous blood that is not shunted through the ductus. It is not receiving any appreciable component from portal venous drainage, and that is the big difference from postnatal life and would apply in the human. As I said, there are clearly going to be species differences in metabolism, but so far the evidence for glutamate being important in the placenta seems to be supported by a number of studies in the human placenta as well. I think the evidence is good. I am also encouraged by the fact that it would not matter whether you studied sheep or human mitochondria from the heart, as they both use glutamate preferentially. I believe that would be true of small bowel in different species as well. So I don't think these cycles are going to be confined to just the ovine species.

Dr. Schneider: In the isolated perfused human placenta, we showed many years ago that there is uptake of glutamate from the fetal circulation and the glutamate is largely metabolized in the placenta. This has been confirmed in blood samples obtained from the umbilical vein and artery at the time of cesarean section. This all supports the view that there is a similar mechanism of glutamate clearance from the umbilical circulation by the placenta in the human.

Dr. Battaglia: The other difference I mentioned relating to the liver was that in fetal life there is no net glucose release. We can't measure net glucose release in the human fetus, but certainly our group and others have looked in the human for evidence of gluconeogenesis and have been unable to demonstrate it. So it seems that those key features of development are similar.

Dr. Milliez: What could be the link between glutamine and parturition? Do you think it is just a coincidence or is there a direct causal relationship?

Dr. Battaglia: We don't know the answer to that. I think this will be linked with parturition and with steroidogenesis in the placenta. The effect may be mediated through glutamate transport into the placenta being turned off. I don't want to focus only on glutamate metabolism; its transport *per se* may be important. But yes, I think that glutamate deprivation of the placenta probably will prove to be important in parturition.

Dr. Chard: But on the same vein, where you showed progesterone going down, presumably you might show other phenomena there, such as estrogens going up and cortisol going up in the same samples. Cortisol might be an even better candidate to control your metabolic processes.

Dr. Battaglia: First of all, let's get rid of the estrogen issue—it's a log order different from progesterone. Steroid output as a whole is decreasing; whether you take progesterone alone or subtract the tiny amount of estrogen, you are not going to affect that statement. As far as cortisol is concerned, I don't know. We haven't studied other tissues in the fetus, and I don't know if there is an effect on the adrenal. There is certainly a possibility of other organ effects. Glutamate is an important signaling compound, that is clear enough, even from studies in postnatal life, and it could affect a multitude of tissues.

Dr. Chard: So your suggestion is that the glutamate is affecting the progesterone, not the reverse.

Dr. Battaglia: What I showed you are the data. The data clearly show, and this is the first demonstration for any aspect of hepatic metabolism, that glutamate fetal hepatic output is changing radically during parturition. I also showed you a correlation with progesterone output by the uterus. I don't know if they are causally related at this stage, but it raises a lot of interesting questions.

Dr. Owens: I am interested in your views on what might be the molecular mechanisms involved in altered steroid exposure modulating hepatic glutamate production. Do you think this is steroid-responsive elements altering gene expression for the relevant enzymes, or do you rather see other endocrine factors or local factors being involved, such as altered IGF-2 or IGF-1 production within the liver?

Dr. Battaglia: We have been talking about that a lot. There is a suggestion in adult hepatocyte cultures that growth hormone triggers a release of glutamate, and that made us interested in whether ovine placental lactogen could be playing such a role, but we have no data for this. To some extent, *in vivo* studies are too laborious and expensive to address endocrine regulation, so you have to do it with *in vitro* cultures.

Dr. Rennie: I think it has been shown that there are at least three different membrane transporters for glutamate that are important in the placenta. There is EAC-1, which is the excitatory amino acid transporter present in the brain; there is the GLUT-1 (GLT-1), which is also present in the brain, and there is the XAG transporter. And those transporters show differential regulation according to the degree of intrauterine growth retardation (IUGR), but the transcription and the protein expression of those transporters go down dramatically in IUGR in rat placenta. And yet the expression of other amino acid transporters does not change to anything like the same extent, so it is obviously crucial.

Dr. Battaglia: There is a problem for us with studying IUGR in this model, because this is a difficult preparation and involves fetal surgery. Many of those fetuses will not tolerate that. The heat stress fetuses will survive if you leave them alone, but if stressed, they don't survive. So we haven't done these kinds of flux studies in growth-retarded animals.

Dr. Marini: The fetus is nourished in the pulsatile way because the mother is eating. Is the level you achieve in the mother equal to the level you can achieve if you feed the animal with a normal meal?

Dr. Battaglia: You are thinking as a clinician. These are ruminants, so you are not going to get anything like the postprandial swings you get in primates. Furthermore, the maternal arterial concentration changes with feeding are quite small for amino acid concentrations.

The Endocrine Function of the Placenta: Interactions Between Trophic Peptides and Hormones

Lise Cedard

U. 361 INSERM, Maternité Baudelocque, 121 Boulevard de Port-Royal, Paris, France

The placenta is classically considered to be a source of hormones that play an important role in the establishment and maintenance of pregnancy. Because of its hemochorial structure, the human placenta produces hormones and easily secretes them into the maternal circulation. They include steroid hormones, such as estrogens and progesterone, and protein hormones, the most important of which are the chorionic gonadotrophins (hCG), discovered in 1927. During the period from 1960 to 1980, the concept of a fetoplacental unit (1) with a complementary role for the fetus in steroid production offered a new approach to steroid metabolism, and since then new proteins and neuropeptides have been discovered (2,3). However, the lack of innervation of placental tissue highlights the importance of understanding neuroendocrine regulation of placental physiology. Sophisticated culture methods enabling the study of biologic phenomena occurring during transformation of cytotrophoblast cells into a syncytiotrophoblast (4) have been combined with electron microscopy and histochemistry. Possibilities offered by molecular biology, including *in situ* hybridization and molecular cloning studies, have also completely modified current knowledge and revealed the presence of a multitude of factors, such as neuropeptides, cytokines, and growth factors, with their own receptors, but the role of these factors is often unclear. Results from these different approaches have recently added a new concept to the classic notion of endocrine production (with hormone secretion into the fetal or maternal circulation, followed by an eventual effect on other organs)—that of paracrine (between cells)/autocrine (into the same cell) regulation, varying at different stages of gestation and under pathologic conditions.

STEROID HORMONES (2,5)

Progesterone

Progesterone clearly plays an important role in enabling implantation. It is necessary for the maintenance of a quiescent myometrium, which is impregnated with this steroid through a process of diffusion from the site of placental insertion. It plays an important role in the development of the mammary gland and exerts a suppressive effect on lymphocyte proliferation and activity. Progesterone is produced by the corpus luteum in early pregnancy, with the relayed production by the placenta (the luteoplacental shift) occurring in the human from day 50 of pregnancy, then increasing in parallel with trophoblast growth (Fig. 1). At the end of pregnancy, the daily production is about 250 mg/d, with maternal blood levels of progesterone reaching 200 ng/mL. Progesterone cannot be synthesized by the trophoblast from acetate, but is derived from maternal cholesterol bound to low-density lipoproteins (LDL) (6) (Fig. 2). The uptake of LDL is accomplished by specific receptors present in the placental microvilli as early as the sixth week of pregnancy. Receptor-mediated endocytosis of LDL is followed by degradation of LDL in lysosomes (7). The presence of scavenger receptors for acetyl-LDL and of specific binding sites for HDL3 increases the possibility of internalization of the huge amount of cholesterol needed for both placenta development and progesterone biosynthesis (8). The placental production of progesterone was formerly considered as autonomous. In fact, its

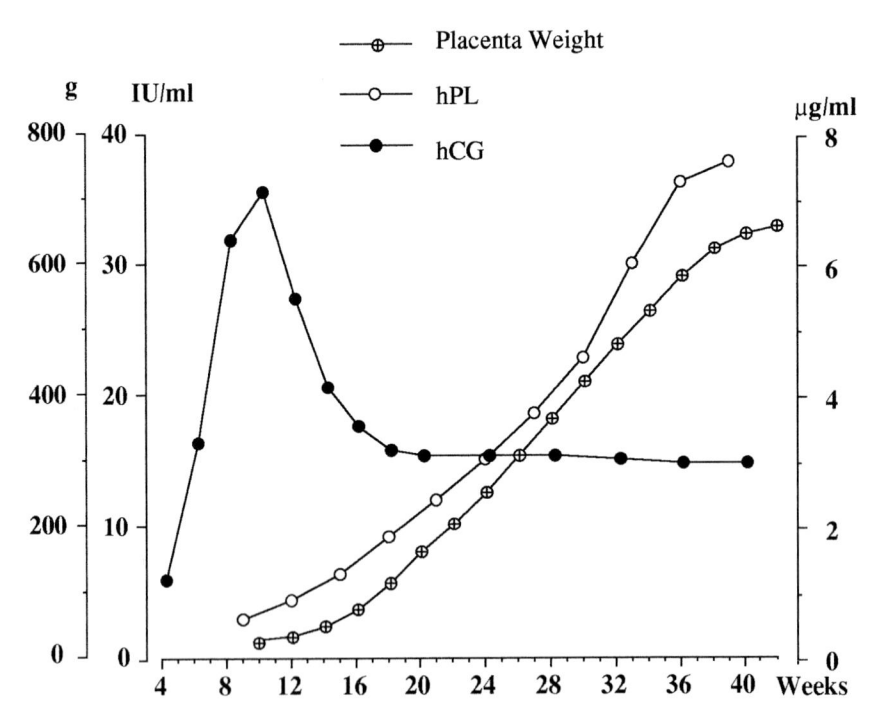

FIG. 1. Evolution of placental weight and levels of hPL and hCG during gestation. The level of hPL rises gradually until term in parallel with the placental growth. The circulating hCG level increases rapidly after implantation and reaches a peak at 8 to 12 weeks. After a drop, a plateau is observed until term.

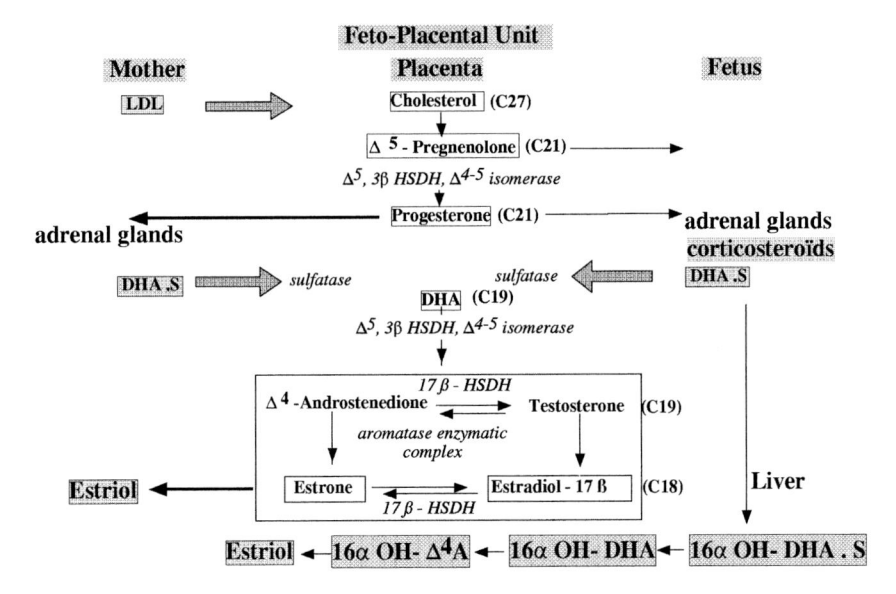

```
                    Feto-Placental Unit
     Mother             Placenta                      Fetus
      LDL    ═══⇒    Cholesterol (C27)
                          ↓
                    Δ 5 - Pregnenolone (C21) ─────────┐
                    Δ⁵, 3β HSDH, Δ⁴⁻⁵ isomerase       │
                          ↓                           ↓
  adrenal glands  ◄─── Progesterone (C21) ──────► adrenal glands
                                                   corticosteroïds
     DHA.S   ═══⇒ sulfatase      sulfatase ⇐═══    DHA.S
                        DHA (C19)
                    Δ⁵, 3β HSDH, Δ⁴⁻⁵ isomerase
                          ↓
                              17β - HSDH
                ┌─ Δ⁴-Androstenedione ──────► Testosterone ─(C19)
                │                  aromatase enzymatic
                │                      complex
                │                      ↓              ↓
   Estriol ◄── │ Estrone ───────► Estradiol - 17β (C18)     Liver
                │         17β - HSDH
                └──────────────────────────────────────┘
       Estriol ◄─ 16α OH- Δ⁴A ◄─ 16α OH- DHA ◄─ 16α OH- DHA.S
```

FIG. 2. Biosynthesis of steroids in women from 10th week of pregnancy until labor. *LDL,* low-density lipoproteins. *DHAS,* dehydroepiandrosterone sulfate.

regulation is extremely complex within the organ. The addition of a synthetic precursor, 25-hydroxycholesterol, increases progesterone production *in vitro* by the presence of a specific cytochrome P_{450} (P_{450} scc). In the baboon, estrogens stimulate key steps in the progesterone biosynthetic pathway, namely LDL receptors and P_{450} scc (9), a process that in the human placenta *in vitro* is stimulated by hCG.

The addition of pregnenolone to different placental preparations increases progesterone production considerably, but the 3-hydroxydehydrogenase 5-4 isomerase (3-HSDH), which is not a rate-limiting factor by itself, can be inhibited by retroaction by 4-3 ketosteroids (androgens, progesterone) (10) and by estrogens. Catecholamines were shown to stimulate progesterone production by the adenylate cyclase protein A system. Activation of adenylate cyclase could also mediate the stimulating effect of luteinizing hormone (LH), hCG, vasoactive intestinal polypeptide (VIP), and prostaglandin E (11). Insulin-like growth factors (IGF-1 and IGF-2) (12) and epidermal growth factor (EGF) stimulate progesterone production *in vitro* by their effect on cytochrome P_{450} scc and 3β-HSDH. Other growth factors, such as transforming growth factor (TGF), platelet-derived growth factor (PDGF), and fibroblast growth factor (FGF), also increase the synthetic capacity of the trophoblast, probably by their role in the regulation of cell growth and differentiation (13).

Apart from low 6-hydroxylation, progesterone cannot be metabolized by the human placenta, and about 25% of the progesterone produced by the placenta is transformed by the fetus into corticosteroids and androgens (Fig. 2).

Estrogens

Estrogens have an important role in implantation and mammary gland development; they induce vasodilation within the maternal uterine vascular bed and enhance uterine contractility by regulating several subcellular mechanisms. The placenta is the main source of estrogen production after the ninth week of pregnancy, but as the human placenta lacks some steroidogenic activity, it has been assumed that steroidogenesis results from the fetoplacental unit. Estrogen production depends on the adrenal gland of the mother or fetus to supply androgens, particularly dehydroepiandrosterone (DHA) sulfate, which is hydrolyzed by a placental sulfatase to produce free DHA. Oxidation by 3-HSDH then forms the 4-androstenedione before aromatization by cytochrome P_{450} aromatase to produce estrone and estradiol, which are interconvertible under the action of a placental 17-dehydrogenase (Fig. 2).

The placenta synthesizes estriol from the 16-DHA sulfate formed in the fetal liver. This steroid circulates in the maternal compartment as a sulfo or glycuro conjugate, whereas in the maternal blood, plasma estradiol (E_2) is mainly in the free form and bound to the sex-binding globulin. The increased E_2-to-progesterone ratio in late gestation is mainly caused by the rise in estrogen production by the placenta, which is itself caused by the development of the fetal adrenal cortex and by the constant increase in placental aromatase activity. Estrogen production by the placenta depends on many factors, such as evolution of the trophoblastic mass and of its blood flow, as well as stimulation by several more or less specific factors (14). Sulfatase, which is the rate-limiting factor in the placental metabolism of the DHA sulfate, is retroinhibited by estrogens and by some progestins. It was initially demonstrated by *in vitro* perfusion that hCG stimulates aromatase activity through the intermediary of an increase in cyclic AMP production; prostaglandins F_2, E_2, and mainly E_1 have the same action. Several clinical conditions occurring in human pregnancy result in subnormal placental estrogen production. For example, in fetal anencephaly there is a decrease in secretion of the fetal adrenal C_{19} steroids, whereas in intrauterine growth retardation, DHA sulfate metabolism is impaired (15). When there is placental sulfatase deficiency, an X-linked error of metabolism, estrogen secretion is very low, but the fetus shows normal development until term, as is the case with the more recently discovered deficiency of placental aromatase. It is thus evident that there is a considerable excess of estrogen production in human pregnancy.

POLYPEPTIDE HORMONES (2,3)

Human Chorionic Gonadotrophins

The placenta is the primary source of hCG in pregnant women. It is essential for maintenance of pregnancy through its actions to increase luteal progesterone production until the placenta is able to produce adequate amounts of progesterone.

The family of glycoprotein hormones to which hCG belongs comprises LH, follicle stimulating hormone (FSH), and thyroid stimulating hormone (TSH). These hormones are heterodimers of α and β subunits noncovalently bound to each other. The α subunits are identical, whereas the β subunits, which confer hormone specificity, are dissimilar among the various hormones. The β subunits of hCG and LH are highly homologous in the N terminal domain, but the hCG subunit has 30 additional amino acids at the C terminus. Both hCG and LH bind to the same receptors and have similar biologic effects.

Before being secreted into the circulation, hCG is synthesized in the form of individual subunits and assembled into the heterodimer. The subunits are encoded by different genes, the α subunit by one single gene on chromosome 6 and the β subunit by a cluster of six genes or pseudogenes on chromosome 19. The production of hCG occurs primarily in the syncytiotrophoblast and to some extent in the cytotrophoblast; messenger RNA for both subunits has been found in those two cellular types.

The secretion pattern of hCG is totally different from that of other well-recognized placental products. The circulating hCG level increases rapidly in the 4 weeks following implantation, doubling every 2 to 3 days. It reaches a peak at 8 to 12 weeks, and then after a fall, a plateau is observed until term (Fig. 1). The β subunit has the same profile, whereas the α subunit steadily increases with advancing gestation.

The primary function of hCG, biologically similar to LH, is to support the so-called corpus luteum rescue characteristic of the beginning of pregnancy. hCG is probably responsible for testosterone secretion by the early fetal testes and stimulates the fetal zone of the adrenal cortex. The activities of the hCG subunit genes are controlled by elements responsive to cyclic AMP (4). We have observed (15) that hCG has a stimulatory effect on placental estrogen production, and that the concomitant increase in glycogen phosphorylase activity is mediated by a rise in cyclic AMP. A wide variety of regulatory agents, including GnRH, TGF, EGF, and dopamine agonists, have been shown to modulate placental hCG synthesis or secretion.

In recent years, the concept of self-regulation of hCG biosynthesis has been developed. Specific receptors have been identified that are modulated by hCG levels and vary as a function of the age of pregnancy (16). The presence of these receptors in different tissues or organs, such as human endometrial or myometrial blood vessels, umbilical cord, and pregnant and nonpregnant myometrium, also suggests that hCG may have a large spectrum of action during pregnancy (17,18). The close temporal relation between the Doppler advent of intervillous maternal blood flow and the hCG peak strongly suggests that the establishment of the intervillous blood flow is associated with the decline in the circulating hCG concentration (19). The yolk sac and the extra-embryonic coelom, two structures that disappear after the 12th week, could also be the principal sources of hCG in the first trimester of pregnancy (20). Strong evidence supports these different hypotheses, and the debate remains open.

Human Placental Lactogen or Somatomammotrophin

The presence of lactogenic hormone in the placenta was suggested by the ability of placental extracts to stimulate secretion from mammary gland explants. Human placental lactogen (hPL) is a single polypeptide having a 96% sequence homology with growth hormone and 67% with prolactin. It has been suggested that these three families of hormones have evolved from a common ancestral gene by repeated gene duplication (21). In the placenta, four genes are expressed on chromosome 17. The hGH-N gene codes for both human growth hormone (hGH) (22 kDa) and a smaller molecular variant of 20 kDa. The hPL-A and hPL-B genes code for a 22-kDa hPL. The messenger RNA for hPL is specifically located in the syncytiotrophoblast and gives rise to a prohormone that is transformed into the mature hormone by removal of a 25-amino acid sequence. It is detected in maternal plasma at 3 weeks of gestation, and its concentration rises gradually up to 10 to 16 g/ml until term. It is the major secretory product of the term placenta, with an output of about 1 g/d, and its secretion parallels that of the placental mass (Fig. 1). The mechanisms by which the hormone is secreted have not been fully elucidated. Cyclic AMP has no regulatory role, whereas the inositol phosphate-phospholipase C system stimulates hPL production (22). Autocrine regulation seems probable because of presence of opioid and angiotensin II receptor sites, the number of which increases during the second part of gestation. Furthermore, interleukin-6 increases the hPL release by human trophoblastic cells (23). In the mother, hPL is an insulin antagonist and has growth hormone-like lipolytic activity. The role of hPL in fetal growth seems to be indirect, through adaptation of maternal intermediary metabolism involved in supplying nutrients to the fetus. Several cases of women in whom normal pregnancy was maintained despite low or undetectable serum concentrations of hPL have been described, caused by a partial or complete deletion of hPL-A and hPL-B genes.

A placental hGH has been purified from placenta and found in the maternal circulation during pregnancy (24). Placental growth hormone is more basic than the pituitary hormone variants with which it competes, with an apparently high potency for binding to liver growth hormone membrane receptors. The hGH-V gene is specifically expressed in the placental villi, and its expression is induced during gestation parallel to hPL secretion. The rate of hGH synthesis increases with the development of the trophoblast, which appears to be a major determinant of the hGH profile in maternal blood. The physiologic role of hGH is not well defined, but a somatogenic effect is likely, as suggested by the parallelism between the gestational profiles of hGH and IGF-1 in women. The regulation of hGH secretion remains unknown, but the presence in the placenta of hGH receptors suggests an autocrine/paracrine regulation.

PLACENTAL NEUROPEPTIDES (3,25,26)

The human placenta contains a number of neuropeptides that are similar to hypothalamic factors; their structure is, however, sometimes slightly different from that of hypothalamic peptides. By analogy with hypothalamic-hypophyseal physiology, it has been suggested that the cytotrophoblast cells are the primary site of the neuropeptide synthesis, whereas the syncytiotrophoblast elaborates the protein hormone.

However, the study of the changes occurring during *in vitro* differentiation of cytotrophoblast attributes a role to the cell aggregation-induced changes mediated by cell adhesion molecules and to membrane fusion-induced regulation of cyclic AMP metabolism (4). True intraplacental neuroendocrine regulation with cell-to-cell interactions and autocrine/paracrine regulatory loops plays a key role.

Gonadotrophin Releasing Hormone

The regulation of gonadotrophin releasing hormone (GnRH) secretion in the human term placenta is illustrated in Fig. 3.

The presence of GnRH activity was demonstrated in 1975 in the human term placenta. GnRH stimulates hCG secretion from placental explants and isolated cultured trophoblasts in a dose-dependent manner at all stages of gestation. GnRH also increases the *in vitro* production of progesterone and prostaglandins (27). Cyclic AMP, prostaglandins E_2 and F_2, epinephrine, insulin, and VIP stimulate GnRH secretion *in vitro*. Inversely, progesterone and estradiol are inhibitors of the hCG secretion provoked by GnRH. GnRH was shown to be present in the cytotrophoblast, villous stroma, and syncytiotrophoblast, but discrepancies in results concerning gestational age-related changes, as well as the localization of pro-GnRH messenger

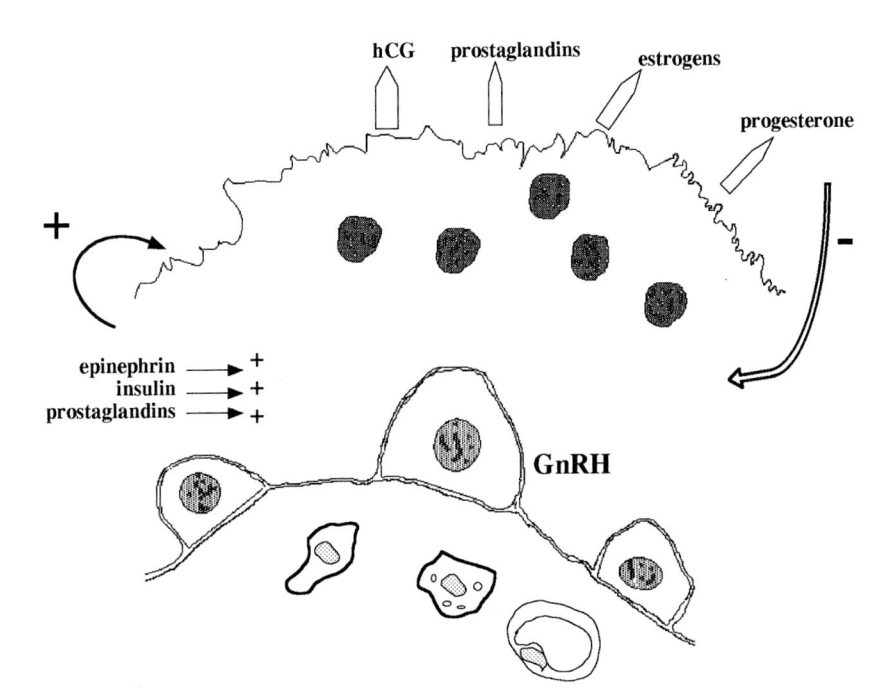

FIG. 3. Schematic drawing of the regulation of GnRH secretion in the human term placenta. GnRH secreted by the cytotrophoblast cells is stimulated by some factors and inhibited by others, such as progesterone produced by the syncytiotrophoblast.

RNA, have been reported. Recently, by means of a sophisticated method of visualization, pro-GnRH was shown to be present in both the cytotrophoblast and syncytiotrophoblast of first-trimester placental villi, but not in cells of fetal connective tissue (28). It has also been demonstrated that the GnRH receptor messenger RNA is expressed in both cytotrophoblast and syncytiotrophoblast and shows changes paralleling the time course of hCG secretion (29). These data provide a mechanistic understanding that the paracrine/autocrine regulation of hCG secretion by placental GnRH is mediated through an increase followed by a decline in GnRH receptor gene expression from first trimester to term placenta.

Corticotrophin Releasing Hormone

Corticotrophin releasing hormone (CRH), a hypothalamic neurohormone that modulates pituitary and adrenal function (hypothalamic-pituitary-adrenal axis), is produced in the placenta and fetal membranes (30). Concentrations of CRH peptide and messenger RNA in the placenta are low in the first trimester and higher during midgestation, and they increase dramatically in the 5 to 6 weeks before term. CRH can first be detected in maternal plasma at about 20 weeks of gestation, and levels rise throughout the latter part of pregnancy, with a rapid increase in the weeks preceding the onset of labor at term. In the human placenta, CRH stimulates the expression of the pro-opiomelanocortin gene and adrenocorticotrophic hormone (ACTH), melanocyte stimulating hormone (MSH), and endorphin trophoblastic production through CRH receptors. Its own secretion is stimulated by prostaglandins, neurotransmitters, neuropeptides, and cytokines. Glucocorticoids increase CRH production, unlike the classic hypothalamic-pituitary-adrenal axis, and the CRH might be able to stimulate the hypothalamic-pituitary-adrenal axis of the fetus, thus increasing glucocorticoid production (26). The bioactivity of circulating CRH is influenced by the CRH binding protein (CRH-BP), which binds to the hormone at an equimolar ratio (31). The exponential rise in CRH with advancing pregnancy is associated with a concomitant fall in CRH-BP at a time that coincides with the onset of parturition (30). It is also known that maternal plasma levels are increased early in pregnancies that are complicated by preterm labor. All these data have led some investigators to speculate that placental CRH may be involved in the mechanism of parturition and that a placental clock controls the length of human pregnancy (32).

Inhibin, Activin, Folliculostatin

The term placenta encompasses immunoactive and bioactive inhibin and immunoactive activin. These glycoproteins, composed of two subunits, were first isolated from the gonads and shown to have opposite effects on FSH production by the pituitary. Their concentrations in maternal circulation increase progressively during

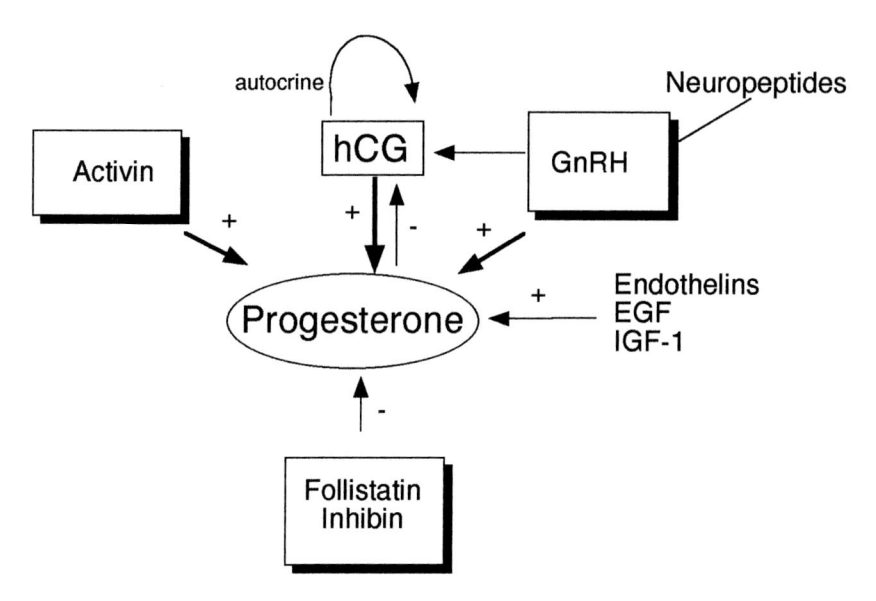

FIG. 4. Modulation of progesterone secretion in human placenta by GnRH, hCG, and various peptides. *hCG*, human chorionic gonadotrophin; *EGF*, epithelial growth factor; *IGF*, insulin-like growth factor.

pregnancy until term. Inhibin, the heterodimer, has an inhibitory effect on GnRH-stimulated hCG secretion by the trophoblast. The activin A dimer of the subunit of inhibin has a stimulatory effect on hCG and progesterone secretion (Fig. 4). The regulation of the secretion and the action of these proteins are very complex (26,33,34). Activin probably acts more as a paracrine regulator of cell growth and function, like TGF-β, than as a regulator of hormone secretion, and its effect is modulated by estrogens and progesterone. The placenta also contains a structurally unrelated protein called *follistatin* or *FSH-suppressing protein* (35), which has the capacity to neutralize the actions of activin. The functional interaction of inhibin, activin, and GnRH in placental cells is supported by the common localization of their messenger RNAs in the placental villi at term. The colocalization of immunoreactive inhibin, activin, and GnRH in the cytoplasm of trophoblast cells further supports the hypothesis of a paracrine/autocrine interaction of these three regulatory factors.

Somatostatin and Growth Hormone Releasing Hormone

Somatostatin and growth hormone releasing hormone (GHRH) could play a role in regulation of the placental growth hormone secretion.

Other neuropeptides, such as neuropeptide Y, thyrotrophin releasing hormone (TRH), neurotensin, and the vasoactive peptides (VIP, AVP, ANP), have also been localized in the placenta, as have been endothelins.

Endothelins

The endothelins are a family of oligopeptides synthesized by endothelial and vascular smooth muscle cells (36). They were first considered as potent endogenous vasoconstrictors, but they also act as growth promoters and mitogenic agents for various types of cells.

Binding sites for endothelin-1 (ET-1) have been characterized in blood vessels of the human placenta, suggesting an important physiologic role for this peptide as a regulator of placental vascular resistance during pregnancy (37). The receptors are coupled with a phospholipase C transducing system (38). The production of ET-1 and ET-3 by trophoblastic cells has been confirmed by the expression of preproendothelin genes in 3-day cell cultures (39). Furthermore, ET-1 and ET-3 increase progesterone release by cultured trophoblast, suggesting an autocrine role in the control of placental steroidogenesis (40) (Fig. 5). As endothelins elicit mitogenic effects toward a variety of cells, it can be postulated that these peptides are potent growth factors in placenta.

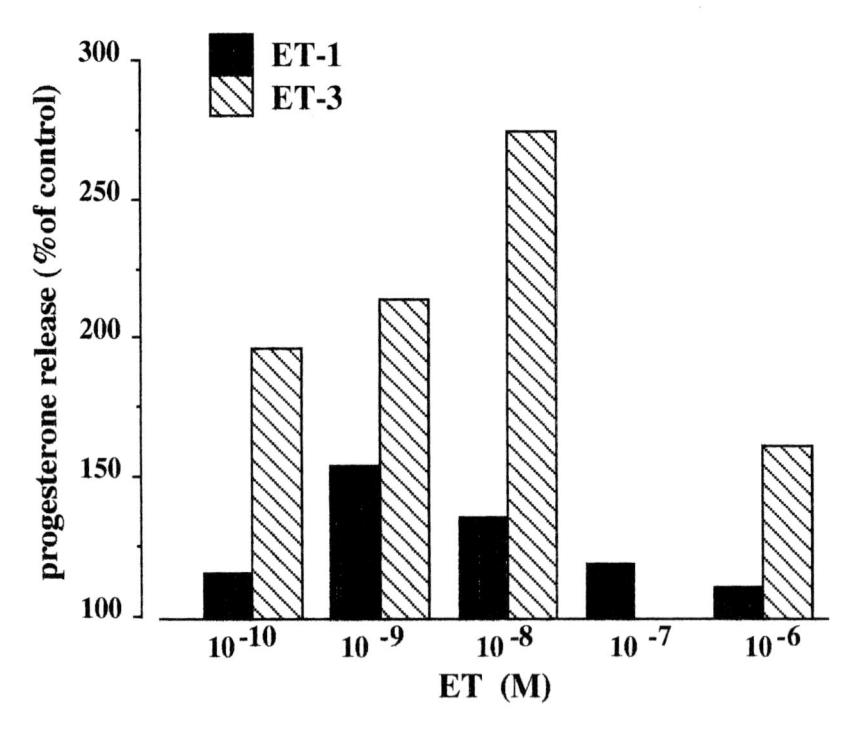

FIG. 5. Action of endothelins (ET) on progesterone synthesis in the human placenta. Concentration-related stimulatory effects of ET-1 and ET-3 on progesterone release are expressed as percentage of control (no addition of peptide) by trophoblasts. After 3 days of culture, cells were incubated for 15 minutes in the presence of increasing concentrations of ET. Each value is the mean of triplicate determinations of a representative experiment. From Mignot et al. (40), with permission.

The placenta also produces some neurotransmitters, such as acetylcholine, catecholamines, and τ-aminobutyric acid (GABA), which are able to act on hormonal secretion.

GROWTH FACTORS AND CYTOKINES

Growth Factors

Growth factors are polypeptides circulating with or without specific binding proteins in an active or inactive form. They bind to specific plasma membrane receptors on their target cells and initiate a rapid series of events that result in the division and differentiation of cytotrophoblastic cells (13). They can be grouped into superfamilies according to their nucleotide and amino acid sequence homologies, as well as by similar binding affinities. Among these, epidermal growth factor (EGF), fibroblast growth factor (FGF), insulin-like growth factors (IGF-1), platelet-derived growth factor (PDGF), insulin, and the different transforming growth factors (TGF) are bound to placental receptors with an intrinsic protein kinase activity and have an important role in the autonomous regulation of placental hormonogenesis. Furthermore, various oncogenes of transforming viruses are related to growth factors and their receptors (41). For example, a close similarity has been noted between thyroid hormone receptor and erb A oncogene protein and between the cytoplasmic domain of EGF receptor and the translated product of erb B oncogene.

Cytokines—Proteins Specific for Pregnancy

Cytokines are proteins that mediate intercellular communication and control growth, cell division, and differentiation. In the human placenta they have multiple immunoendocrine or immunosuppressive functions (42, 43). The most important are probably colony stimulating factors (CSF-1, GM-CSF), interleukins (IL-2, IL-4, IL-6), and interferons-α and -τ. The placenta also produces a series of *proteins specific for pregnancy* detected in the maternal blood (44), such as Schwangershafts protein-1 (SP-1), which may be involved in the control of fetal growth, and the so-called pregnancy-associated proteins. PP-5 is an antithrombin that prevents coagulation in the intervillous space, PP-12 is an IGF-binding protein that probably plays a role in insulin-glucose homeostasis, and PP-14 is a lactoglobulin. PAPPA is an inhibitor of the protease involved at the maternoplacental interface.

Enzymes

Some enzymes are also produced. *Renin*, which converts angiotensinogen to angiotensin, is also secreted by the human chorion, and this enzyme plays a role in implantation and in vascular changes occurring during pregnancy. The role of heat-stable *alkaline phosphatase* is unknown, whereas *cystine aminopeptidase* degrades oxytocin, a potent myometrial contractile agent.

CONCLUSION

The hormonal production of the placenta is fundamental for the establishment and maintenance of pregnancy. The trophoblast secretes into the maternal circulation steroids and trophic peptides that are essential for fetal development. They are modulators of uteroplacental blood flow and regulators of myometrial contractility. Because of its lack of innervation, the placenta requires an autonomous regulatory system, which appears to be very complex (Fig. 6). Thus, locally produced hormones regulate the secretion of other placental hormones or their own production through specific binding proteins and receptors. However, the placenta is a unique organ from many points of view. It contains a series of hormones and neuropeptides that are distributed in different organs, such as the hypothalamus, the hypophysis, the gonads, and the adrenals. It is constantly remodeling, and the classic distinction between cytotrophoblast cells and syncytiotrophoblast is obsolete. Hormone and peptide production is modified during the cell adhesion and membrane fusion processes, which occur with syncytiotrophoblast formation under the influence of cyclic

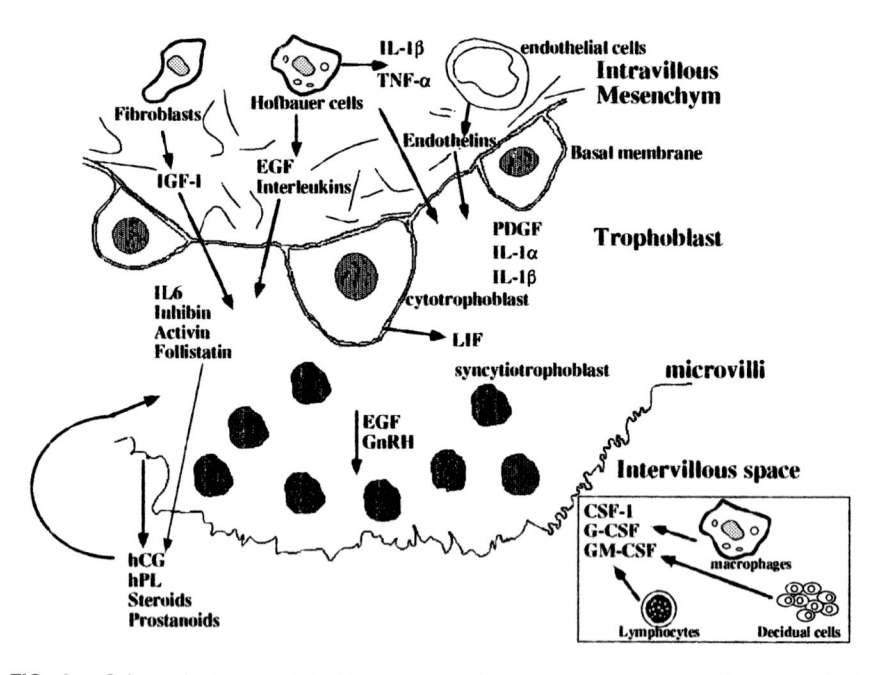

FIG. 6. Schematic drawing of the interactions between trophic peptides and hormones in the human placenta. Neuropeptides, growth factors, and cytokines produced by the different cellular structures modulate the hormonal production by the trophoblast.

AMP, growth factors, and cytokines produced by other cells, such as macrophages. For ethical and practical reasons, it is impossible to study the normal placenta during the second part of gestation, when hormone production is maximal, and it is well-known that the full-term placenta obtained at cesarean section and *a fortiori* after vaginal delivery (45) is not comparable with the midterm organ. The cytotrophoblast cells of the anchoring villi, which adhere to the uterine epithelium, migrate to the endometrium, and invade the spiral arteries, are also difficult to use for biochemical studies. The use of choriocarcinoma or transfected cells for *in vitro* studies is an alternative, but the regulation of hormonal secretion by these cells is not the same. The difference between the results obtained by *in vivo* analysis of circulating hormones or peptides and those from various *in vitro* models has provoked controversy, and some observations remain unexplained. In particular, the variations in hCG secretion during pregnancy could be a consequence either of physiologic temporal changes, or of paracrine/autocrine autoregulation.

ACKNOWLEDGMENT

I thank T. M. Mignot and M. Verger for secretarial assistance.

REFERENCES

1. Diczfalusy E. Endocrine functions of the human feto-placental unit. *Fed Proc* 1964;23:791–798.
2. Martal J, Cedard L. Endocrine functions of the placenta. In: Thibault C, Levasseur MC, Hunter RHF, eds. *Reproduction in Mammals and Man*. Paris: Editions Ellipes; 1993:435–459.
3. Ogren L, Talamantes F. The placenta as an endocrine organ: polypeptides. In: Knobil E, Neill J, eds. *The Physiology of Reproduction*. 2nd ed. New York: Raven Press; 1994: 875–946 (vol 2).
4. Kliman HJ, Nestler JE, Sermasi E, et al. Purification, characterization, and *in vitro* differentiation of cytotrophoblasts from human term placentae. *Endocrinology* 1986;118:1567–1582.
5. Solomon S. The placenta as an endocrine organ: steroids. In: Knobil E, Neill J, eds. *The Physiology of Reproduction*. 2nd ed. New York: Raven Press; 1994: 863–875 (vol 2).
6. Winkel CA, Snyder JM, MacDonald PC, et al. Regulation of cholesterol and progesterone synthesis in human placental cells in culture by serum lipoprotein. *Endocrinology* 1980;106:1054–1060.
7. Alsat E, Malassiné A, Cedard L. Low density lipoprotein receptor function. *Trophoblast Res* 1991; 5:127–149.
8. Alsat E, Mondon F, Malassiné A, et al. Identification of distinct receptors for native and acetylated low density lipoprotein in human placental microvilli. *Trophoblast Res* 1987;2:17–27.
9. Pepe GJ, Albrecht ED. Actions of placental and fetal adrenal steroid hormones in primate pregnancy. *Endocr Rev* 1995;16:608–648.
10. Ferré F, Breuiller M, Cedard L, et al. Human placental $\Delta 5$-3β hydrosteroid dehydrogenase activity ($\Delta 5$-3β HSDH): intracellular distribution, kinetic properties, retroinhibition and influence of membrane delipidation. *Steroids* 1975;26:551–570.
11. Strauss JF, Kido S, Sayegh R, et al. The cAMP signalling system and human trophoblast function. *Placenta* 1992;13:389–403.
12. Nestler J. Insulin and insulin-like growth factor-I stimulate the 3β-hydroxysteroid dehydrogenase activity of human placental cytotrophoblasts. *Endocrinology* 1989;125:2127–2133.
13. Evain-Brion D. Growth factors and trophoblast differentiation. *Trophoblast Res* 1992;6:1–18.
14. Bedin M, Ferré F, Alsat E, et al. Regulation of steroidogenesis in the human placenta. *J Steroid Biochem* 1980;12:17–24.
15. Cedard L, Bedin M, Leblond J, Tanguy G. Maternal plasma total oestriol and dehydroepiandrosterone

sulfate loading test as indicators of feto-placental function or placental sulfatase deficiency. *J Steroid Biochem* 1979;11:501–507.
16. Licht P, Cao H, Lei ZM, Rao CV, Merz WE. Novel self-regulation of human chorionic gonadotropin biosynthesis in term pregnancy human placenta. *Endocrinology* 1993;133:3014–3025.
17. Lei ZM, Reshef E, Rao CV. The expression of human chorionic gonadotrophin/luteinizing hormone receptors in human endometrial and myometrial blood vessels. *J Clin Endocrinol Metab* 1992;75: 651–659.
18. Zuo J, Lei ZM, Rao CV. Human myometrial chorionic gonadotrophin/luteinizing hormone receptors in preterm and term deliveries. *J Clin Endocrinol Metab* 1994;79:907–911.
19. Meuris S, Nagy AM, Delogne-Desnoeck J, Jurkovic D, Jauniaux E. Temporal relationship between the human chorionic gonadotropin peak and the establishment of intervillous blood flow in early pregnancy. *Hum Reprod* 1995;10:947–950.
20. Chard T, Iles R, Wathen N. Why is there a peak of human chorionic gonadotrophin (HCG) in early pregnancy? *Hum Reprod* 1995;10:1837–1840.
21. Walker WH, FitzPatrick SL, Barrera-Saldana HA, Resendez-Perez D, Saunders GF. The human placental lactogen genes: structure, function, evolution and transcriptional regulation. *Endocr Rev* 1991;12:316–327.
22. Petit A, Guillon G, Tence M, *et al.* Angiotensin II stimulates both inositol phosphate production and human placental lactogen release from human trophoblastic cells. *J Clin Endocrinol Metab* 1989; 69:280–286.
23. Stephanou A, Handwerger S. Interleukin-6 stimulates placental lactogen expression by human trophoblast cells. *Endocrinology* 1994;135:719–723.
24. Frankenne F, Scippo ML, Van Beeumen J, Igout A, Hennen G. Identification of placental human growth hormone as the growth hormone-V gene expression product. *J Clin Endocrinol Metab* 1990; 71:15–18.
25. Petraglia F, Volpe A, Genazzani AR, *et al.* Neuroendocrinology of human placenta. *Front Neuroendocrinol* 1990;11:6–37.
26. Petraglia F, De Micheroux A, Florio P, Salvatori M, Gallinelli A, Cela V, *et al.* Steroid-protein interaction in human placenta. *J Steroid Biochem* 1995;5:1–6.
27. Siler-Khodr TM, Kang IA, Khodr GS. Current topic: Symposium on placental endocrinology. 1. Effects of chorionic GnRH on intrauterine tissues and pregnancy. *Placenta* 1991;12:91–103.
28. Duello TM, Tsai SJ, Van Ess PJ. *In situ* demonstration and characterization of progonadotropin-releasing hormone messenger ribonucleic acid in first trimester human placenta. *Endocrinology* 1993; 133:2617–2623.
29. Lin L-S, Roberts VJ, Yen SS. Expression of human gonadotropin-releasing hormone receptor gene in the placenta and its functional relationship to human chorionic gonadotropin secretion. *J Clin Endocrinol Metab* 1995;80:580–584.
30. Challis JRG, Matthews SG, Van Meir G, Ramirez MM. Current topic: the placental corticotrophin-releasing hormone-adrenocorticotrophin axis. *Placenta* 1995;16:481–502.
31. Petraglia F, Potter E, Cameron VA, Sutton S, Behan DP, Woods RJ, et al. Corticotropin-releasing factor-binding protein is produced by human placenta and intrauterine tissues. *J Clin Endocrinol Metab* 1993;77:919–924.
32. McLean M, Bisits A, Davies J, Woods R, Lowry P, Smith R. A placental clock controlling the length of human pregnancy. *Nat Med* 1995;1:460–461.
33. Qu J, Thomas K. Regulation of inhibin secretion in human placental cell culture by epidermal growth factor, transforming growth factors, and activin. *J Clin Endocrinol Metab* 1993;77:925–931.
34. Keelan J, Song Y, France JT. Comparative regulation of inhibin, activin and human chorionic gonadotropin production by placental trophoblast cells in culture. *Placenta* 1994;15:803–818.
35. Petraglia F, Gallinelli A, Grande A, Florio P, Ferrari S, Genazzani AR, et al. Local production and action of follistatin in human placenta. *J Clin Endocrinol Metab* 1994;78:205–210.
36. Yanagisawa M, Kurihara H, Kimura S, *et al.* A novel potent vasoconstrictor peptide produced by vascular endothelial cells. *Nature* 1988;332:411–415.
37. Mondon M, Malassiné A, Robaut C, *et al.* Biochemical characterization and autoradiographic localization of [^{125}I] endothelin-1 binding sites on trophoblast and blood vessels of human placenta. *J Clin Endocrinol Metab* 1993;76:237–244.
38. Mondon F, Doualla-Bell Kotto Maka F, Sabry S, Ferré F. Endothelin-induced phosphoinositide hydrolysis in the muscular layer of stem villi vessels of human term placenta. *Eur J Endocrinol* 1995;133:606–612.

39. Robert B, Malassiné A, Bourgeois C, Mignot TM, Cronier L, Ferré F, et al. Expression of endothelin precursor genes in human trophoblast in culture. *Eur J Endocrinol* 1996;134:490–496.
40. Mignot TM, Malassiné A, Cronier L, Ferré F. Endothelin increases progesterone release by human trophoblast in culture. *Front Endocrinol* 1995;15:277–283 (Baldi E, Maggi M, Cameron IT, Dunn MJ, eds. *Endothelins in Endocrinology: New Advances*).
41. Sugawara T, Maruo T, Otani T, Mochizuki M. Increase in the expression of c-erb A and c-erb B mRNAs in the human placenta in early gestation: their role in trophoblast proliferation and differentiation. *Endocr J* 1994;41:S127–S133.
42. Duc-Goiran P. Expression of cytokines in human pregnancy. *Arta IV* 1993;Issues 1–2:61–69.
43. Feinberg BB, Anderson DJ, Steller MA, Fulop V, Berkowitz RS, Hill JA. Cytokine regulation of trophoblast steroidogenesis. *J Clin Endocrinol Metab* 1994;73:586–591.
44. Chard T. Placental hormones and metabolism. In: Reece LA, Hobbins JC, Mahoney MJ, Petrie RH, eds. *Medicine of the Fetus and Mother*. London: Lippincott; 1992:88–96.
45. Ferré F, Alsat E, Breuiller M, et al. Placental steroid hormones and parturition in the human. In: Monset-Couchard M, Minkowsky A, eds. *Physiological and Biochemical Basis of Perinatal Medicine*. Basel: S Karger; 1981:274–283.

DISCUSSION

Dr. Page: We know that there is a wide range of putative hormones in the placenta, peptides in particular, and they seem in many cases to have a simple proportionality with placental mass. Can we say that this is a controlling factor, or is it more likely that the placenta is an organ that is under very tight hormonal control? Can we go as far as making that distinction yet?

Dr. Cedard: Some substances, like hPL, which has no particular action, have no apparent regulation, but as far as the active hormones are concerned there is regulation. I have been interested for a long time in the synthesis of estrogen, and it is striking that this is very well regulated. There are factors that increase the production of estrogen from androgen—hCG is very important in that field like prostaglandin or adrenaline—but the estrogens by themselves have no toxicity because free estradiol is present in very small amounts, mostly protein-bound in conjugated form, which prevents it from entering cells. Maternal liver transforms estrone into its conjugated form with glucuronyl sulfate. Estriol has practically no action, since the liver transforms all the estrogen into conjugated estriol. So the secretion of estrogen has no toxicity. There is also control of androgen production. Sulfatase, which is the first enzyme, is blocked by the free compound. If you have an excess of androgen, the sulfatase is inhibited, and there are some other substances that can mimic that. Overall, the control of androgen synthesis is very well regulated.

Dr. Boyd: I was interested to see that both EGF and endothelin have a role in progesterone release, and in the stomach endothelin affects the activity of maxi chloride channels and EGF also affects chloride transport. I wonder if there is a cross-link between subjects there. How far is there pulsatility in release of the different hormones from placenta? And what is the mechanism of release from syncytial trophoblast into villous space of the different categories of hormones?

Dr. Cedard: Pulsatility has been studied, particularly by Barnea (1), who made superfusions of explants and showed pulsatility to be present. There is no study on the release of hCG. What is known is that there are no granules, unlike in the hypophysis. In the placenta you generally find what you are looking for! But the regulation seems to be simpler, and hCG is secreted free. The placenta is not a storage organ.

Dr. Talamantes: Pulsatility depends on the hormone. Placental growth hormone variant loses its pulsatility in pregnancy. So it depends very much on a hormone as to whether there is pulsatility or not. hCG is not the only hormone in pregnancy.

Dr. Boyd: You said that Barnea had shown the pulsatile release of protein hormones. You also said that there is no storage of protein hormone products in placenta. Am I right to conclude from that that there must be pulsatile amino acid transport into syncytiotrophoblast to sustain the hormone secretion you are talking about?

Dr. Chard: The random fluctuations that have been documented by many people over the years take place in the order of minutes or even seconds; they are very very rapid indeed. It seems to me that they would be much too fast to involve complete synthesis or switching off of synthesis of any of these proteins. Now to come back to your perfectly reasonable logical point: If that is the case and they are not stored, then how does it happen? One possibility could be variation of peripheral metabolism; if there are fast variations in peripheral metabolism, they could create the appearance of fluctuations.

Dr. Boyd: Mrs. Cedard touched on one important point, which is that the placenta does not store its protein hormones. You would expect the organ of origin to be a storage site; for example, you would expect to find a lot of hCG in the placenta, but this is not the case. The level of hCG in placental extracts is about the same as the circulating level.

Dr. Talamantes: Henry Friesen in Canada has shown that in hPL there are two pools—a readily releasable pool that turns over very fast and a storage pool. So there *is* a small storage pool for hPL. In placental growth hormone variant, you can notice in the first half of pregnancy that pituitary prolactin has episodic and circadian rhythms, as one would expect, but as soon as you get into the last trimester of pregnancy, the placental growth hormone variant is turned on and released, and it is released in a very constant way. The matter of secretory granules and how the hormone gets out is very questionable; for example, some people have shown secretory granules in the placenta in the past. However, there do seem to be two pools in the human, although we have not found this in mice, and we have not seen secretory granules in mice.

Dr. Anthony: In the sheep, placental lactogen and many other peptide hormones are definitely stored in secretory granules.

Dr. Owens: Could you comment perhaps on placental CRH as the time clock for parturition in the human? I wondered if you were aware of direct experimental evidence for this—for example, by giving CRH to the sheep or other species to induce parturition.

Dr. Cedard: There is a suggestion that CRH has an action on the fetal hypophysis, but the level is very low during pregnancy. Earlier work showed that the pre-CRH and the peptide increase between the 36th and 40th week of pregnancy. This is a very striking phenomenon. There is also a decrease in the protein binding. So I think it is possible that this has an important role in initiating labor. There appear also to be different curves between patients who have normal term pregnancy and preterm pregnancy.

Dr. Chard: It is my understanding that that particular situation is unique to the human. Unfortunately, the experiments that one would like to see done are probably not going to be done on ethical grounds, because one would have to think of some therapeutic indication to enable one to carry out such an experiment.

REFERENCE

1. Barnea ER, Kaplan M. Spontaneous, gonadotropin-releasing hormone-induced and progesterone-inhibited pulsatile secretion of human chorionic gonadotropin in the first trimester placenta *in vitro*. *J Clin Endocrinol Metab* 1989;69:215–217.

Placental Function and Fetal Nutrition,
edited by Frederick C. Battaglia,
Nestlé Nutrition Workshop Series, Vol. 39.
Nestec Ltd., Vevey/Lippincott-Raven Publishers,
Philadelphia, © 1997.

The Endocrine Function of the Placenta: Human Placental Growth Hormone Variant

Frank Talamantes

Sinsheimer Laboratories, University of California, Santa Cruz, California 95064, USA

The placenta of mammals is a very adaptable organ that accomplishes many critical functions necessary for the well-being of the host and developing fetus. For example, the placenta serves as an attachment site to secure the developing fetus to the uterus, and it transports nutrients from the maternal to the fetal compartment. During the evolution of viviparity, the placenta has assumed various morphologies and a diverse set of endocrine functions. As an endocrine organ, it is very versatile. Its versatility arises from its ability to produce a wide array of protein and steroid hormones. The protein hormones that are elaborated by the placenta share structural and functional overlap with those produced by the hypothalamus and the anterior pituitary gland. The structural and biologic features of the various protein hormones produced by the placenta are very species-dependent. For example, in humans the placenta produces human chorionic gonadotrophin (hCG), a hormone that shares structural and functional properties with pituitary luteinizing hormone; decidual prolactin and chorionic somatomammotrophin (hCS) (also referred to as *human placental lactogen*), which share structural and functional overlap with pituitary growth hormone (hGH) and prolactin; and human placental growth hormone (human growth hormone variant, hGH-V), which shares structural and functional overlap with pituitary growth hormone (reviewed in ref. 1). In this review, I will limit my discussion to the knowledge that is available on the structure and function of hGH-V.

The human growth hormone locus (Fig. 1) contains five structurally related genes spanning 47 kB (2,3) and located on chromosome 17q22-q24 (4). The five growth hormone genes are all organized in the same transcriptional orientation and are each composed of five exons. From 5' to 3' these genes are as follows: growth hormone (hGH-N), chorionic somatomammotrophin-like (hCS-L), chorionic somatomammotrophin-A (hCS-A), growth hormone variant (hGH-V), and chorionic somatomammotrophin-B (hCS-B) (5). Interestingly, despite linkage and homology, the growth hormone genes are expressed in two mutually exclusive tissue-specific patterns. The hGH-N gene is expressed solely in the somatotrophs and lactosomatotrophs of the anterior pituitary, whereas hCS-L, hCS-A, hGH-V, and hCS-B are specifically expressed in the syncytiotrophoblastic layer of the placenta (reviewed in ref. 6). Each

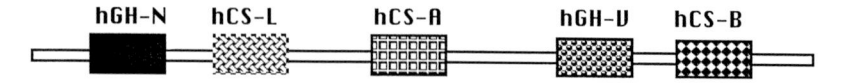

FIG. 1. Organization of the growth hormone gene family containing the five genes located on chromosome 17q22-24.

of the genes can use one or more alternative splicing pathways during RNA processing (6,7).

GROWTH HORMONE VARIANT

The presence of hGH-V in the blood and placenta was originally suggested by the observation that when two different monoclonal antibodies were used to measure the concentration of GH-like immunoreactivity in the serum, the resulting gestational profiles were very similar until about week 25, but differed considerably thereafter (8,9). After week 25, increasing concentrations of GH-like immunoreactivity were detected with one of the antibodies, whereas declining concentrations of GH-like activity were detected with the other. GH-like activity was also detected in term placental extracts with the former antibody, but not the latter, which suggested that the placenta contains GH-like activity that is not related to the presence of pituitary hGH (9). Further evidence to substantiate the presence of a placental growth hormone included the binding of an hGH-V probe to placental RNA by dot-blot analysis (10), and the cloning of a complementary DNA (cDNA) for placental growth hormone from a placental cDNA library (11). Placental growth hormone was then purified (12), and sequence analysis of its cDNA and the purified protein showed that it was the product of the hGH-V gene.

GENE STRUCTURE

The hGH-V gene was discovered when the entire hGH cluster was sequenced (3). Originally, it was speculated that it was a pseudogene. The primary transcript of the hGH-V gene undergoes alternative splicing to yield hGH-V and hGH-V2 messenger RNAs. Messenger RNA for hGH-V conforms to the predominant splicing pattern of other members of the gene family and contains the five complete exons of the gene and no intron sequences. On the other hand, the hGH-V2 messenger RNA contains five exons and all of intron 4 (13). Both messenger RNAs are present in the placenta, with hGH-V2 messenger RNA accounting for about 5% and 15% of hGH-V gene transcripts in the first and third trimesters, respectively (14). Unlike the primary transcript of the hGH-N gene, which undergoes alternative splicing in exon 3 to yield a messenger RNA in which the first 15 codons of exon 3 are deleted, the primary transcript of the hGH-V does not appear to undergo alternative splicing at this site (15). The nucleotide differences between the hGH-N and hGH-V genes that are responsible for this difference in splicing patterns have been identified (16). The transcription start site of the hGH-V gene is 30 nucleotides downstream of a TATAAA sequence (16). The 5'-flanking region of the hGH-V gene contains the distal, but not the proximal, binding site for GHF-1 (17,18).

PROTEIN STRUCTURE

The hGH-V protein consists of 191 amino acids. The hormone is glycoslated (5,11,12,19) and contains two disulfide bonds linking *cys*-53 with *cys*-165 and *cys*-182 with *cys*-189. Interestingly, the amino acid sequence of hGH-V differs from the pituitary-derived growth hormone by 15 amino acids (Fig. 2). Thirteen of the amino acid differences reside in the mature protein and are located throughout the sequence. Two of three amino acid residues in the PRL receptor binding domain of pituitary hGH that have been shown to be involved in coordinating zinc in the hGH-PRL receptor complex (20) are not conserved in hGH-V (positions 18 and 21). The ability to bind zinc in this region appears to be important for binding of hGH and hCS to the extracellular domain of the human PRL receptor but not for the binding of PRL to the same receptor (20,21). Consequently, the binding of hGH-V to the human PRL receptor may occur by a mechanism that is more readily compared with that used by hPRL than with that used by hGH and hCS. When the hGH-V messenger RNAs were cloned from the placenta, it was observed that the hGH-V gene encodes two alternatively spliced messenger RNAs, hGH-V and hGH-V2 (13). Although the actual protein of the hGH-V2 has not been found to be sequenced, its predicted structural sequence and the presence of a hydrophobic domain in the novel C terminus have led to suggestions that hGH-V2 could be an integral membrane protein (13).

```
                    (10)              (20)             (30)             (40)
hGH      F P T I P L S R L F D N A M L R A H R L H Q L A F D T Y Q E F E E A Y I P K E Q
hGH-V    F P T I P L S R L F D N A M L R R R R L Y Q L A Y D T Y Q E F E E A Y I L K E Q

                    (50)              (60)             (70)             (80)
hGH      K Y S F L Q N P Q T S L C F S E S I P T P S N R E E T Q Q K S N L E L L R I S L L
hGH-V    K Y S F L Q N P Q T S L C F S E S I P T P S N R V K T Q Q K S N L E L L R I S L L

                    (90)             (100)            (110)            (120)
hGH      L I Q S W L E P V Q F L R S V F A N S L V Y G A S D S N V Y D L L K D L E E G I
hGH-V    L I Q S W L E P V Q L L R S V F A N S L V Y G A S D S N V R H L L K D L E E G I

                   (130)             (140)            (150)            (160)
hGH      Q T L M G R L E D G S P R T G Q I F K Q T Y S K F D T N S H N D D A L L K N Y G
hGH-V    Q T L M W R L E D G S P R T G Q I F N Q S Y S K F D T K S H N D D A L L K N Y G

                   (170)             (180)            (190)
hGH      L L Y C F R K D M D K V E T F L R I V Q C R S V E G S C G F
hGV-V    L L Y C F R K D M D K V E T F L R I V Q C R S V E G S C G F
```

FIG. 2. Amino acid sequence of hGH and hGH-V. Numbering for the hGH sequences is shown above the sequence. Helical segments in hGH amino acids are 9-34, 38-47, 64-70, 72-92, 94-100, 106-138, and 155-184.

LOCALIZATION

The expression of the hGH-V gene has been sublocalized within the placenta by Northern blot analysis and *in situ* hybridization. Northern analysis of messenger RNA isolated from four placental layers—amnion, chorion, decidua, and villi—showed specific expression localized only to the villi (13). Expression of the hGH-V was sublocalized within the villi to the syncytiotrophoblast epithelium by histohybridization using a cDNA probe specific for intron 4 of the hGH-V gene (22).

GESTATIONAL PROFILE

The gestational profile of hGH-V in maternal serum and its presence in other body compartments (e.g., amniotic fluid) has been determined as the difference in growth hormone values obtained with assays using two monoclonal antibodies, one of which recognizes hGH-V and the other of which does not (9,23). A difference in growth hormone values measured with these two antibodies appears between weeks 21 and 26 of pregnancy, suggesting that hGH-V appears in maternal serum in detectable concentrations during this period. Its concentration increases until about week 36 and then remains relatively constant for the remainder of pregnancy (9,23,24). However, hGH-V may be present in maternal serum much earlier than week 21, as messenger RNAs for hGH-V and hGH-V2 are present in the placenta by week 9 (22). The apparent absence of hGH-V in serum in early pregnancy probably reflects the relative insensitivity of the assay used. At term, hGH-V has not been detected in amniotic fluid or fetal serum (24).

The gestational profile of hGH-V in maternal blood parallels changes in the level of hGH-V messenger RNA in the placenta (14), suggesting that the rate of hormone synthesis could be a major determinant of the hGH-V gestational profile in maternal blood. The retention of intron 4 in the hGH-V2 messenger RNA by alternative splicing is regulated during the development of the placenta, resulting in a threefold increase of hGH-V2 messenger RNA between weeks 10 and 38 of gestation. This regulation of hGH-V intron 4 splicing suggests that synthesis of hGH-V2 might be important for placental function (13).

BIOLOGIC FUNCTION

In an attempt to understand the biologic function of hGH-V, the activity of the hormone has been analyzed in various bioassays and according to its ability to bind to both PRL and growth hormone receptors. In the rat NB2 lymphoma cells, hGH-V has been shown to be mitogenic, as are hGH and PRLs (25,26). It has also been shown that hGH-V binds to PRL binding sites on the lymphoma cells and in rat liver (27). Its affinity for the rat PRL receptor and its potency in the NB2 cell assay are significantly less than that of pituitary hGH (26,27). This suggests that hGH-V is not as potent a lactogen as hGH in the rat. Like pituitary growth hormone, hGH-V has been shown to have somatogenic activity in that it stimulates body weight gain in the hypophysectomized rat (26). In addition, it has been shown to stimulate glucose oxidation and lipolysis in rat adipose tissue (28). In both systems, the potency of hGH-V is comparable with that of pituitary hGH. Although the somatogenic biologic activity of hGH-V has not been examined in human tissue, the hormone has been shown to bind to the circulating human growth hormone binding protein with an affinity similar to that of pituitary growth hormone (29). Given that human growth hormone binding protein is structurally similar to the extracellular binding domain of the human growth hormone receptor (30), the affinities of hGH-V and pituitary growth hormone for the growth hormone receptor are probably very similar. Based on the findings described above, it has been hypothesized that the expression of hGH-V during middle to late gestation, coupled with its preference for the somatogenic receptor, may be responsible for the acromegaloid facial features detected in some women during pregnancy (29). The replacement of hGH-N by hGH-V in maternal serum at midgestation (9) suggests that hGH-V might have a role in mediating the metabolic demands of pregnancy. Examination of the gestational profiles of hGH-V and insulin-like growth factor-1 (IGF-1) in women has revealed a significant correlation between them, suggesting a possible role for hGH-V in regulating IGF-1 production in the second half of pregnancy (23). Additional observations provide evidence that hGH-V may also have a role in preparing the breast for lactation. For example, somatogen receptor messenger RNA has been observed in breast tissue (31,32), growth hormone binding protein has been found in milk (33), and precocious mammary development and lactation have been demonstrated in transgenic mice expressing growth hormone locally in mammary gland tissue. In addition, it has been observed that growth hormone has a potent effect on mammary gland development by acting through the somatogen receptor (34). Thus, given this set of data, one can hypothesize that hGH-V encodes an important gestational hormone whose action might be important for the mother, the developing fetus, or both. Specific binding of hGH-V to human placental membranes (35), expression of hGH receptor messenger RNA (36), and immunoreactivity (37) in human placenta raises the possibility that hGH-V could have an autocrine function in the placenta.

WHAT REMAINS TO BE DISCOVERED

Although a considerable amount of information has accumulated about the structure of the protein and gene for placental growth hormone-V, more effort has to be directed at understanding what regulates the expression of this hormone and what are its relevant functions during pregnancy. To begin to appreciate its function, better discrimination of the circulating forms of hGH is needed through the development of specific methods for measuring hGH-V alone and not hormones like hGH-N. The ability to generate sizable quantities of highly purified hGH-V will permit further detailed studies characterizing its biologic properties. The majority of studies examining the biologic activity of hGH-V have used heterologous systems. Although much useful information can be generated by cross-species analysis, it is of the utmost importance that attempts be made to sort out the biologic activities of hGH-V on human tissue. To date, very little information exists about the secretagogues that may be important in regulating the expression of hGH-V. One has to be able to verify the hypotheses that have been generated about the role of the hGH-V2 gene product. The maintenance of "normal" pregnancies does not appear to require the presence of hGH-V. This raises the interesting question about the potential compensatory mechanisms that may exist in such cases. Although care has to be used in extrapolating data generated from nonprimate species to the primate species, it may be possible to learn a significant amount about placental growth hormone if one examines whether other species (e.g., mice) produce a placental growth hormone. If this turns out to be the case, it would be easier to design experiments that would shed light on the function and regulation of expression of placental growth hormone.

REFERENCES

1. Ogren L, Talamantes F. The placenta as an endocrine organ: polypeptides. In: Knobil E, Neill JD, eds. *The Physiology of Reproduction*. 2nd ed. New York: Raven Press; 1994:875–945.
2. Barsh GS, Seeburg PH, Gelinas RE. The human growth hormone gene family: structure and evolution of the chromosomal locus. *Nucleic Acids Res* 1983;11:3939–3958.
3. Chen EY, Liao Y- C, Smith DH, Barrera-Saldana HA, Gelinas RE, Seeburg PH. The human growth hormone locus: nucleotide sequence, biology, and evolution. *Genomics* 1989;4:479–497.
4. George DL, Phillips JA, Francke U, Seeburg PH. The genes for growth hormone and chorionic somatomammotropin are on the long arm of human chromosome 17 in region Q21-qter. *Hum Genet* 1981;57:138–141.
5. Seeburg PH. The human growth hormone gene family: nucleotide sequences show recent divergence and predict a new polypeptide hormone. *DNA* 1982;1:239–249.
6. Cooke NE, Liebhaber SA. Molecular biology of the growth hormone-prolactin gene system. *Vitam Horm* 1995;50:385–459.
7. Cooke NE, Jones BK, Urbanek M, Misra-Press A, Lee AK, Russell JE, et al. Placental expression and function of the human growth hormone gene cluster. In: Soares MJ, Handwerger S, Talamantes F, eds. *Trophoblast Cells: Pathways for Maternal-Embryonic Communications*. New York: Springer-Verlag; 1993:222–239.
8. Hennen G, Frankenne F, Pirens G, et al. New chorionic GH-like antigen revealed by a monoclonal antibody radioimmunoassays. *Lancet* 1985:1:399–400.
9. Hennen G, Frankenne F, Closset J, Gomez F, Pirens G, El Khayat N. A human placental growth hormone: increasing levels during second half of pregnancy with pituitary growth hormone suppression as revealed by monoclonal antibody radioimmunoassays. *Int J Fertil* 1985;30:27–33.
10. Frankenne F, Rentier-Delrue F, Scippo M-L, Martial J, Hennen G. Expression of the growth hormone variant gene in human placenta. *J Clin Endocrinol Metab* 1987;64:635–637.
11. Igout A, Scippo M-L, Frankenne F, Hennen G. Cloning and nucleotide sequence of placental hGH-V cDNA. *Arch Int Physiol Biochim* 1988;96:63–67.
12. Frankenne F, Scippo M-L, van Beeumen J, Igout A, Hennen G. Identification of placental human growth hormone as the growth hormone-V gene expression product. *J Clin Endocrinol Metab* 1990;71:15–18.
13. Cooke NE, Ray J, Emery JG, Liebhaber SA. Two distinct species of human growth hormone-variant mRNA in the human placenta predict the expression of novel growth hormone proteins. *J Biol Chem* 1988;263:9001–9006.
14. MacLeod JN, Lee AK, Liebhaber SA, Cooke NE. Developmental control and alternative splicing of the placentally expressed transcripts from the human growth hormone gene cluster. *J Biol Chem* 1992;267:14219–14226.

15. Cooke NE, Ray J, Watson MA, Estes PA, Kuo BA, Liebhaber SA. Human growth hormone gene and the highly homologous growth hormone variant gene display different splicing patterns. *J Clin Invest* 1988;82:270–275.
16. Estes PA, Cooke NE, Liebhaber SA. A difference in the splicing patterns of the closely related normal and variant human growth hormone gene transcripts is determined by a minimal sequence divergence between two potential splice-acceptor sites. *J Biol Chem* 1990;265:19863–19870.
17. Nickel BE, Kardami E, Cattini PA. Differential expression of human placental growth hormone variant and chorionic somatomammotrophin in culture. *Biochem J* 1990;267:653–658.
18. Nickel BE, Nachtigal MW, Bock ME, Cattini PA. Differential binding of rat pituitary-specific nuclear factors to the 5'-flanking region of the pituitary and placental members of the human growth hormone gene family. *Mol Cell Biochem* 1991;106:181–187.
19. Ray R, Jones BK, Liebhaber SA, Cooke NE. Glycosylated human growth hormone variant. *Endocrinology* 1989;125:566–568.
20. Cunnigham BC, Bass S, Fuh G, Wells JA. Zinc mediation of the binding of human growth hormone to the human prolactin receptor. *Science* 1990;250:1709–1712.
21. Lowman HB, Cunningham BC, Wells JA. Mutational analysis and protein engineering of receptor-binding determinants in human placental lactogen. *J Biol Chem* 1991;266:10982–10988.
22. Liebhaber SA, Urbanek M, Ray J, Tuan R, Cooke NE. Characterization and histologic localization of human growth hormone-variant gene expression in the placenta. *J Clin Invest* 1989;83:1985–1991.
23. Caufriez A, Frankenne F, Englert Y, et al. Placental growth hormone as a potential regulator of maternal IGF-I during human pregnancy. *Am J Physiol* 1990;258:E1014–E1019.
24. Frankenne F, Closset J, Gomez F, Scippo M-L, Smal J, Hennen G. The physiology of growth hormones (GHs) in pregnant women and partial characterization of the placental growth hormone variant. *J Clin Endocrinol Metab* 1988;66:1171–1180.
25. Nickel BE, Kardami E, Cattini PA. The human placental growth hormone variant is mitogenic for rat lymphoma NB2 cells. *Endocrinology* 1990;126:971–976.
26. MacLeod JN, Worsley I, Ray J, Friesen HG, Liebhaber SA, Cooke NE. Human growth hormone variant is a biologically active somatogen and lactogen. *Endocrinology* 1991;128:1298–1302.
27. Ray J, Okamura H, Kelly PA, Cooke NE, Liebhaber SA. Human growth hormone-variant demonstrates a receptor binding profile distinct from that of normal pituitary growth hormone. *J Biol Chem* 1990;265:7939–7944.
28. Goodman HM, Tai L-R, Ray J, Cooke NE, Liebhaber SA. Human growth hormone variant produces insulin-like and lipolytic responses in rat adipose tissue. *Endocrinology* 1991;129:1779–1783.
29. Baumann G, Davila N, Shaw MA, Ray J, Liebhaber SA, Cooke NE. Binding of human growth hormone (growth hormone)-variant (placental growth hormone) to growth hormone-binding proteins in human plasma. *J Clin Endocrinol Metab* 1991;73:1175–1179.
30. Cramer SD, Talamantes F. The growth hormone receptor and binding protein: structure, function and regulation. In: Pang PKT, Schreibman MP, eds. *Vertebrate Endocrinology: Fundamentals and Biomedical Applications*. New York: Academic Press; 1992:117–149.
31. Jammes H, Gaye P, Belair I, Dijane J. Identification and characterization of growth hormone receptor mRNA in the mammary gland. *Mol Cell Endocrinol* 1991;75:27–35.
32. Thordarson G, Jin E, Guzman R, Swanson SM, Nandi S, Talamantes F. Refractoriness to mammary tumorigenesis in parous rats. Is it caused by persistent changes in the hormonal environment or permanent biochemical alterations in the mammary epithelia? *Carcinogenesis* 1995;16:2847–2853.
33. Postel-Vinay M-C, Belair L, Kayser C, Kelly PA, Dijane J. Identification of prolactin and growth hormone binding proteins in rabbit milk. *Proc Natl Acad Sci U S A* 1991;88:6687–6690.
34. Feldman M, Ruan W, Cunningham BC, Wells JA, Kleinberg DL. Evidence that the growth hormone receptor mediates differentiation and development of the mammary gland. *Endocrinology* 1993;133:1602–1608.
35. Frankenne F, Alsat E, Scippo M-L, Igout A, Hennen G, Evain-Brion, D. Evidence for the expression of growth hormone receptor in human placenta. *Biochem Biophys Res Commun* 1992;182:481–486.
36. Urbanek M, MacLeod JN, Cooke NE, Liebhaber SA. Expression of a human growth hormone (hGH) receptor isoform is predicted by tissue-specific alternative splicing of exon 3 of the hGH receptor gene transcript. *Mol Endocrinol* 1992;6:279–287.
37. Hill DJ, Riley SC, Bassett NS, Waters MJ. Localization of the growth hormone receptor, identified by immunocytochemistry, in second trimester human fetal tissues and in placenta throughout gestation. *J Clin Endocrinol Metab* 1992;75:646–650.

DISCUSSION

Dr. Chard: Perhaps I could start off on the functional aspect. I believe that pregnancies with a gene deletion have been described but that fetal growth was effectively normal in those pregnancies.

Dr. Talamantes: That is true, but we don't know whether it was compensatory mechanisms that had taken over in those particular cases. It's the same with placental lactogen. It is true that there have been cases in which the genes have not produced the product and we have had a "healthy birth."

Dr. Anthony: Am I correct in remembering that hGH-V does not get into the fetal circulation?

Dr. Talamantes: Yes, it is not found in the amniotic fluid or in the fetal circulation.

Dr. Milliez: Do you have any data on twin pregnancies, and do you have any data on trophoblastic disease?

Dr. Talamantes: I have not seen anything on twin pregnancies. It does not make a difference if you have a male or a female fetus, and there is only one paper that I know of looking at pathologic pregnancies. I think only in diabetes was there a hint that there might be an alteration. But this is based on only one study. There have not been enough good studies to look at this carefully.

Dr. Ogata: What is the relationship between hGH-V and IGF? You showed plasma concentrations, but is there any information concerning molecular secretion?

Dr. Talamantes: The only data looking at this have examined correlations between the amount of hGH-V and IGF-1. What I neglected to say is that hGH-V has the same affinity for the growth hormone binding protein as does normal growth hormone. In humans and in rodents, there is a circulating binding protein for growth hormone. In the case of the human, the growth hormone binding protein is the hormone binding domain of the receptor once it anchors itself into the cell. The same affinity exists for hGH-V, and it may well be circulating with a binding protein in the pregnancy, but that has not been checked.

Dr. Owens: What is the cross-reactivity of hPL on the somatogenic receptors, given the much higher concentration in the circulation? Is it able to compete effectively?

Dr. Talamantes: No, these assays are really specific. The cross-reactivity was quite low.

Dr. Owens: How do you envisage this growth hormone variant having any real role in control of fetal growth if, for example, it is present in very low concentrations in fetal blood. You have talked about the evidence for a role in mammary development, but do you see it being important in terms of the fetus? Is it simply that it is concerned with maternal adaptation? This would be consistent with its absence not having a great impact on the fetus.

Dr. Talamantes: My feeling is that the hormone need not be in the fetus but could affect transport of all kinds of things across the placenta. It is a unique receptor for growth hormone in the placenta. It is structurally quite different from the growth hormone receptor on the maternal side, in liver or wherever. We don't know yet know whether growth hormone might not be important in causing transport of important nutrients across the placenta.

Dr. Chard: David Hill published data suggesting that the fetal liver has a specific hPL receptor and is therefore much more sensitive to hPL than adult tissues (1). The same has not been shown for the hGH variant, but it is another hypothesis.

Dr. Boyd: I think when we are looking for *purposes* for hormones one has to put it in a biologic context. I remember that two to three generations ago epiphyses weren't fused until the early or middle 20s, and yet people started reproducing in their middle teens. I wonder whether your human growth hormone variant could be an emergency pelvic growth hormone—whether in the pregnant women with unfused epiphyses it could have an evolutionary drive around that sort of function. You could put it to the test by looking in deprived populations at whether the achieved pelvic growth is bigger in people who have early pregnancies.

Dr. Talamantes: I am not a clinician, so I don't know. I think that sometimes we may be looking at the wrong thing in relation to the issue of hormones and their function. For example, let's talk about rodents, which I can deal with in more detail. If one looks at the function of growth hormone (and I am convinced that hGH-V is also very important for the human mammary gland), many years ago Roberto Ceriani at Berkeley took fetal rat skin from day 10 and organ-cultured it to see what kind of hormones were necessary to get the gland to look like that of a 20-day-old rat fetus. And what it needed was growth hormone and prolactin. However, the rat fetal pituitary does not make growth hormone until near term. So it was a question of where that hormone was coming from. That prompted us to look in the amniotic fluid, and the amniotic fluid, at least in mice, contains lots of growth hormone. Obviously, if you make an observation like this *in vitro*, you need to see what happens *in vivo*.

Dr. Milliez: I might have missed the point, but can you tell me again how early in pregnancy this hormone is produced by the placenta?

Dr. Talamantes: Circulating hormone begins at about 25 weeks. But if you look at Northern blots, you can see quite a lot of message in the first trimester. The question is whether it is not being expressed at that time. People who work in the field are convinced that at 25 weeks they can see hGH-V from the placenta.

Dr. Milliez: It is definitely not produced in pre-embryo culture?

Dr. Talamantes: They have not looked at that.

REFERENCE

1. Hill DJ, Freemark M, Strain AJ, Handwerger S, Milner RDG. Placental lactogen and growth hormone receptors in human fetal tissues: relationship to fetal plasma hPL concentrations and fetal growth. *J Clin Endocrinol Metab* 1988;66:1283–1290.

Development of Hormone Receptors Within the Fetus

R. V. Anthony, M. D. Fanning, and L. C. Richter

Animal Reproduction and Biotechnology Laboratory, Department of Physiology, Colorado State University, Fort Collins, Colorado 80523-1683, USA

Many factors affect the rate of fetal growth and development in addition to overall fetal well-being. In eutherian mammals, the placenta serves as the primary mediator and modulator of those factors that ultimately determine development rate. The placenta accomplishes this task in the following ways: (a) by serving as the site of nutrient and waste transfer between the mother and fetus; (b) by serving as a barrier against the maternal immune system and pathogens; and (c) by functioning as an endocrine organ. Regarding this latter function, the placenta is capable of synthesizing and secreting a plethora of protein and steroid hormones, growth factors, cytokines, and other bioactive molecules (1–3), many of which are produced at extraplacental sites as well. However, some are synthesized only by the placenta and are "true" placental hormones, such as the placental lactogens (1–3).

Assigning specific biologic roles to any placental hormone is difficult, because classic ablation-replacement experiments are not feasible. Emphasis has therefore been placed on identifying the receptor for each placental hormone—its location and mechanism of action. Considerable effort has been expended on determining whether or not the placental lactogens act through structurally distinct receptors, or if they act through the growth hormone or prolactin receptor. As yet, firm conclusions cannot be drawn about the existence of distinct placental lactogen receptors, which has hampered our understanding of the function of this placental hormone. In some species (human and sheep), it has been suggested (4) that placental lactogen serves to modulate maternal and fetal metabolism, possibly by stimulating the expression of the insulin-like growth factors (IGFs). If this hypothesis is correct, it provides a direct link between placental hormone production and fetal growth regulation, because evidence now in hand clearly shows the importance and developmental pattern of the IGF system within the fetus (2). This chapter focuses on our current knowledge of the development of fetal growth hormone/placental lactogen receptors and their mechanism of action, with emphasis on humans and sheep.

STRUCTURE AND FUNCTION OF PLACENTAL LACTOGEN

Placental lactogens are members of the growth hormone/prolactin gene family, but they differ considerably from species to species in their primary structure. Primate placental lactogens are structurally more similar to growth hormone than they are to prolactin, with human placental lactogen (hPL) showing 87% amino acid sequence identity with pituitary-derived human growth hormone and only 23% amino acid sequence identity with human prolactin (1,2). In rodents, the placental members of this family are structurally more similar to prolactin than they are to growth hormone (5), and in the species examined thus far, there are two major types of placental lactogen (PL-1 and PL-2), which differ in structure and secretion pattern (1,5). As for rodents, the placental lactogens synthesized by domestic ruminants are structurally more similar to prolactin than they are to growth hormone, but as in primates, only a single structural type of placental lactogen has been identified (6).

The exact biologic role of the placental lactogens is not well defined for any species, and the diversity shown between species in primary structure may impart diverse biologic functions. As shown in Fig. 1, there may be multiple sites of action for placental lactogens within the maternal system, and the importance of the various sites is likely to be different between species. For example, there appears to be direct luteotropic actions by one or more of the mouse placental lactogens (7) and by bovine placental lactogen (8), whereas evidence for direct luteal support by human or sheep placental lactogens is lacking. This example of functional diversity may result from the gestational requirement for corpus luteum-derived progesterone in the former species, or the lack of a requirement for it in the latter. Species divergence in the structure-function relationship for placental lactogens may be a reflection of evolutionary adaptation. Bovine and ovine placental lactogens are structurally more similar to each other (approximately 66%) (6) than they are to other members of this gene family, yet the divergence in primary structure between the ruminant placental lactogens is greater than the divergence in primary structure between bovine and ovine growth hormone or between bovine and ovine prolactin (approximately 99% amino acid sequence identity). Comparison of the sequence similarities between

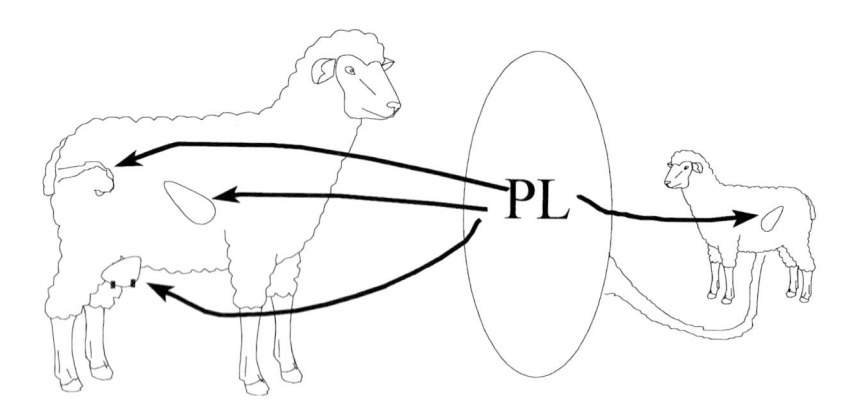

FIG. 1. Schematic diagram depicting potential sites of action for placental lactogen within the maternal and fetal systems. These include luteotropic and mammotropic actions within the mother and metabolic actions within the mother and fetus.

these ruminant placental lactogens revealed a non-synonymous substitution rate greater than the synonymous substitution rate (9), suggesting that the more rapid rate of evolution between bovine and ovine placental lactogens may have resulted from adaptive rather than neutral mutations. On the other hand, there appear to be interspecific commonalties in function, as there is direct and indirect evidence of mammotropic actions for placental lactogens in primates, rodents, and ruminants (1,10,11).

As implied in Fig. 1, placental lactogens may modulate maternal and fetal metabolism by exerting action on maternal and fetal liver, as well as other metabolic tissues. Grumbach *et al.* (12) initially proposed that placental lactogen serves as an insulin antagonist, thereby inducing peripheral tissue insulin resistance and increased lipolysis and proteolysis within the mother, with the net result of providing additional glucose and amino acids for transport to the fetus. All these responses are normal adaptations in metabolism that occur in pregnant women, and there is experimental evidence (13) to support Grumbach's hypothesis (12). However, for obvious reasons, *in vivo* data from humans to support this hypothesis are lacking, and many of the data acquired *in vitro* were obtained using heterologous systems. Even in the pregnant sheep model, in which *in vivo* approaches are feasible, there is a dearth of experimental evidence supporting the role of placental lactogen as a major modulator of maternal and fetal metabolism (6).

As alluded to in the introductory section, our lack of understanding of the specific biologic role of placental lactogen is at least in part a consequence of the inability to use classic ablation-replacement approaches in defining the function of placental hormones. Further exacerbating the difficulty in defining specific functions is the fact that in both humans and sheep, the endogenous concentration of placental lactogen (2,13) is quite high relative to the K_d of the placental lactogen binding sites described in maternal and fetal tissues. Therefore, administration of additional placental lactogen into what may already be a saturated or near-saturated system is unlikely to yield easily interpretable results. There have been cases in which deletions within the human growth hormone-placental lactogen gene cluster resulted in low to undetectable concentrations of human placental lactogen and human placental growth hormone (hGH-V), yet by all indications pregnancy outcome was normal (13). These data imply that production of placental lactogen is not an absolute requirement for normal pregnancy outcome. It is entirely possible that placental lactogen, hGH-V, and fetal pituitary-derived growth hormone serve within a redundant system aimed at providing the homeorrhetic environment required during pregnancy. Such redundancy is becoming more commonplace as the "true" biology of various systems is described, and definition of the location, mechanism of action, and structural identity of the receptor through which each hormone acts may help determine the role of each hormone within this potentially redundant system.

GROWTH HORMONE / PLACENTAL LACTOGEN RECEPTORS

Many of the placental lactogens were originally purified using heterologous growth hormone or prolactin receptor assays, and both human placental lactogen (hPL) and ovine placental lactogen (oPL) will bind the growth hormone receptor of their species (14,15). This has led to the suggestion that, at least in these species, placental lactogen exerts its actions through the growth hormone receptor. As yet, no specific placental lactogen receptor has been structurally characterized, and it is likely that in humans and sheep the placental lactogen receptor is either closely related to the growth hormone receptor, or indeed is the growth hormone receptor. Therefore, a brief description of this receptor and its mechanism of action is warranted before the available information related to the existence of fetal growth hormone/placental lactogen receptors is examined.

The growth hormone receptor is a member of the cytokine receptor superfamily, and is comprised of three domains: a 246-amino acid extracellular domain that binds to and is dimerized by a single molecule of growth hormone; a short transmembrane segment; and a 350-amino acid intracellular domain required for signal transduction events (16,17). A single molecule of growth hormone is bound by two molecules of the growth hormone receptor (1:2 stoichiometry) (17), and dimerization of the receptor is essential for signal transduction to take place. Binding of growth hormone to its receptor initiates a signal transduction pathway that involves tyrosine phosphorylation of multiple cellular peptides (Fig. 2). The identification of Janus kinase 2 (JAK2) as a growth hormone receptor-associated, growth hormone-activated tyrosine kinase, established tyrosine phosphorylation as the initial step in the signal transduction of growth hormone (18).

Growth hormone has been observed to stimulate phosphorylation of tyrosine residues within insulin receptor substrate-1 (IRS-1) (19), which is critical not only in insulin signaling but also in providing a binding site for the regulatory subunit of phosphatidylinositol 3'-kinase. Additionally, growth hormone stimulates tyrosine

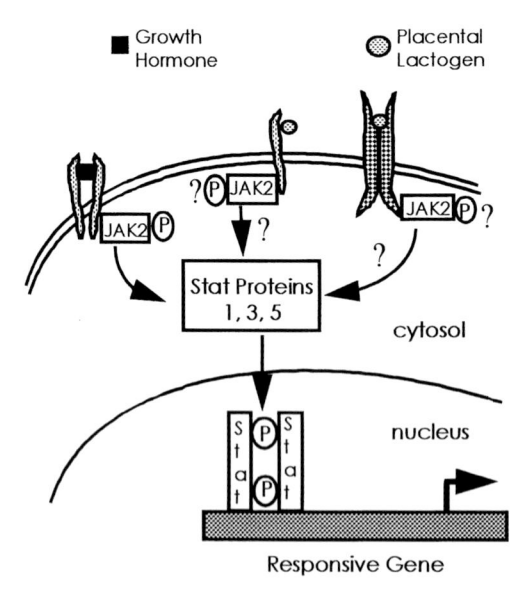

FIG. 2. Schematic diagram of the signal transduction cascade induced by growth hormone binding to its receptor. The signal transduction cascade is also depicted as to how it may be activated by placental lactogen. *JAK2*, Janus kinase 2; *Stat*, signal transducer/activator of transcription protein.

phosphorylation of latent cytoplasmic transcription factors designated as signal transducer/activator of transcription (Stat) proteins-1 (Stat-1) and -3 (Stat-3), and their activation (Fig. 2) leads to transactivation of target genes (20–22). These Stat proteins mediate the transcriptional response stimulated by multiple growth factors and cytokines. Co-precipitation and growth hormone receptor mutagenesis experiments indicate that growth hormone activation of Stat-1, Stat-3, and IRS-1 require their interaction with JAK2 rather than growth hormone receptor, supporting the hypothesis that JAK2 is the initial signaling molecule for growth hormone. It has recently been shown that intermittent pulses of growth hormone stimulate the tyrosine phosphorylation, translocation to the nucleus, and activation of DNA binding of Stat-5, suggesting that Stat-5 is an additional intracellular mediator of the stimulatory effects of growth hormone (23). As yet, the signal transduction pathways induced by placental lactogen binding to its target tissues have not been examined (Fig. 2).

Fetal Growth Hormone Receptors

The lack of effect of growth hormone deficiency on human fetal growth rate resulting from anencephaly or congenital absence of the pituitary gland led to the conclusion that fetal development occurs independently of fetal pituitary-derived growth hormone (24). This has been thought to result from a lack of growth hormone receptor within the fetus, but the growth hormone receptor or its messenger RNA has now been identified in fetal tissues from a variety of species. These more recent data, coupled with clinical data inferring impaired *in utero* growth of infants with idiopathic growth hormone deficiency (25) or growth hormone receptor dysfunction (26), suggest that in fact growth hormone has actions within some fetal tissues.

Hill *et al.* (27) showed specific binding of growth hormone to human fetal liver microsomes obtained at midgestation, but could not demonstrate specific binding to the microsomal fraction of fetal skeletal muscle. However, specific binding sites for hPL were identified in both fetal liver and skeletal muscle (27). The growth hormone binding sites in fetal liver showed a sixfold greater affinity for growth hormone than for placental lactogen, and the placental lactogen binding sites showed a ninefold greater affinity for placental lactogen than for growth hormone, suggesting that the respective binding sites (receptors) are different. These results were supported by the immunohistochemical localization of the growth hormone receptor in fetal liver, pancreas, kidney, skin, and cerebral cortex, but not in fetal skeletal or cardiac muscle, adrenal gland, intestine, lung, or epiphyseal growth plate (28).

The messenger RNA encoding the human growth hormone receptor was recently identified (29) in the same tissues in which the growth hormone receptor was immunolocalized (28), as well as in tissues in which the growth hormone receptor could not be immunolocalized (muscle, adrenal gland, intestine, and lung). Both exon 3-retaining and exon 3-deleted transcripts were detected, and the relative expression pattern of the two growth hormone receptor isoforms appeared to be individual-specific rather than tissue-specific and may be developmentally regulated (29), with exon 3-retaining transcripts predominating in later gestation. Deletion of exon 3 from the growth hormone receptor messenger RNA results in a 22-amino acid deletion at the amino terminus of the growth hormone receptor, but this deletion does not alter the binding affinity of the growth hormone receptor for growth hormone (30), such that its deletion probably does not account for the absence of detectable growth hormone receptor (28) or growth hormone binding (27) in some tissues (e.g., skeletal muscle). The growth hormone receptor messenger RNA identified in various fetal tissues (29) was not examined for the potential variation in exon 1 sequences that exists in human growth hormone receptor messenger RNA transcripts (16,31). Eight different sequences have been described (31) for the exon 1 region of the human growth hormone receptor messenger RNA, and although exon 1 contains only 5'-untranslated sequence (5'-UTR), it is possible that use of one or more of these variant 5'-UTRs could provide for posttranscriptional regulation (inhibition of translation) of the growth hormone receptor in tissues like fetal skeletal muscle.

A different scenario appears to exist in fetal mice and rats. Messenger RNA encoding the growth hormone receptor or the growth hormone binding protein (GHBP) have been identified in fetal mouse (32) and rat (33) tissues as early as embryonic days 12 and 14, and the amount of growth hormone receptor/GHBP immunolocalized in fetal rat tissues increased from day 12 to 18 of gestation (33). However, the identity of the ligand for fetal mouse and rat growth hormone receptor remains in question, as fetal pituitary-derived growth hormone does not appear until very late in gestation (about day 19) (34). It appears unlikely that the ligand is mouse or rat placental lactogen, at least not PL-2, as mouse growth hormone does not compete for mouse PL-2 binding sites on hepatic membranes (35). Recently, Southard *et al.* (36) showed that mouse growth hormone receptor messenger RNA contains two different 5'-UTRs (exon 1 sequences): one (L1) was preferentially used in pregnant maternal liver transcripts, whereas the other (L2) was predominant in nonpregnant and fetal tissues. The L2 5'-UTR contains an AUG translation initiation codon with features of a preferred start site (37), followed by a stop codon generating a short open reading frame preceding the "normal" growth hormone receptor open reading frame. The GC-rich content of the L2 5'-UTR, coupled with the short open reading frame encoded within L2, may potentially inhibit translation (38) of the growth hormone receptor, which begins within the exon 2-derived sequence. Therefore, the growth hormone receptor messenger RNA found in mouse fetal liver (day 16), as early as embryonic day 14 (32), may not be efficiently translated into the growth hormone receptor, because only L2-containing growth hormone receptor messenger RNA was detected (36). Posttranscriptional regulation of the growth hormone receptor messenger RNA, as a function of the particular 5'-UTR within the messenger RNA, has yet to be demonstrated.

Fetal sheep have long been considered to be growth hormone receptor-deficient until the immediate periparturient period (1,2,6). However, recent cross-linking and immunoprecipitation data indicate that the ovine growth hormone receptor is present in fetal liver between 125 to 135 days of gestation (39). The amount of specific ovine growth hormone binding to fetal hepatic microsomes was still quite low in these samples (1.2 ± 0.4%), and others (40) have concluded from saturation analyses of day 105 to 120 fetal liver microsomes that specific binding of growth hormone is nonexistent. Growth hormone receptor messenger RNA has been detected in fetal liver and skeletal muscle tissues as early as day 60 of gestation (41,42), but the major growth hormone receptor messenger RNA transcript present during midgestation is about 300 base pairs larger (Fig. 3) than the growth hormone receptor messenger RNA expressed in maternal liver (42). This difference in growth hormone receptor messenger RNA size appears to result from use of a variant 5'-UTR up through 120 days of gestation (42), in that the 5'-UTR encoded by the adult liver, specifically exon 1A (43), was not detectable until after day 120 (42). Recently, exon 1B was isolated and characterized from postnatal skeletal muscle, another tissue that does not appear to express exon 1A (44). Two of the authors (L. C. Richter and R. V. Anthony, *unpublished data*) have determined, using reverse transcriptase polymerase chain reactions and Southern hybridizations, that the 5'-UTR sequence present in fetal liver and skeletal muscle, as well as the placenta, is derived from exon 1B. Exon 1B sequence is detectable in fetal liver messenger RNA on days 60, 90, 105, 120, and 135 of gestation, which coincides with our earlier detection of exons 2 to 10 from day 60 on (42). In contrast to our earlier results (42), some individual samples obtained at 120 days of gestation have been found to express exon 1A, suggesting that a developmental switch in ovine growth hormone receptor gene transcription or primary transcript splicing occurs around 120 days of gestation.

Combined, the available information on growth hormone receptor gene transcription in human, rodent, and ruminant fetal tissues indicates that developmental

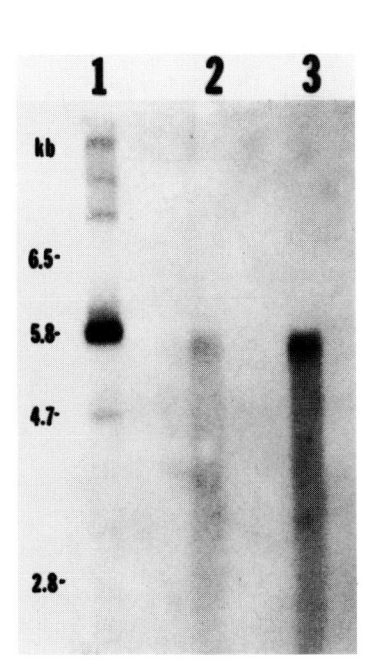

FIG. 3. Northern hybridization analysis of poly(A)+ RNA obtained from day 105 fetal liver (*lane 1*), day 135 fetal liver (*lane 2*), and day 100 maternal liver (*lane 3*). The electrophoretic gel was blotted onto a nylon membrane and hybridized to a bovine growth hormone receptor complementary DNA. From Pratt and Anthony (42), with permission.

switches occur in growth hormone receptor gene transcription or in subsequent splicing events. As discussed earlier, in the human fetus there appears to be an individual-dependent switch between exon 3-deleted and exon 3-retaining growth hormone receptor messenger RNA as gestation progresses (29). Whether or not there is a developmental switch in the use of the various 5'-UTRs transcribed from the human growth hormone receptor gene (16,31) has yet to be determined. There appears to be a commonality between mice (36) and sheep (42) in the use of 5'-UTR sequences in the growth hormone receptor messenger RNA expressed in fetal liver. As depicted in Fig. 4 for fetal sheep liver, exon 1B (analogous to L2 in mice) (36) is expressed throughout most of gestation and into adult life (44), but exon 1A is not expressed until around 120 days of gestation. Both exon 1B in sheep (44) and L2 in mice (36) contain a translation initiation codon that meets the requirements of a preferred site (37). This initiation codon is followed by a translation stop codon, creating an autonomous open reading frame that precedes the "normal" growth hormone receptor open reading frame. Within the sheep exon 1A sequence (Fig. 4) lie two potential initiation codons, but neither conforms to the requirements (a purine at position -3 and a G at position -4) of a preferred initiation site (37) and are probably not used. Additionally, both exons 1B and L2 have a high GC content,

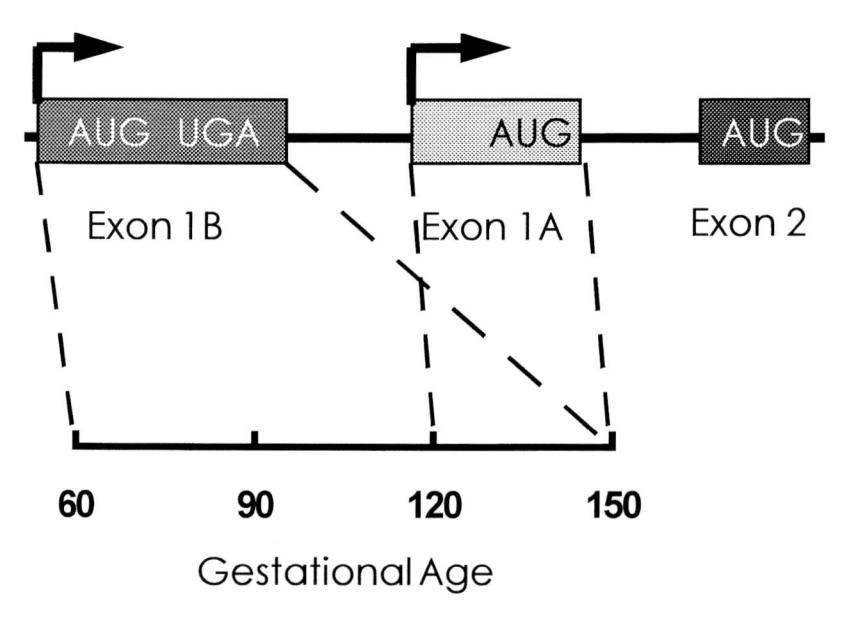

FIG. 4. Diagrammatic representation of the developmentally regulated transcription of the ovine growth hormone receptor gene. Exon 1B is transcribed throughout gestation, but it is not until approximately 120 days of gestation that exon 1A is transcribed. Exon 1B contains an autonomous open reading frame that may inhibit translation initiation of the growth hormone receptor within exon 2. The translation initiation sites within exon 1A do not conform to the conditions of a preferred site, and do not appear to be used. The *bent arrows* indicate the transcriptional start sites for exons 1B and 1A, respectively.

which could create sufficient secondary structure to interfere with the assembly of the preinitiation complex for translation (38). Both an autonomous open reading frame and excessive secondary structure within the 5'-UTR probably hinder the efficient translation of growth hormone receptor messenger RNA, a common occurrence in proto-oncogenes, growth factors, and growth factor receptor genes (38). Cell lines need to be established that express growth hormone receptor messenger RNA containing this type of 5'-UTR (e.g., exon 1B or L2) to examine the effect on translation efficiency. If these messenger RNAs are not efficiently translated into a functional growth hormone receptor, it could explain why it is difficult to show specific growth hormone binding to fetal liver microsomes in species such as the sheep. Additionally, the transcriptional regulation involved in these apparent developmental switches needs to be examined.

Fetal Placental Lactogen Receptors

Specific binding sites for hPL have been identified in fetal liver and skeletal muscle (27) that appear to be distinct from the hGH binding sites identified in fetal liver. Although hPL and hGH share 87% primary amino acid sequence identity, hPL binds the hGH receptor with 2300-fold lower affinity (14), indicating that the fetal liver and skeletal muscle hPL binding sites are not the growth hormone receptor. As yet, no attempts at purification or structural characterization of the fetal hPL binding sites have been reported.

Numerous studies have examined the binding of oPL to maternal and fetal hepatic microsomes (2,6). Specific high-affinity binding ($K_d \approx 0.12$ to 0.5 nM) of oPL to fetal liver microsomes has been demonstrated (40,45), whereas ovine growth hormone or prolactin shows negligible specific binding to these membranes (40,46). During quantification of oPL binding sites by saturation analyses (40), the concentration of the fetal liver binding site did not change with increasing gestational age when data were expressed per milligram of microsomal protein. However, when the concentration was expressed per milligram of DNA (i.e., per cell), the concentration did increase with increasing gestational age, indicating that as the fetus ages and develops there are increased numbers of oPL binding sites per cell. Additionally, saturation analyses using radiolabeled oPL, prolactin, or growth hormone as the ligand (40) and fetal hepatic microsomes (days 105 to 120 gestational age) as the source of receptors show saturable binding kinetics for oPL, but no specific binding of oPRL or growth hormone. Although a partial purification of this binding site has been reported (45), no amino acid sequence data are available on this receptor.

Recent cross-linking and immunoprecipitation studies indicate that oPL and ovine growth hormone are able to bind an identical or quite similar receptor present in fetal liver at 125 to 135 days of gestation (39). However, the amount of specific binding of ovine growth hormone to these microsomes (1.2 ± 0.4%) was considerably less than the amount of specific binding of oPL (7.6% ± 2.4%). These investigators (39) suggested that the difference in the amount of specific binding between oPL and ovine growth hormone might be explained by oPL interacting with the growth hormone receptor in a 1:1 stoichiometry rather than the 1:2 stoichiometry shown by growth hormone binding the growth hormone receptor. Precedence for placental lactogen binding in a 1:1 stoichiometry with the growth hormone receptor was provided by the data of Staten et al. (47) using bovine placental lactogen (bPL) and the bovine growth hormone receptor. It was observed that bPL bound the bovine growth hormone receptor in a 1:1 stoichiometry rather than the 1:2 stoichiometry shown with bovine growth hormone (47). Additionally, a monoclonal antibody raised against the extracellular domain of the bovine growth hormone receptor competes with bovine growth hormone binding to the growth hormone receptor, but does not compete with bPL binding to the growth hormone receptor, suggesting that the binding sites of the two ligands are not exactly the same. However, when the ovine growth hormone receptor was expressed in CHO cells, growth hormone showed a greater affinity (K_d = 0.30 nM) than did oPL (K_d = 0.76 nM) for this receptor, yet both ligands bound approximately the same number of ovine growth hormone receptor molecules per cell (15). These latter data are not consistent with the suggestion (39) that oPL is binding the growth hormone receptor within fetal liver in a 1:1 stoichiometry. In other words, if the common receptor for ovine growth hormone and oPL present in late-gestation fetal liver (39) is the ovine growth hormone receptor, then one must ask why ovine growth hormone is not bound with affinity equal to or greater than that of oPL.

As yet, firm conclusions cannot be drawn about the structural identity of the receptor in fetal tissues through which placental lactogen acts. There are several possibilities related to the identity of the fetal placental lactogen receptor, as shown in Fig. 5. One possibility is that placental lactogen acts by binding to a single monomer of the growth hormone receptor (Fig. 5A) in a 1:1 stoichiometry, as has been demonstrated for bPL (47). If this is the case, it is not clear why it has been difficult to show significant specific binding of growth hormone to fetal liver microsomes until late gestation, as this hypothesis assumes that functional growth hormone receptors are present. Furthermore, activation of the signal transduction pathways of the human growth hormone receptor (see above) requires growth hormone-induced dimerization (17) of the growth hormone receptor, and preliminary evidence (48) suggests that when bPL binds the growth hormone receptor in a 1:1 stoichiometry (Fig. 2), JAK2 does not undergo tyrosyl phosphorylation. The requirement for dimerization could be met by placental lactogen inducing a heterodimer between a growth hormone receptor monomer and an as yet to be described placental lactogen-specific monomer (Fig. 5B). However, this hypothesis again assumes the availability of growth hormone receptor monomers in fetal tissues, which would also allow specific binding of growth hormone to occur. In short, the hypotheses as to the identity of the fetal placental lactogen receptor depicted in Fig. 5 A,B do not coincide with the lack of specific growth hormone binding in sheep fetal liver and human fetal skeletal muscle.

Another possibility is that the placental lactogen receptor is a modified form of

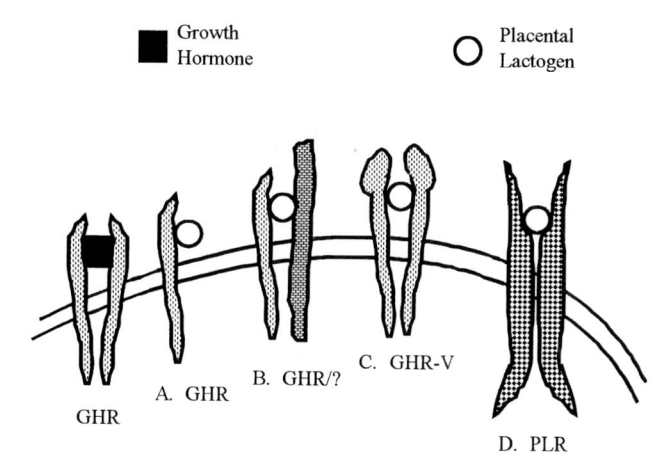

FIG. 5. Diagrammatic representation of the potential identity of the placental lactogen (*PL*) receptor found in fetal tissues. **A:** Placental lactogen may act by binding to one monomer of the growth hormone receptor (*GHR*). **B:** Placental lactogen may act by binding to one monomer of the growth hormone receptor and to a placental lactogen-specific monomer, generating a heterodimer. **C:** Placental lactogen may act by binding to two monomers of a growth hormone receptor variant (*GHR-V*) resulting from an amino terminal extension encoded by a variant 5'-UTR in the growth hormone receptor messenger RNA. **D:** Placental lactogen may act through binding a structurally distinct receptor (*PLR*).

the growth hormone receptor (GHR-V) (Fig. 5C). As discussed earlier, variant 5'-UTRs of the growth hormone receptor messenger RNA are expressed in fetal tissues. Both the mouse L2 5'-UTR and the sheep 5'-UTR encoded by exon 1B contain preferred translation initiation sites that precede the initiation site used in translating the growth hormone receptor (36,44). However, these "upstream" initiation sites are followed by translation stop codons, forming an autonomous open reading frame. It is possible that as yet undescribed 5'-UTRs exist in fetal tissues possessing similar upstream translation initiation sites that are in-frame with the initiation site in exon 2, and in the absence of an intervening stop codon, a growth hormone receptor could be translated that possesses an amino terminal extension. Such an amino terminal extension (Fig. 5C) could alter the conformation of the growth hormone receptor such that it no longer recognizes growth hormone with high affinity, but rather preferentially binds placental lactogen. As yet, no such growth hormone receptor 5'-UTR has been described in any species.

The final possibility (Fig. 5D) is that the placental lactogen receptor is a structurally distinct receptor and is not directly derived from either the growth hormone receptor or prolactin receptor genes but rather from a closely related gene. This is an inherently attractive hypothesis that coincides with most of the receptor binding data obtained with human and sheep fetal tissues. The structural characterization of such a receptor awaits its purification or complementary DNA isolation by expression cloning methods. Insight into the identity of the fetal placental lactogen binding site may be gained by examining the ability of placental lactogen to activate the

JAK2/Stat signal transduction pathway (Fig. 2). The ability of placental lactogen to activate this system in cells expressing the "normal" growth hormone receptor, or growth hormone receptor encoded by messenger RNA containing the various 5'-UTRs, could be compared with the ability of placental lactogen to activate this system in primary fetal cell cultures. If placental lactogen activates the signal transduction cascade coupled to the growth hormone receptor—and the same pathway in fetal cells—it would be important to ascertain if the activation of fetal cells could be blocked with antibodies raised against the growth hormone receptor. In short, if the ability of placental lactogen to activate cells expressing the growth hormone receptor could be blocked by antibodies raised against the growth hormone receptor, but its ability to activate fetal cells could not be blocked with these same antibodies, strong evidence would be provided for a structurally distinct receptor.

SUMMARY

Placental-fetal hormonal interactions play an important role in determining fetal growth rate and overall well-being. Placental lactogen is a member of the growth hormone/prolactin gene family that is thought to serve as an important mediator of the *in utero* environment, but it may be only one component of a redundant system that includes fetal pituitary-derived growth hormone. As yet, a specific placental lactogen receptor has not been structurally characterized, but the available evidence in humans and sheep indicates that such a receptor exists in fetal tissues. Additional effort needs to be directed toward the isolation and structural characterization of the fetal placental lactogen receptor to clarify the role of placental lactogen in fetal development. Furthermore, more evidence is becoming available to suggest that fetal development is not entirely independent of fetal pituitary-derived growth hormone, and that transcription of the growth hormone receptor gene may be a developmentally regulated event. What appears to be developmentally regulated use of various growth hormone receptor 5'-UTRs, on further analysis should provide insight into the developmental switches that are important for the transition from fetal to postnatal life. A thorough understanding of the transcriptional regulation of these developmental switches will provide new insight into fetal growth regulation, and could provide the basis for future interventions to treat intrauterine growth retardation or care for premature infants.

REFERENCES

1. Talamantes F, Ogren L. The placenta as an endocrine organ: polypeptides. In: Knobil E, Neill J, eds. *The Physiology of Reproduction.* New York: Raven Press; 1988:2093–2144.
2. Anthony RV, Pratt SL, Liang R, Holland MD. Placental-fetal hormonal interactions: impact on fetal growth. *J Anim Sci* 1995;73:1861–1871.
3. Roberts RM, Anthony RV. Molecular biology of trophectoderm and placental hormones. In: Findlay JK, ed. *Molecular Biology of the Female Reproductive System.* San Diego: Academic Press; 1994: 395–440.

4. Handwerger S. Clinical counterpoint: the physiology of placental lactogen in human pregnancy. *Endocr Rev* 1991;12:329–336.
5. Soares MJ, Faria TN, Roby KF, Deb S. Pregnancy and the prolactin family of hormones: coordination of anterior pituitary, uterine, and placental expression. *Endocr Rev* 1991;12:402–423.
6. Anthony RV, Liang R, Kayl EP, Pratt SL. The growth hormone/prolactin gene family in ruminant placentae. *J Reprod Fertil Suppl* 1995;49:83–95.
7. Galosy SS, Talamantes F. Luteotropic actions of placental lactogens at midpregnancy in the mouse. *Endocrinology* 1995;136:3993–4003.
8. Lucy MC, Byatt JC, Curran TL, Curran DF, Collier RJ. Placental lactogen and somatotropin: hormone binding to the corpus luteum and effects on growth and function of the ovary in heifers. *Biol Reprod* 1994;50:1136–1144.
9. Wallis M. Remarkably high rate of molecular evolution of ruminant placental lactogens. *J Mol Evol* 1993;37:86–88.
10. Forsyth IA. The biology of the placental prolactin/growth hormone gene family. In: Milligan SR, ed. *Oxford Reviews of Reproductive Biology*. Oxford: Oxford University Press; 1991;13:97–148.
11. Byatt JC, Eppard PJ, Veenhuizen JJ, Curran TL, Curran DF, McGrath MF, et al. Stimulation of mammogenesis and lactogenesis by recombinant bovine placental lactogen in steroid-primed dairy heifers. *J Endocrinol* 1994;140:33–43.
12. Grumbach MM, Kaplan SL, Sciarra JJ, Burr IM. Chorionic growth hormone-prolactin (CGP): secretion, disposition, biological activity in man, and postulated function as the "growth hormone" of the second half of pregnancy. *Ann N Y Acad Sci* 1968;148:501–531.
13. Ogren L, Talamantes F. The placenta as an endocrine organ: polypeptides. In: Knobil E, Neill JD, eds. *The Physiology of Reproduction*. New York: Raven Press; 1994:875–945.
14. Lowman HB, Cunningham BC, Wells JA. Mutational analysis and protein engineering of receptor-binding determinants in human placental lactogen. *J Biol Chem* 1991;266:10982–10988.
15. Fiddes RJ, Brandon MR, Adams TE. Functional expression of an ovine growth hormone receptor in transfected Chinese hamster ovary cells. *Mol Cell Endocrinol* 1992;86:883–889.
16. Leung DW, Spencer SA, Cachianes G, Hammonds RG, Collins C, Henzel WJ, et al. Growth hormone receptor and serum binding protein: purification, cloning and expression. *Nature* 1987;330:537–543.
17. Cunningham BC, Ultsch M, de Vos AM, Mulkerrin MG, Clausser KR, Wells JA. Dimerization of the extracellular domain of the human growth hormone receptor by a single hormone molecule. *Science* 1991;254:821–825.
18. Argetsinger LS, Campbell GS, Yang X, Witthuhn BA, Silvennoinen O, Ihle JN, et al. Identification of JAK2 as a growth hormone receptor-associated tyrosine kinase. *Cell* 1993;74:237–244.
19. Argetsinger LS, Hsu GW, Myers MG, Billestrup N, White MF, Carter-Su C. Growth hormone, interferon-τ, leukemia inhibitory factor promoted tyrosyl phosphorylation of insulin receptor substrate-1. *J Biol Chem* 1995;270:14685–14692.
20. Silva CM, Lu H, Weber MJ, Thorner MO. Differential tyrosine phosphorylation of JAK1, JAK2, and Stat 1 by growth hormone and interferon-τ in IM-9 cells. *J Biol Chem* 1994;269:27532–27539.
21. Meyer DJ, Campbell GS, Cochran BH, Argetsinger LS, Larner AC, Finbloom DS, et al. Growth hormone induces DNA binding factor related to the interferon-stimulated 91 kDa transcription factor. *J Biol Chem* 1994;269:4701–4704.
22. Gronowski AM, Rotwein P. Rapid changes in nuclear protein tyrosine phosphorylation after growth hormone treatment *in vivo*. *J Biol Chem* 1994;269:7874–7878.
23. Waxman DJ, Prabha AR, Park S-H, Choi HK. Intermittent plasma growth hormone triggers tyrosine phosphorylation and nuclear translocation of a liver-expressed, Stat 5 related DNA binding protein. *J Biol Chem* 1995;270:13262–13270.
24. Browne CA, Thorburn GD. Endocrine control of fetal growth. *Biol Neonate* 1989;55:331–346.
25. Gluckman PD, Gunn AJ, Wray A, Cutfield WS, Chatelain PG, Guilbaud O, et al. Congenital idiopathic growth hormone deficiency associated with prenatal and early postnatal growth failure. *J Pediatr* 1992;121:920–923.
26. Rosenfeld RG, Rosenbloom AL, Guevara-Aguirre J. Growth hormone (GH) insensitivity due to primary growth hormone receptor deficiency. *Endocr Rev* 1994;15:369–390.
27. Hill DJ, Freemark M, Strain AJ, Handwerger S, Milner RDG. Placental lactogen and growth hormone receptors in fetal tissues: relationship to fetal plasma human placental lactogen concentrations and fetal growth. *J Clin Endocrinol Metab* 1988;66:1283–1290.
28. Hill DJ, Riley SC, Bassett NS, Waters MJ. Localization of the growth hormone receptor, identified

by immunocytochemistry, in second trimester human fetal tissues and placenta throughout gestation. *J Clin Endocrinol Metab* 1992;75:646–650.
29. Zogopoulos G, Figueiredo R, Jenab A, Ali Z, Lefebvre Y, Goodyer CG. Expression of exon 3-retaining and -deleted human growth hormone receptor messenger ribonucleic acid isoforms during development. *J Clin Endocrinol Metab* 1996;81:775–782.
30. Urbanek M, Russell JE, Cooke NE, Liebhaber SA. Functional characterization of the alternatively spliced, placental human growth hormone receptor. *J Biol Chem* 1993;268:19025–19032.
31. Pekhletsky RI, Chernov BK, Rubstov PM. Variants of the 5'-untranslated sequence of human growth hormone receptor mRNA. *Mol Cell Endocrinol* 1992;90:103–109.
32. Ilkbahar YN, Wu K, Thordarson G, Talamantes F. Expression and distribution of messenger ribonucleic acids for growth hormone (GH) receptor and GH-binding protein in mice during pregnancy. *Endocrinology* 1995;136:386–392.
33. Garcia-Aragon J, Lobie PE, Muscat GE, Gobius KS, Norstedt G, Waters MJ. Prenatal expression of the growth hormone (GH) receptor/binding protein in the rat: a role for GH in embryonic and fetal development. *Development* 1992;114:869–876.
34. Strasser MT, Mialhe P. Growth hormone secretion in the rat as a function of age. *Horm Metab Res* 1975;7:275–278.
35. Harigaya T, Smith WC, Talamantes F. Hepatic placental lactogen receptors during pregnancy in the mouse. *Endocrinology* 1988;122:1366–1372.
36. Southard JN, Barrett BA, Bikbulatova L, Ilkbahar Y, Wu K, Talamantes F. Growth hormone (GH) receptor and GH-binding protein messenger ribonucleic acids with alternative 5'-untranslated regions are differentially expressed in mouse liver and placenta. *Endocrinology* 1995;136:2913–2921.
37. Kozak M. An analysis of vertebrate mRNA sequences: intimations of translational control. *J Cell Biol* 1991;115:887–903.
38. Geballe AP, Morris DR. Initiation codons within 5'-leaders of mRNAs as regulators of translation. *Trends Biochem Sci* 1994;19:159–164.
39. Breier BH, Funk B, Surus A, Ambler GR, Wells CA, Waters MJ, *et al.* Characterization of ovine growth hormone (oGH) and ovine placental lactogen (oPL) binding to fetal and adult hepatic tissue in sheep: evidence that oGH and oPL interact with a common receptor. *Endocrinology* 1994;135:919–928.
40. Pratt SL, Kappes SM, Anthony RV. Ontogeny of a specific high-affinity binding site for ovine placental lactogen in fetal and postnatal liver. *Domest Anim Endocrinol* 1995;12:337–347.
41. Klempt M, Bingham B, Breier BH, Baumbach WR, Gluckman PD. Tissue distribution and ontogeny of growth hormone receptor messenger ribonucleic acid and ligand binding to hepatic tissue in the midgestation sheep fetus. *Endocrinology* 1993;132:1071–1077.
42. Pratt SL, Anthony RV. The growth hormone receptor messenger ribonucleic acid present in ovine fetal liver is a variant form. *Endocrinology* 1995;136:2150–2155.
43. O'Mahoney JV, Brandon MR, Adams TE. Identification of a liver-specific promoter for the ovine growth hormone receptor. *Mol Cell Endocrinol* 1994;101:129–139.
44. Adams TE. Differential expression of growth hormone receptor messenger RNA from a second promoter. *Mol Cell Endocrinol* 1995;108:23–33.
45. Freemark M, Comer M. Purification of a distinct placental lactogen receptor, a new member of the growth hormone/prolactin receptor family. *J Clin Invest* 1989;83:883–889.
46. Freemark M, Comer M, Handwerger S. Placental lactogen and growth hormone receptors in sheep liver: striking differences in ontogeny and function. *Am J Physiol* 1986;251:E328–E333.
47. Staten MR, Byatt JC, Krivi GG. Ligand-specific dimerization of the extracellular domain of the bovine growth hormone receptor. *J Biol Chem* 1993;268:18467–18473.
48. Warren WC, Sweeny CA, Hunyh MS, Staten NR, McGrath MF. Binding alone to the bovine somatotropin receptor does not always stimulate known somatotropin cellular responses. *J Anim Sci* 1995;73(Suppl 1):47.

DISCUSSION

Dr. Soothill: One aspect of concern relating to growth hormone in the fetus is the Laron type of growth hormone receptor deficiency syndrome, in which the babies have apparently almost normal weight. Do you have any idea about the switching of the growth hormone receptor variants in such cases?

Dr. Anthony: The 5'-UTR variants have not been looked at to any extent in the fetus. The exon 3 deletion has been looked at, and you find both exon 3-containing and exon 3-deleted forms within fetal tissues, and there is some indication that there may be some developmental switching going on there; however, it appears to be almost an individual-specific phenomenon rather than a tissue-specific phenomenon. The exon 3-deleted form has the same affinity for growth hormone or growth hormone variant as does the exon 3-containing form, so there doesn't seem to be a functional problem with that form of the receptor. But with these 5'-UTR variants, we don't yet know if any one of those are expressed proportionally more in fetal life in humans.

Dr. Soothill: I mentioned families with Laron syndrome specifically because if you found that they did produce one of the variants in pregnancy, that might be the explanation why those children have normal birth weight; until we have an explanation for that, we have to assume that growth hormone is not very important in the fetus.

Dr. Anthony: I agree with you. But I am not sure we have necessarily found all the variants. I can't rule out the possibility that there are other variants.

Dr. Battaglia: I have been pushing my obstetrical colleagues in Colorado to look at epiphyseal growth. You know that obstetricians measure femur length, which is really looking at the solid bone, but all the trophic peptides seem to act on the epiphyses, and with new imaging, you can look at epiphyseal growth in much more detail. So my question is, in terms of receptor development in fetal tissues, were you talking only about liver, or is this a broader phenomenon of growth hormone action? What is the developmental sequence if you take several target tissues? Is the developmental sequence always the same?

Dr. Anthony: From the standpoint of the growth hormone receptor, it seems that we see the same thing in fetal skeletal muscle, although we don't see the onset of exon 1A in skeletal muscle. That seems to be a liver-specific exon that is produced late in gestation and in adult life. We also see this in the placenta, but we haven't had a chance to go back and look at some of the other tissues that we have in the freezer, and I don't know about bone. Almost all David Hill's work was done in fetal liver and skeletal muscle; there hasn't been a broad-spectrum examination of other tissues. Mike Freemark at Duke is doing that with the prolactin receptor in the fetal rat, and Caroline McMillen's laboratory in Adelaide is doing it with the prolactin receptor (1), and I think they have planned to do it with the growth hormone receptor. I think we will know more about the distribution across tissues within the next year or two.

Dr. Chard: Can we assume from what you and others have said that there is general agreement that a growth hormone or growth hormone-like compound plays a key role in the intrauterine growth of the *sheep* fetus? We have heard all the reservations and doubts about that in the human. Is it clearer in the sheep? What about the hypophysectomized sheep?

Dr. Anthony: Unfortunately, it is probably not clear in the sheep! The hypophysectomized fetus does grow, but not totally normally. It is interesting that one of the things you see with those is a higher fat deposition. There was some work done several years ago in primary cultures; they challenged fetal sheep adipocytes with growth hormone and in fact they were responsive. In the fetal sheep you tend to see subcutaneous fat deposition until almost the analogous time when we start to pick up the adult exon 1A form of the growth hormone receptor, so possibly the fat is a target tissue that most of us have overlooked. There is plenty of fetal pituitary-derived growth hormone in the fetal sheep, and I think that many of us who may have discounted its role are rethinking that to some extent, especially late in gestation.

I think there is evidence of early placentally derived growth hormone, but that is in the first 50 days of gestation, so it is not as clear.

Dr. Girard: The receptor is there, but you need to have the protein in the phosphorylation cascade to be present and to be capable of doing the job.

Dr. Anthony: I can state that from the standpoint of placental lactogen, steps 1 and 3 are activated as early as 100 days of gestation. We have not collected hepatocytes earlier than that, and we tried to sort that out with growth hormone as well. One problem is that we know that placental lactogen will bind to growth hormone receptor and *vice versa*, so when you do those experiments, sorting that out is not easy. So our approach is to take the adult form of the growth receptor message and the fetal form and make cell lines of those, and then we're doing challenges with growth hormone and placental lactogen. At the same time, we are doing the same experiments with cultured fetal hepatocytes. If we can block the action with an antibody against the growth hormone receptor (which might block the action of growth hormone but not of placental lactogen in the fetal hepatocyte), then hopefully we will be able to sort some of these things out. But I don't believe that the limiting step will be some of the signal transduction cascade components, because many of these are used in other systems that are probably active much earlier in gestation.

Dr. Soares: You mentioned some experiments done with bovine placental lactogen showing that it failed to activate the cascade. What sort of system were they working on? In that system, does bovine placental lactogen actually have an effect, or is it just able to bind to receptors?

Dr. Anthony: In 1993, Staten showed that in the case of bovine placental lactogen when it bound to bovine growth hormone receptor you didn't get receptor dimerization. They followed this up by making a stable cell line expressing growth hormone receptor in BHK21 cells and then challenged them with both growth hormone and placental lactogen, looking for phosphorylation by Western blotting.

Dr. Godfrey: I think there are human data indicating that growth hormone may play a role in fetal growth; they come from a large Scandinavian series of children with growth hormone deficiency who, although they were of normal birth weight, were short at birth. So I think it is very important that we address the effects on specific fetal compartments.

Dr. Anthony: I think we are dealing with a redundant system that shows up in a lot of biologic systems. If you lack of one or other hormone, you may see some subtle changes or some important things may take place, but if you lack a single hormone you are not going to have severe intrauterine growth retardation.

Dr. Owens: There are two studies that may cast light on the importance of growth hormone or placental lactogen-like protein for growth in the fetal sheep. One is by Alan Bell at Ithaca, who a number of years ago had a graduate student who infused purified ovine placental lactogen into fetal sheep for several weeks and wrote it up as a thesis. I have seen the data in abstract form only, but apparently there was no effect on fetal growth, which was a bit disappointing. That may just be telling us that increasing placental lactogen above normal levels cannot promote growth, but placental lactogen may still be required. The other is a more recent study by Michael Bauer in Aukland (2); he infused bovine growth hormone into fetal sheep for 10 days and found a marked increase in placental weight and fetal weight at the end of the treatment. What would be interesting to know there is to what extent bovine growth hormone is growth hormone-like or prolactin-like in the sheep.

Dr. Anthony: The data from Alan Bell were in abstract form. The one thing that they did see and reported in that abstract was that there was about a 40% increase in fetal circulating IGF-1, but there was no effect on IGF binding protein. Alan told me they also saw a 40%

increase in IGF-2. There were some effects on the placenta, but it was very hard to sort out exactly what they were. That infusion was for 14 days and started at 122 days of gestation, and I think that by that point you may be too late to show really dramatic effects. In contrast, if you look at the 10-day infusion from the Aukland group's experiments, I would like to think it was given at a window of opportunity at which growth hormone may begin to be quite important. I think timing is very important. What stage of gestation are you at, and is it the proper stage to address what is going on?

Dr. Ogata: You haven't mentioned the insulin receptors. IGF acts in part through insulin receptors in the fetus, at least in the rat. Is there a role here for the insulin receptor? In the old days, we would say that insulin is the growth hormone of the fetus.

Dr. Anthony: I think undoubtedly there is a role for the insulin receptor. I am not sure if there is any developmental regulation of the insulin receptor in this situation. I don't think so.

Dr. Marini: It is very important that we should think of the very preterm fetus as suffering from a syndrome of placental deprivation from an endocrinologic point of view. We neonatologists tend to think only in terms of the placenta carrying nutrients to the fetus and cleaning the fetus, but the placenta has an important endocrine role in the formation of receptors in the fetus. For instance, if you think about the high incidence of osteopenia in the very small preterm baby, and if you realize the role that estrogen plays in bone mineralization, then the fact that these babies are deprived of estrogen for about 3 months when they should have been supplied with it by the placenta in fetal life is an important practical point.

REFERENCES

1. Phillips ID, Anthony RV, Butler TG, *et al.* Hepatic prolactin receptor gene expression increases in the sheep fetus before birth and after cortisol infusion. *Endocrinology* 1997;138:1351–1354.
2. Bauer MK, Harding JE, Breier BH, *et al.* Treatment of fetal sheep with growth hormone for 10 days results in increased placental and fetal weights. *Proc Aust Perinat Soc* 1996;14(A51):21.

Placental Function and Fetal Nutrition,
edited by Frederick C. Battaglia,
Nestlé Nutrition Workshop Series, Vol. 39.
Nestec Ltd., Vevey/Lippincott-Raven Publishers,
Philadelphia, © 1997.

Regulation of Gene Expression by Nutrients During the Perinatal Period

Jean Girard, Sylvie Hauguel-de Mouzon, Florence Chatelain, Pascal Boileau, Stéphane Thumelin, and Jean-Paul Pégorier

Centre de Recherche sur l'Endocrinologie Moléculaire et le Développement, Centre National de la Recherche Scientifique, 9 Rue Jules Hetzel, Meudon, France

The regulation of specific gene expression in response to changes of nutrition has become a major focus of modern nutritional research, owing to the emergence of techniques of molecular biology that have allowed the cloning of a number of genes involved in the regulation of carbohydrate and fat metabolism. It has been shown that major (glucose, fatty acids, amino acids) or minor (iron, vitamins) dietary constituents participate, in conjunction with many hormones, in the regulation of gene expression in response to nutritional changes (1–4). When we initiated the investigations summarized below, our long-term objectives were (a) to identify plasma hormones and substrates that signal to liver, muscle, adipose, and placental cells that the nature of alimentation has changed, and (b) to understand, at a molecular level, each of the events that intervened between the binding of the hormone to its cellular receptor, the uptake and metabolism of substrates, and the altered expression of specific enzymes or nutrient transporters. Two different experimental models will be discussed: (a) the fetus of a diabetic mother who receives a large amount of glucose through the placenta, and (b) the nutritional transition from the high-carbohydrate, low-fat environment of the fetus to the low-carbohydrate, high-fat environment (milk) of the suckling rat.

REGULATION OF GLUCOSE TRANSPORTER AND HEXOKINASE EXPRESSION IN FETAL TISSUES AND THE PLACENTA

Fetal growth and metabolism require a continuous flow of energy substrates from the mother to the fetus through the umbilical circulation. Glucose provides the major part of the energy needed for fetal growth and metabolism (5,6) and is the primary energy substrate of the placenta (7–11).

Glucose enters the cells through a facilitative diffusion process mediated by a family of proteins, the glucose transporters (GLUTs). Glucose is then rapidly phosphorylated into glucose-6-phosphate by hexokinases and metabolized in the glycolytic or lipogenic pathways, or stored as glycogen. In adult tissues, four major isoforms of facilitative glucose transporters have been described: GLUT-1 through GLUT-4 (12). GLUT-1 is expressed in all cells and is considered as the ubiquitous isoform of facilitative glucose transporters. GLUT-2 is specifically expressed in liver and pancreatic β cells. GLUT-3 is an isoform specifically expressed in neurons. GLUT-4 has been shown to be specifically expressed in insulin-sensitive tissues (skeletal muscle, heart, and adipose tissues) and to be regulated by insulin. Once inside the cell, glucose is rapidly phosphorylated into glucose-6-phosphate by a family of proteins, the hexokinases (HK). In adult tissues, four major isoforms of hexokinases have been described: HK-1 through HK-4 (13,14). HK-1 is expressed in all tissues and is considered to be the ubiquitous isoform of hexokinases. HK-2 has been shown to be specifically expressed in insulin-sensitive tissues (skeletal muscle, heart, and adipose tissues) and to be regulated by insulin. HK-3 is an isoform mostly expressed in fetal tissues. HK-4 (glucokinase) is specifically expressed in liver and pancreatic β cells. The coupling of glucose transport and glucose phosphorylation is of cardinal importance, as it allows the maintenance of a negative glucose gradient between the cell and the plasma, a condition required for a continuous glucose uptake.

ONTOGENESIS OF GLUCOSE TRANSPORTERS AND HEXOKINASES IN THE PLACENTA

The expression of genes involved in placental glucose transport and phosphorylation has been examined in the rat placenta. Several studies have reported that glucose transport in hemochorial placenta is mainly mediated by two facilitative glucose transporters, GLUT-1, the ubiquitous isoform, and GLUT-3, the brain-type isoform (15–18). GLUT-1 and GLUT-3 messenger RNAs are differentially expressed in the rat placenta during the last week of gestation (days 15 to 21). GLUT-1 messenger RNA expression remains steady, whereas the expression of GLUT-3 shows a threefold increase (Fig. 1). The rat placenta expresses messenger RNA for the low-K_m hexokinases (HK-1, HK-2, and HK-3), whereas the high-K_m hexokinase (HK-4, or glucokinase) is not detected in this tissue (data not shown). During the last week of gestation, the concentrations of HK-1, -2, and -3 messenger RNA isoforms do not change (data not shown). This suggests that a functional coupling of glucose transport and phosphorylation is not a prerequisite for the regulation of placental glucose utilization.

IMPACT OF MATERNAL DIABETES ON GLUCOSE TRANSPORTER EXPRESSION IN THE PLACENTA

To investigate the impact of maternal diabetes on glucose transporter expression in the placenta, we have used control or diabetic pregnant rats. In these experiments,

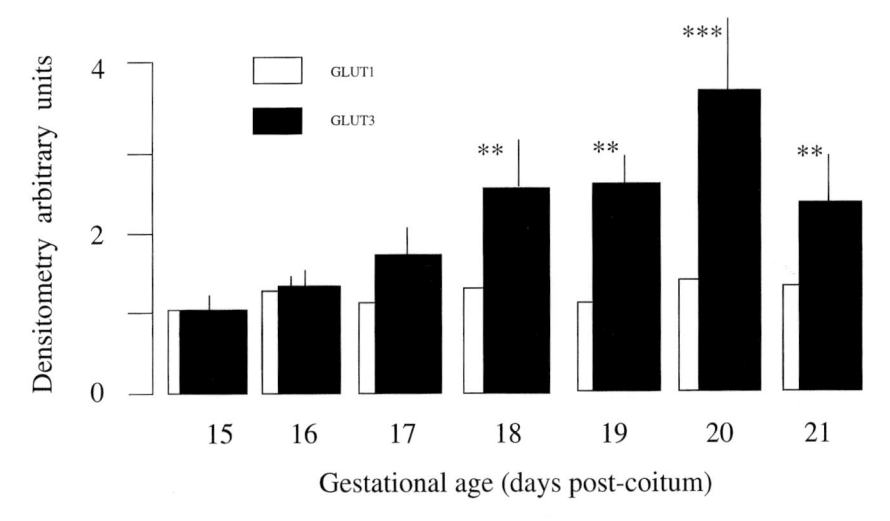

FIG. 1. GLUT-1 and GLUT-3 glucose transporter expression in the rat placenta during the last week of gestation. Placentae were obtained from pregnant rats on days 15 to 21 of gestation. Total RNA samples were prepared using one placenta from each gestational age and analyzed by Northern blotting. The blots were sequentially hybridized with rat GLUT-1 and GLUT-3 complementary DNA probes and then exposed to autoradiography. Results are means ± SE of scanning densitometry data obtained from three independent Northern blots. $^{**}p<.002$ and $^{***}p<.001$ vs. controls. From Boileau et al. (17).

severe insulinopenic maternal diabetes was induced by intraperitoneal injection of streptozotocin (65 mg/kg body weight) to rats on the first day of pregnancy (17). Throughout gestation, diabetic mothers were markedly hyperglycemic (460 mg/dl), and insulinopenic (43 μU/ml) compared with controls (90 mg/dl and 45 μU/ml). Near the term, fetuses were hyperglycemic (344 mg/dl), and their plasma insulin levels were decreased by 50%. Because maternal insulin does not cross the placental barrier, this suggested that the pancreas of the fetuses exposed to chronic hyperglycemia presented a defect in insulin secretion. Severe maternal diabetes was associated with a reduction in fetal weight (-25% at term) and an increase in placental weight (+40% at term) (17). In some experiments, phlorizin was infused to diabetic mothers from day 15 to day 20 of gestation to reduce their hyperglycemia (248 mg/dl) and to lower the glucose levels of fetuses (129 mg/dl), without improving their insulinopenia. This treatment did not correct the reduced fetal weight and the increased placental weight (17).

In the placenta of diabetic mothers, GLUT-1 and HK-1, -2, and -3 messenger RNA levels remained unchanged, whereas GLUT-3 messenger RNA levels were increased fourfold (17) (Fig. 2). This reinforced the idea that the regulation of placental glucose utilization did not necessarily involve a functional coupling of glucose transport and phosphorylation.

The localization of the two major glucose transporter isoforms, GLUT-1 and GLUT-3, was studied in the placenta of 20-day pregnant rats. Immunocytochemical

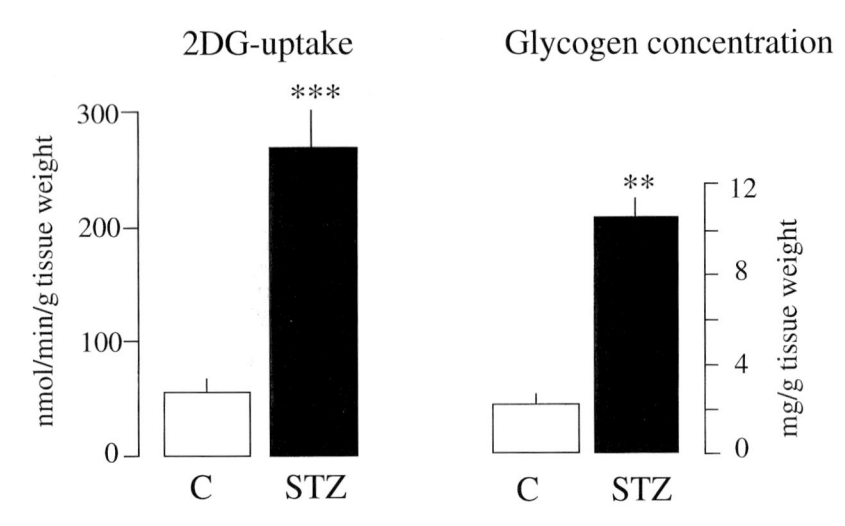

FIG. 2. Glucose uptake and glycogen concentration in placenta of diabetic rats. Placentae were obtained from 20-day pregnant control or diabetic rats. They were analyzed individually for 2-deoxy-^{3}H-glucose uptake and glycogen content. $^{**}p<.002$ and $^{***}p<.001$ vs. controls. From Boileau et al. (17).

study revealed that GLUT-1 protein was expressed both in the junctional zone (maternal side) and the labyrinthine zone (fetal side) of the placenta. In contrast, expression of GLUT-3 protein was restricted to the labyrinthine zone, specialized in nutrient transfer (17). The regulation of placental glucose utilization in conditions of severe hyperglycemia was further assessed by studying the modifications of GLUT-1 and GLUT-3 protein concentrations. Following 19 days of severe maternal insulinopenic diabetes, GLUT-3 protein levels were increased fourfold to fivefold compared with those of nondiabetic rats, whereas GLUT-1 protein levels remained unchanged. Placental 2-deoxyglucose uptake and glycogen concentrations were also increased fivefold in diabetic rats (Fig. 2). This suggested that GLUT-3 plays a major role in placental glucose uptake and metabolism.

The specific effect of hyperglycemia in the regulation of GLUT-3 expression was assessed by lowering the glucose levels of diabetic pregnant rats. After phlorizin infusion to pregnant diabetic rats from day 15 to day 19, placental GLUT-3 messenger RNA and protein levels returned to levels similar to those observed in nondiabetic rats (Fig. 3).

To further demonstrate that placental GLUT-3 expression is controlled by hyperglycemia, we performed studies with prolonged euglycemic-hyperinsulinemic (96 ± 4 mg/dl, 4820 ± 204 µU/ml) and hyperglycemic-hyperinsulinemic (613 ± 45 mg/dl, 450 ± 30 µU/ml) clamps in nondiabetic pregnant rats. At the end of 12-hour euglycemic-hyperinsulinemic clamps, GLUT-3 messenger RNA levels remained unchanged (Fig. 4). In contrast, after 12-hour hyperglycemic-hyperinsulinemic clamps, placental GLUT-3 messenger RNA levels were increased fourfold,

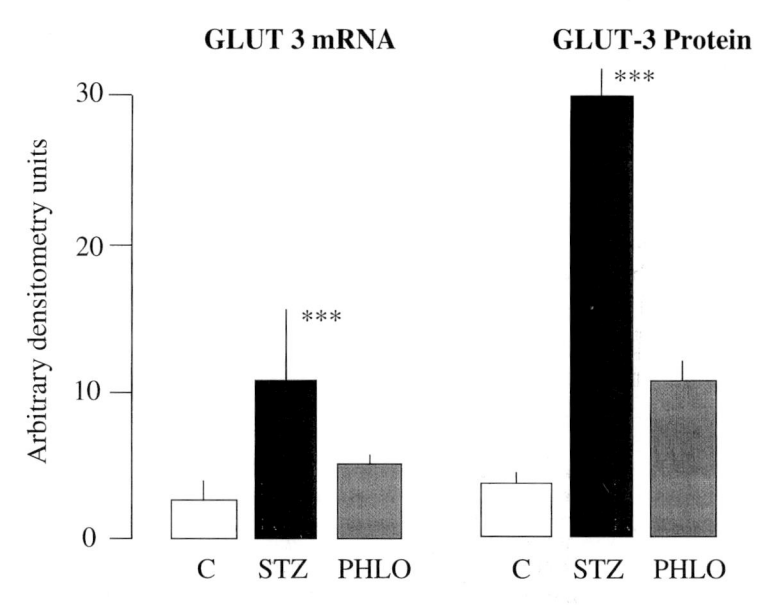

FIG. 3. Regulation of placental GLUT-3 messenger RNA and protein levels in diabetic rats. Diabetes was induced by administration of streptozotocin (65 mg/kg body weight) to pregnant rats on day 1 of gestation. Diabetic rats were infused with phlorizin from day 15 to day 20 of gestation. Placentae were obtained on day 20 of gestation. Northern blots were performed with 30 μg total RNA per lane and hybridized with a GLUT-3 complementary DNA probe. Western blots were performed with 100-μg crude placental membranes and electrophoresis was done on 10% sodium dodecylsulfate polyacrylamide gels. After electrotransfer, the filters were hybridized with anti-GLUT-3 antibody and exposed to autoradiography. Results are means ± SE of scanning densitometry data. Tissue was sampled from pregnant control (*C*), pregnant diabetic (*STZ*), and pregnant diabetic rats treated with phlorizin (*PHLO*). Difference is statistically significant for ***$p < .002$ compared with controls. From Boileau et al. (17).

a level similar to that observed in diabetic rats (Fig. 4). Under those experimental conditions, there was no change in GLUT-1 messenger RNA levels (Fig. 4).

This study provided the first evidence that placental GLUT-3 messenger RNA and protein expression was stimulated *in vivo* under hyperglycemic conditions. Thus, GLUT-3 transporter isoform appears to be highly sensitive to ambient glucose levels, and it may play a pivotal role in the severe alterations of placental function observed in diabetic pregnancies.

REGULATION OF THE EXPRESSION OF ENZYMES CONTROLLING FATTY ACID OXIDATION AND KETOGENESIS IN NEONATAL RAT LIVER

The perinatal period is attended by marked changes of nutrition. *In utero*, the fetus is continuously supplied through the placenta with a diet rich in carbohydrate and amino acids and poor in fat (6). Immediately after birth, the maternal supply

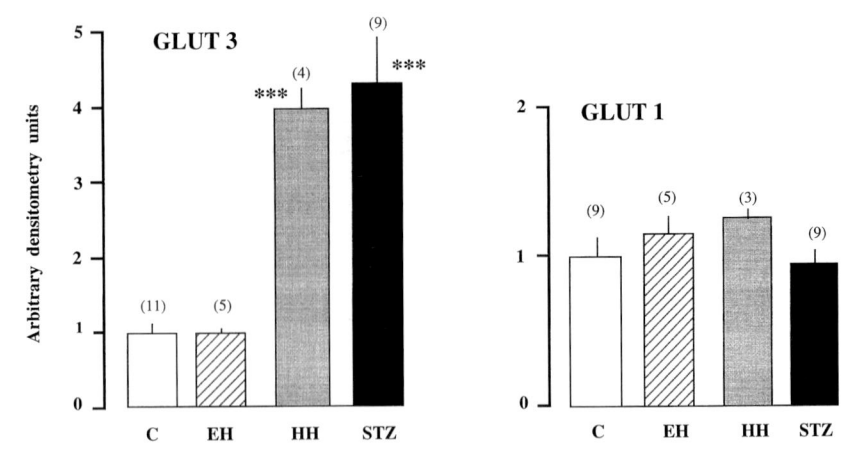

FIG. 4. Effect of euglycemic-hyperinsulinemic and hyperglycemic-hyperinsulinemic clamps on placental GLUT-1 and GLUT-3 messenger RNA levels in nondiabetic pregnant rats. Euglycemic-hyperinsulinemic and hyperglycemic-hyperinsulinemic clamp studies were performed during 12 hours in 20-day nondiabetic pregnant rats. Shown are scanning densitometry data obtained from two individual Northern blots. Results are expressed as means ± SE. (*n*) represents the number of placentae sampled from each rat. *C*, control (89 ± 4 mg/dl, 30 ± 3 μU/ml); *EH*, euglycemic-hyperinsulinemic clamps (96 ± 4 mg/dl, 4820 ± 204 μU/ml); *HH*, hyperglycemic-hyperinsulinemic clamps (613 ± 45 mg/dl, 450 ± 30 μU/ml); *STZ*, streptozotocin-induced diabetic rats (440 ± 11 mg/dl, 5 ± 1 μU/ml). Differences are statistically significant for $^{***}p<.002$ compared with controls. From Boileau et al. (17).

of substrates ceases abruptly, and the newborn has to withstand a brief period of starvation before being fed at intervals with milk that constitutes a high-fat (70% of energy) and low-carbohydrate (10% of energy) diet. To meet the energy needs of the newborn, the capacity for long-chain fatty acid (LCFA) oxidation increases rapidly in many tissues (liver, heart, skeletal muscle, lung, kidney cortex, small intestine, brown adipose tissue) (6). In the liver, the increased oxidation of LCFA results in an enhanced rate of ketone body production.

The postnatal development of hepatic LCFA oxidation and ketogenesis are closely related to the increase in the activities of the carnitine palmitoyltransferase (CPT) system and of the mitochondrial 3-hydroxy-3-methylglutaryl-CoA (HMG-CoA) synthase. The CPT system allows the transfer of LCFA into mitochondria and is composed of three distinct entities: CPT-1, localized in the outer mitochondrial membrane, and carnitine-acylcarnitine translocase and CPT-2, localized in the inner mitochondrial membrane (Fig. 5). In this system, CPT-1 represents the main site of control for the entry of LCFA into the mitochondria (19), and mitochondrial HMG-CoA synthase is the rate-limiting enzyme of the ketogenesis pathway (conversion of acetyl-CoA into ketone bodies) (20–22). However, if one considers ketogenesis as the metabolic pathway converting LCFA into ketone bodies, then the CPT system is the rate-limiting step, as it controls the supply of acyl-CoA for β oxidation and acetyl-CoA for ketogenesis (19).

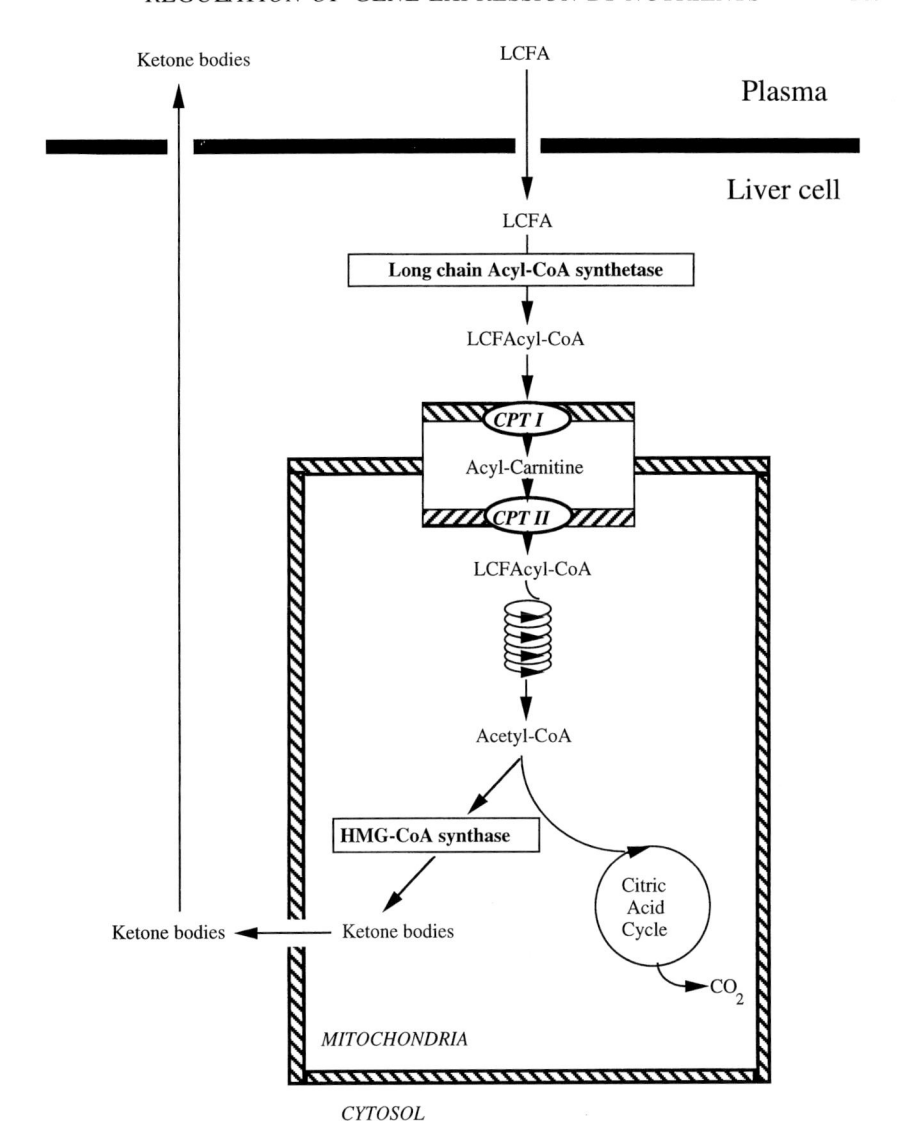

FIG. 5. Schematic representation of hepatic fatty acid oxidation and ketogenesis. *LCFA*, long-chain fatty acids; *CPT-1, CPT-2*, carnitine palmitoyltransferase-1 and -2; *HMG-CoA synthase*, hydroxymethylglutaryl-CoA synthase.

Liver CPT-1 and Mitochondrial HMG-CoA Synthase Gene Expression During the Perinatal Period

The complementary DNAs of CPT-1 (23), CPT-2 (24), and mitochondrial HMG-CoA synthase (25) have been recently cloned, and the antibodies directed against

CPT-1, CPT-2 (23,26), and mitochondrial HMG-CoA synthase (20) are available. This allowed the study of the molecular mechanisms controlling the changes in CPT-1, CPT-2, and mitochondrial HMG-CoA synthase activities during the postnatal period.

Changes in Hepatic CPT-1 and CPT-2 Gene Expression

The activity of CPT-1 is very low in the fetal rat liver and increases markedly during the first 24 hours of extrauterine life (27–29). In contrast, the activity of CPT-2 is already high in the fetal rat liver and does not change after birth (27,29). This strengthens the idea that CPT-1 is the rate-limiting step of the CPT system and of liver LCFA oxidation. The changes in maximal activities of CPT-1 and CPT-2 parallel those observed for immunoreactive CPT-1 and CPT-2 protein concentrations (29). The postnatal increase in the amount of CPT-1 protein results from a stimulation of CPT-1 gene transcription, as shown by run-on studies on isolated liver nuclei (30). This leads to a sevenfold increase in CPT-1 messenger RNA concentration in liver during the first 24 hours after birth (29,31) (Fig. 6). Thus, the changes in the activity of CPT-1 after birth result from a stimulation of CPT-1 gene transcription.

The liver CPT-2 messenger RNA and protein concentrations remain remarkably constant during development and are not influenced by the nutritional and hormonal changes (29,31) (Fig. 6). This is in agreement with previous studies concerning changes in CPT-2 protein levels (26) and CPT-2 activity (27) during the perinatal period.

Changes in Hepatic Mitochondrial HMG-CoA Synthase Gene Expression

Once inside the mitochondria, LCFA are rapidly oxidized into the β oxidation pathway, but the metabolic fate of the acetyl-CoA produced (Krebs cycle *vs.* ketone body production) partly depends on the activity of mitochondrial HMG-CoA synthase, the rate-limiting enzyme in the HMG-CoA pathway. As reported above, the activity of mitochondrial HMG-CoA synthase increases during the immediate postnatal period (20,32–37). We have thus examined the mechanisms responsible for regulation of the synthesis of this protein during development of the rat.

In the fetal rat liver, the messenger RNA coding for mitochondrial HMG-CoA synthase is not detectable before the 18th day of pregnancy. The concentrations increase slightly until the 21st day of pregnancy (38). This increase could result from a progressive demethylation of the mitochondrial HMG-CoA synthase gene, as demethylation has been reported to be one of the factors responsible for the activation of the transcription of this gene (39). During the first 24 hours after birth, the concentration of mitochondrial HMG-CoA synthase messenger RNA increases markedly (38,40) (Fig. 6).

Relative CPT I and CPT II mRNA levels

Relative HMG-CoA synthase mRNA levels

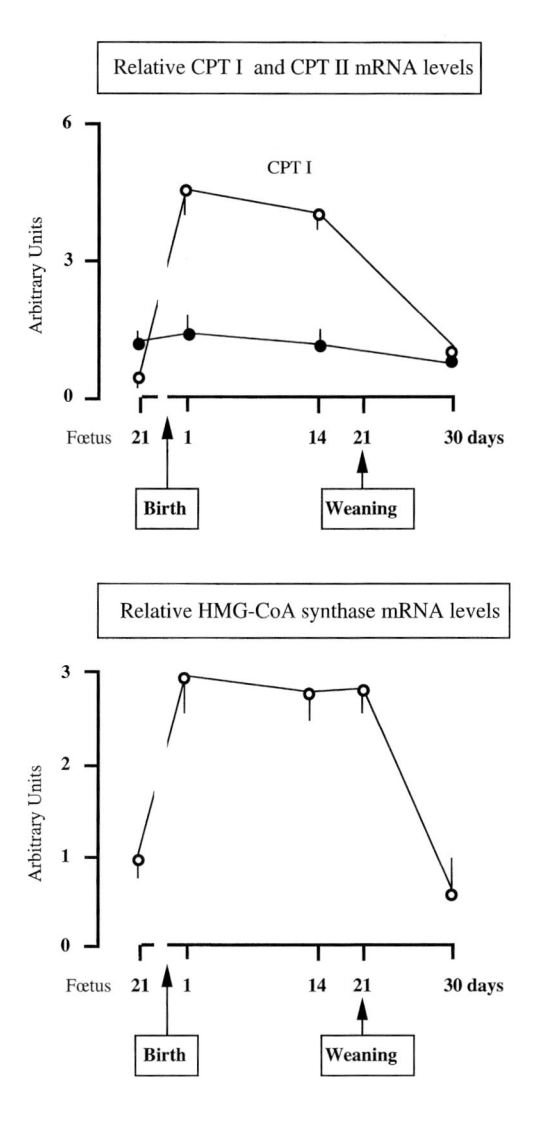

FIG. 6. Developmental changes in hepatic CPT-1, CPT-2, and HMG-CoA synthase messenger RNA concentrations. The levels of hepatic CPT-1, CPT-2, and HMG-CoA synthase were determined from densitometric analysis of six different Northern blots. Results are expressed as arbitrary units, the reference value (1) being the concentration of messenger RNA in the liver of 30-day-old rats. Results are expressed as means ± SEM of six different experiments. From Chatelain et al. (30) and Thumelin et al. (38).

Control of Hepatic Fatty Acid Oxidation and Ketogenesis by Hormones and Nutrients

The modifications of fatty acid metabolism in the postnatal period are attended by changes in plasma nonesterified fatty acid, carnitine, and pancreatic hormones (6). Immediately after birth, plasma insulin concentrations fall, whereas plasma nonesterified fatty acid (NEFA), carnitine, and glucagon concentrations dramatically increase (6). The effects of glucagon and insulin in the induction of hepatic fatty acid oxidation were demonstrated using cultured fetal hepatocytes (41,42). However, the possible role of nonesterified fatty acids and carnitine in the regulation of hepatic fatty acid oxidation was unknown. The individual role of hormones and nutrients in the regulation of CPT-1, CPT-2, and mitochondrial HMG-CoA synthase genes was studied using cultured hepatocytes from 18- to 20-day-old fetal rats (30). The hepatocytes were cultured for 48 hours in serum-free media containing the substances to be tested (30).

Regulation of CPT-1 Gene Expression

Addition of dibutyryl cyclic AMP increased the accumulation of CPT-1 messenger RNA in cultured hepatocytes from 20-day-old fetal rats in a dose-dependent manner, and insulin antagonized the effects of dibutyryl cyclic AMP (30). The effects of dibutyryl cyclic AMP resulted from a fourfold stimulation of CPT-1 gene transcription (30). The half-life of CPT-1 messenger RNA was unaffected by dibutyryl cyclic AMP (30). Insulin counteracted the accumulation of CPT-1 messenger RNA in response to dibutyryl cyclic AMP in a dose-dependent manner, suggesting that the decrease in plasma insulin levels potentiates the effects of increased plasma glucagon and liver cyclic AMP concentrations.

Addition of carnitine in cultured hepatocytes from fetal rats did not increase the concentration of CPT-1 messenger RNA (data not shown).

Addition of fatty acids, bound to albumin, in cultured hepatocytes from fetal rats had different effects on the concentration of CPT-1 messenger RNA (30) (Fig. 7). Medium-chain fatty acids (octanoate, decanoate) did not increase the concentration of CPT-1 messenger RNA (30). In contrast, LCFAs induced a twofold to fourfold increase in the concentration of CPT-1 messenger RNA (30). The effects of fatty

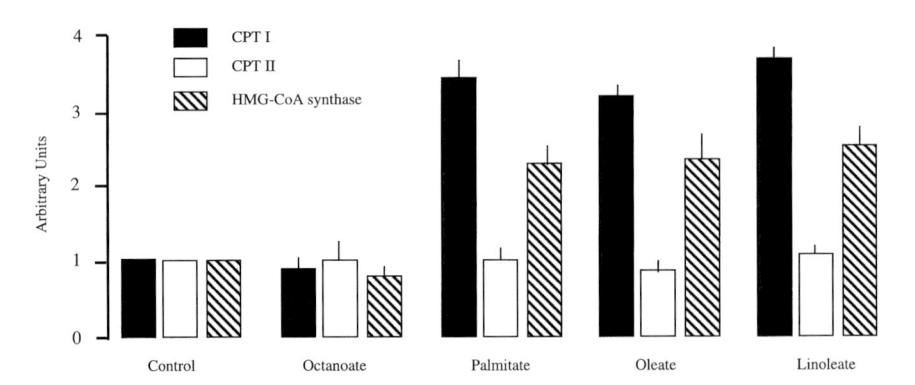

FIG. 7. Effects of various fatty acids on CPT-1, CPT-2, and HMG-CoA synthase messenger RNA gene expression in cultured fetal rat hepatocytes. Hepatocytes from 20-day-old fetuses were cultured for 48 hours in the absence (control) or in the presence of various fatty acids at a concentration of 0.5 mM bound to fat-free albumin (0.2% final concentration). Results are expressed as relative messenger RNA level, the reference value (1) being the level of CPT-1, CPT-2, or HMG-CoA synthase messenger RNAs in control conditions. Results are means ± SEM of six different cultures. From Chatelain *et al.* (30) and *unpublished data*.

acids on CPT-1 messenger RNA were observed with both saturated (palmitate), monounsaturated (oleate), and polyunsaturated (linoleate, eicosapentenoate, docosahexaenoate) LCFAs (30). The effects of linoleate resulted from a twofold stimulation of CPT-1 gene transcription (30). The half-life of CPT-1 messenger RNA was increased by 50% by linoleate (30). This strongly supports the view that the postnatal induction of CPT-1 gene expression is under the control of LCFAs, both at transcriptional and posttranscriptional levels. The increase in liver CPT-1 messenger RNA was faster in suckling than in fasting neonates (31), suggesting that some factors contained in milk activate CPT-1 gene transcription. As plasma NEFA levels did not increase in fasting neonates, but markedly increased in suckling neonates as a result of the hydrolysis of milk triglycerides (35), NEFA could potentiate the effects of increased liver cyclic AMP levels on CPT-1 messenger RNA by stabilizing messenger RNA.

It then became important to know whether the effects of cyclic AMP and LCFAs on CPT-1 gene transcription were not mediated by the same intracellular mechanisms. Indeed, dibutyryl cyclic AMP could have stimulated triglyceride breakdown and increased intracellular fatty acids, and fatty acids could have increased intracellular cyclic AMP levels. Several lines of evidence suggested that the effects of cyclic AMP and LCFAs on CPT-1 gene transcription were not mediated by the same intracellular mechanisms (30). First, LCFAs did not increase phosphoenolpyruvate carboxykinase (PEPCK) messenger RNA in cultured fetal rat hepatocytes. This should have occurred if LCFAs had increased cyclic AMP levels, as this gene is exquisitely sensitive to cyclic AMP in cultured fetal rat hepatocytes (43). Second, inhibitors of lysosomal acid lipase (glycodiazine, chloroquine) suppressed lipolysis and ketogenesis in response to dibutyryl cyclic AMP but did not impair the effects of dibutyryl cyclic AMP on CPT-1 messenger RNA accumulation. Third, half-maximal concentrations of dibutyryl cyclic AMP and linoleate produced an additive effect on CPT-1 messenger RNA accumulation.

Two lines of evidence suggested that LCFAs must be transformed to their respective CoA esters to be active in the induction of CPT-1 messenger RNA (30). First, the addition of 2-bromopalmitate—an analogue of palmitate that is transported into the liver cells, transformed to 2-bromopalmitoyl-CoA, but not further metabolized—was highly active on CPT-1 messenger RNA accumulation in cultured fetal rat hepatocytes. Second, the inhibition of LCFA oxidation by tetradecylglycidic acid, which at the concentration used did not itself influence CPT-1 messenger RNA, enhanced the accumulation of CPT-1 messenger RNA in response to linoleate. Under these conditions, linoleyl-CoA markedly accumulated in the cells, because fetal hepatocytes have a low capacity for esterification (44).

Regulation of CPT-2 Gene Expression

Following the addition of dibutyryl cyclic AMP, medium- or long-chain fatty acids did not increase CPT-2 messenger RNA in cultured hepatocytes from fetal rats (30) (Fig. 7). This strongly supports the view that the effects of cyclic AMP and LCFAs on CPT-1 gene transcription were quite specific.

Regulation of Mitochondrial HMG-CoA Synthase Gene Expression

When hepatocytes from rat fetuses were cultured in the presence of glucagon, mitochondrial HMG-CoA synthase messenger RNA accumulates in a dose-dependent manner, with a half-maximal concentration of glucagon (100 nM) close to the one found in the plasma of newborn rats (38). These results are consistent with the finding that a cyclic AMP-responsive element is present in the promoter region of mitochondrial HMG-CoA synthase gene (45).

The level of mitochondrial HMG-CoA synthase gene expression is also regulated by the nutrients contained in the diet. Addition of fatty acids, bound to albumin, in cultured hepatocytes of fetal rats had different effects on the concentration of mitochondrial HMG-CoA synthase messenger RNA (F. Chatelain *et al., unpublished data*) (Fig. 7). Medium-chain fatty acids (octanoate, decanoate) did not increase the concentration of HMG-CoA synthase messenger RNA (F. Chatelain *et al., unpublished data*). In contrast, LCFAs induced a twofold to fourfold increase in the concentration of HMG-CoA synthase messenger RNA (F. Chatelain *et al., unpublished data*). The effects of fatty acids on HMG-CoA synthase messenger RNA were observed with both saturated (palmitate), monounsaturated (oleate), and polyunsaturated (linoleate, eicosapentenoate, docosahexaenoate) LCFAs (F. Chatelain *et al., unpublished data*). The absorption of large amounts of fats immediately after birth could promote the transcription of hepatic mitochondrial HMG-CoA synthase, as fatty acids have been shown to stimulate mitochondrial HMG-CoA synthase gene expression in hepatoma cells (46).

CONCLUSION AND PERSPECTIVES

The regulation of specific gene expression in response to changes in nutrition has become a major focus of modern nutritional research. Nutrients such as glucose and fatty acids have been shown to participate, in conjunction with hormones, in the regulation of gene expression of several transporters and enzymes involved in the control of metabolic pathways (2–4). Here, we report that glucose and LCFA constitute important regulatory factors for the transcriptional control of glucose transporter GLUT-3 in the placenta and CPT-1 and HMG-CoA synthase in neonatal liver.

The molecular mechanisms by which glucose, glucagon (cyclic AMP), insulin, and LCFA regulate gene expression remain to be established. Further investigations will be necessary to characterize the intracellular metabolites, transcription factors, and DNA sequence responsible for the transcriptional activation of the GLUT-3 gene by glucose and the CPT-1 and HMG-CoA synthase genes by LCFAs. It has been suggested that glucose-6-phosphate (47) or xylulose-5-phosphate (48) could be the metabolites involved in the regulation of glycolytic (pyruvate kinase) and lipogenic enzyme (fatty acid synthase) gene transcription. Upstream stimulatory factor (USF) has also been suggested as the transcription factor involved in the effects of glucose on glycolytic and lipogenic enzyme gene transcription. Concerning LCFAs, it has been suggested that they act through nuclear receptors of the steroid-thyroid superfamily, the peroxisome proliferator-activated receptors (PPAR) (49). The regulation of fatty acid oxidative enzyme and mitochondrial HMG-CoA synthase gene expression by fatty acids has been suggested to be mediated by PPARs (46,50). What is not clear is whether acyl-CoA is capable of binding to a homologue of PPAR (51) or whether it acts, as in bacteria, through distinct entities, such as acyl-CoA binding proteins (52,53).

REFERENCES

1. Goodridge AG. Dietary regulation of gene expression: enzymes involved in carbohydrate and lipid metabolism. *Annu Rev Nutr* 1987;7:157–185.
2. Clarke S, Abraham S. Gene expression. Nutrient control of pretranscriptional and posttranscriptional events. *FASEB J* 1992;6:3146–3152.
3. Girard J, Perdereau D, Foufelle F, Prip-Buus C, Ferré P. Regulation of lipogenic enzyme gene expression by nutrients and hormones. *FASEB J* 1994;8:36–42.
4. Vaulont S, Kahn A. Transcriptional control of metabolic regulation genes by carbohydrates. *FASEB J* 1994;8:28–35.
5. Battaglia FC, Meschia G. Principal substrates of fetal metabolism. *Physiol Rev* 1978;58:499–527.
6. Girard J, Ferré P, Pégorier JP, Duée PH. Adaptations of glucose and fatty acid metabolism during the perinatal period and the suckling-weaning transition. *Physiol Rev* 1992;72:507–562.
7. Battaglia FC. Fetal metabolism. In: Van Assche FA, Robertson WB, eds. *Fetal Growth Retardation.* Edinburgh: Churchill Livingstone; 1981:3–12.
8. Hauguel S, Challier JC, Cedard L. Metabolism of the human placenta perfused *in vitro*: glucose transfer and utilization, oxygen consumption, lactate and ammonia production. *Pediatr Res* 1983; 17:729–732.
9. Hay WWJ, Sparks JW, Wilkening RB, Battaglia FC, Meschia G. Partition of maternal glucose production between conceptus and maternal tissues in sheep. *Am J Physiol* 1983;245:E347–E350.
10. Leturque A, Revelli JP, Hauguel S, Kandé J, Girard J. Hyperglycemia and hyperinsulinemia increase glucose utilization in fetal rat tissues. *Am J Physiol* 1987;253:E616–E620.
11. Hauguel S, Leturque A, Gilbert M, Girard J. Effects of pregnancy and fasting on muscle glucose utilization in the rabbit. *Am J Obstet Gynecol* 1988;158:1215–1218.
12. Bell GI, Kayano T, Buse JB, Burant CF, Takeda J, Lin D, Fukumoto H, Seino S. Molecular biology of mammalian glucose transporters. *Diabetes Care* 1990;13:198–208.
13. Grossbard L, Schimke RT. Multiple hexokinases of rat tissues. Purification and comparison of solubles forms. *J Biol Chem* 1966;241:3546–3550.
14. Wilson JE. Hexokinases. *Rev Physiol Biochem Pharmacol* 1995;126:65–198.
15. Zhou J, Bondy C. Placental glucose transporter gene expression and metabolism in the rat. *J Clin Invest* 1993;91:845–852.
16. Devaskar SU, Devaskar UP, Schroeder RE, Demello D, Fiedorek FT, Mueckler M. Expression of genes involved in placental glucose uptake and transport in the nonobese diabetic mouse pregnancy. *Am J Obstet Gynecol* 1994;171:1316–1323.
17. Boileau P, Mrejen C, Girard J, Hauguel-De Mouzon S. Overexpression of GLUT 3 placental glucose transporter in diabetic rats. *J Clin Invest* 1995;96:309–317.
18. Hahn T, Hartmann M, Blaschitz A, Skofitsch G, Graf R, Dohr G, Desoye G. Localisation of the high affinity facilitative glucose transporter protein GLUT 1 in the placenta of human, marmoset monkey (*Callithrix jacchus*) and rat at different developmental stages. *Cell Tissue Res* 1995;280: 49–57.

19. McGarry JD, Woeltje KF, Kuwajima M, Foster DW. Regulation of ketogenesis and the renaissance of carnitine palmitoyltransferase. *Diabetes Metab Rev* 1989;5:271–284.
20. Quant PA, Robin D, Robin P, Ferré P, Brand MD, Girard J. Control of hepatic mitochondrial 3-hydroxy-3-methylglutaryl-CoA synthase during the foetal/neonatal transition, suckling and weaning in the rat. *Eur J Biochem* 1991;195:449–454.
21. Quant PA. The role of mitochondrial HMG-CoA synthase in regulation of ketogenesis. *Essays Biochem* 1994;28:13–25.
22. Valera A, Pelegrin M, Asins G, Fillat C, Sabater J, Pujol A, Hegardt FG, Bosch F. Overexpression of mitochondrial 3-hydroxy-3-methylglutaryl-CoA synthase in transgenic mice causes hepatic hyperketogenesis. *J Biol Chem* 1994;269:6267–6270.
23. Esser V, Britton CH, Weis BC, Foster DW, McGarry JD. Cloning, sequencing, and expression of a cDNA encoding rat liver carnitine palmitoyltransferase-I. Direct evidence that a single polypeptide is involved in inhibitor interaction and catalytic function. *J Biol Chem* 1993;268:5817–5822.
24. Woeltje KF, Esser V, Weis BC, Sen A, Cox WF, McPhaul MJ, Slauther CA, Foster DW, McGarry JD. Cloning, sequencing, and expression of a cDNA encoding rat liver mitochondrial carnitine palmitoyltransferase II. *J Biol Chem* 1990;265:10720–10725.
25. Ayte J, Gil-Gomez G, Haro D, Marrero PF, Hegardt F. Rat mitochondrial and cytosolic 3-hydroxy-3-methylglutaryl-CoA synthases are encoded by two different genes. *Proc Natl Acad Sci U S A* 1990;87:3874–3878.
26. Kolodziej MP, Crilly PJ, Corstorphine CG, Zammit VA. Development and characterization of a polyclonal antibody against rat liver mitochondrial overt carnitine palmitoyltransferase (CPT I). *Biochem J* 1992;282:415–421.
27. Saggerson ED, Carpenter CA. Regulation of hepatic carnitine palmitoyltransferase activity during the foetal-neonatal transition. *FEBS Lett* 1982:150:177–180.
28. Chalk PA, Higham FC, Caswell AM, Bailey E. Hepatic mitochondrial fatty acid oxidation during the perinatal period in the rat. *Int J Biochem* 1983;15:531–538.
29. Thumelin S, Esser V, Charvy D, Kolodziej M, Zammit V, McGarry JD, Girard J, Pégorier JP. Expression of liver carnitine palmitoyltransferase I and II genes during development in the rat. *Biochem J* 1994;300:583–587.
30. Chatelain F, Kohl C, Esser V, McGarry JD, Girard J, Pégorier JP. Cyclic AMP and fatty acids increase carnitine palmitoyltransferase I gene transcription in cultured fetal rat hepatocytes. *Eur J Biochem* 1996;235:789–798.
31. Asins G, Serra D, Arias G, Hegardt F. Developmental changes in carnitine palmitoyltransferase I and II gene expression in intestine and liver of suckling rats. *Biochem J* 1995;306:379–384.
32. Lockwood EA, Bailey E. The course of ketosis and the activity of key enzymes of ketogenesis and ketone body utilization during development of the postnatal rat. *Biochem J* 1971;124:249–254.
33. Hipolito-Reis C, Bailey E, Bartley W. Factors involved in the control of the activity of enzymes of hepatic ketogenesis during development of the rat. *Int J Biochem* 1974;5:31–39.
34. Shah J, Bailey E. Changes in the activities of the enzymes of hepatic ketogenesis in the rat between late fetal and weaning. *Enzyme* 1977;22:35–40.
35. Ferré P, Pégorier JP, Williamson DH, Girard J. The development of ketogenesis at birth in the rat. *Biochem J* 1978;176:759–765.
36. Caswell AM, Bailey E. Studies of rat hepatic mitochondrial hydroxymethylglutaryl-CoA synthase during the perinatal period. *Biol Neonate* 1983;43:263–268.
37. Decaux JF, Robin D, Robin P, Ferré P, Girard J. Intramitochondrial factors controlling hepatic fatty acid oxidation at weaning in the rat. *FEBS Lett* 1988:232:156–158.
38. Thumelin S, Forestier M, Girard J, Pégorier JP. Developmental changes in mitochondrial 3-hydroxy-3-methylglutaryl-CoA synthase gene expression in rat liver, intestine and kidney. *Biochem J* 1993;292:493–496.
39. Ayte J, Gil-Gomez G, Hegardt FG. Methylation of the regulatory region of the mitochondrial 3-hydroxy-3-methylglutaryl-CoA synthase gene leads to its transcriptional inactivation. *Biochem J* 1993;295:807–812.
40. Serra D, Casals N, Asins G, Royo T, Ciudad CJ, Hegardt FG. Regulation of mitochondrial 3-hydroxy-3-methylglutaryl-CoA synthase protein by starvation, fat feeding, and diabetes. *Arch Biochem Biophys* 1993;307:40–45.
41. Pégorier JP, Garcia-Garcia MV, Prip-Buus C, Duée PH, Kohl C, Girard J. Induction of ketogenesis and fatty acid oxidation by glucagon and cyclic AMP in cultured hepatocytes from rabbit fetuses.

Evidence for a decreased sensitivity of carnitine palmitoyltransferase I to malonyl-CoA inhibition after glucagon or cyclic AMP treatment. *Biochem J* 1989;264:93–100.
42. Prip-Buus C, Pégorier JP, Duée PH, Kohl C, Girard J. Evidence that the sensitivity of carnitine palmitoyltransferase I to inhibition by malonyl-CoA is an important site of regulation of hepatic fatty acid oxidation in the fetal and newborn rabbit. Perinatal development and effects of pancreatic hormones in cultured rabbit hepatocytes. *Biochem J* 1990;269:409–415.
43. Pégorier JP, Salvado J, Forestier M, Girard J. Dominant role of glucagon in the initial induction of phosphoenolpyruvate carboxykinase (PEPCK) mRNA in cultured hepatocytes from fetal rats. *Eur J Biochem* 1992:210:1053–1059.
44. Ferré P, Satabin P, Decaux JF, Escriva F, Girard J. Development and regulation of ketogenesis in hepatocytes isolated from newborn rats. *Biochem J* 1983;214:937–942.
45. Gil-Gomez G, Ayte J, Hegardt FG. The rat mitochondrial 3-hydroxy-3-methylglutaryl-CoA synthase gene contains elements that mediate its multihormonal regulation and tissue specificity. *Eur J Biochem* 1993;213:773–779.
46. Rodriguez JC, Gil-Gomez G, Hegardt FG, Haro D. Peroxisome proliferator-activated receptor mediates induction of the mitochondrial 3-hydroxy-3 methylglutaryl-CoA synthase gene by fatty acids. *J Biol Chem* 1994;269:18767–18772.
47. Foufelle F, Gouhot B, Pégorier J, Perdereau D, Girard J, Ferré P. Glucose stimulation of lipogenic enzyme gene expression in cultured white adipose tissue—a role for glucose 6-phosphate. *J Biol Chem* 1992;267:20543–20546.
48. Doiron B, Cuif MH, Chen R, Kahn A. Transcriptional glucose signaling through the glucose response element is mediated by the pentose phosphate pathway. *J Biol Chem* 1996;271:5321–5324.
49. Keller H, Wahli W. Peroxisome proliferator-activated receptors. A link between endocrinology and nutrition? *Trends Endocrinol Metab* 1993;4:291–296.
50. Gulick T, Cresci S, Caira T, Moore D, Kelly D. The peroxisome proliferator-activated receptor regulates mitochondrial fatty acid oxidative enzyme gene expression. *Proc Natl Acad Sci U S A* 1994;91:11012–11016.
51. Amri EZ, Bonino F, Ailhaud G, Abumrad NA, Grimaldi PA. Cloning a protein that mediates transcriptional effects of fatty acids in preadipocytes. Homology to peroxysome proliferator-activated receptors. *J Biol Chem* 1995;270:2367–2371.
52. Black P, DiRusso C. Molecular and biochemical analysis of fatty acid transport, metabolism and gene regulation in *Escherichia coli*. *Biochim Biophys Acta* 1994;1210:123–145.
53. Raman N, DiRusso C. Analysis of acyl-CoA binding to the transcription factor FadR and identification of amino acid residues in the carboxyl terminus required for ligand binding. *J Biol Chem* 1995;270: 1092–1097.

DISCUSSION

Dr. Rennie: I wonder if you could tell me how quickly the protein comes. The messenger RNA for the glucose transporters appears within 6 hours. How quickly after that do you think the protein comes, because that's a very rapid switch on, isn't it?

Dr. Girard: The messenger RNA appears between 6 and 12 hours in the clamp experiments, and the protein follows within 12 hours. There is a delay of 6 hours between the messenger RNA and the appearance of the protein.

Dr. Rennie: Have you looked at other glucose transporters, like GLUT-5?

Dr. Girard: We have not found any GLUT-2, GLUT-4, or GLUT-5 in the placenta.

Dr. Sibley: It is probably worth pointing out at this point the species differences. There is no good evidence that GLUT-3 is expressed at protein level in the human placenta, although you obviously get effects in the rat. In the human placenta, GLUT-1 is the major glucose transporter.

Dr. Girard: One very important aspect is that in the placenta the localization of the GLUT transporter varies. One problem may be the antibody used. It must be very specific for GLUT-3, and some of the antibodies against GLUT-3 cross-react with actin in the human, so we have to be very careful in that respect. But in the rat it is clear that GLUT-3 is considerably increased.

Dr. Rennie: In our laboratory we have found GLUT-3 in human placenta.

Dr. Girard: I am not surprised, since the GLUT-3 messenger RNA is highly expressed in the human placenta. I am not aware of a lot of situations in which a messenger RNA is highly expressed and there is no protein produced, but we have not worked with the human placenta yet.

Dr. Battaglia: In your model, how long does the hyperglycemic infusion go on for?

Dr. Girard: Six or 12 hours.

Dr. Battaglia: With streptozotocin, you have an effect that goes on throughout gestation, in contrast to your hyperglycemia model, in which you probably don't end up by doubling the size of the placenta, as you do with streptozotocin. All the graphs you showed were in arbitrary units. It seems to me that in comparing hyperglycemia and the streptozotocin model, you are comparing apples with oranges. In one case the organ is double the size. How did you correct for that?

Dr. Girard: We don't correct for that. What we have done in normal pregnant rats is to show that hyperglycemia has a very important effect on GLUT-3 messenger RNA concentration. Our purpose was not to reproduce the effect of diabetes in pregnancy but to discover whether in a normal placenta, in a normal milieu, glucose was able to increase GLUT-3 transcription. We tried to demonstrate that glucose alone was capable of increasing the transcription of GLUT-3.

Dr. Battaglia: I guess it is the question of how you define up-regulation. I assume you mean that per cell you are getting more expression of the transporters, and I couldn't tell that from the data as they were presented.

Dr. Girard: The protein concentration per organ weight is exactly the same in diabetic and nondiabetic rats. So if we express the GLUT-3 per unit of protein concentration, which is similar in control and diabetic rats, there is always a threefold or fourfold increase in GLUT-3 messenger RNA.

Dr. Ogata: I know your work is consistent with observations in the nonobese diabetic mouse (1), and as I understand that mouse model, there are mild, moderate, and severe expressions of hyperglycemia basically. In the severe expression, GLUT-3 messenger RNA in the placenta is increased, and GLUT-1 is reduced. There are no protein data. We have measured GLUT-3 messenger RNA in rat placenta, but—and this may be our technique—we have not been able to find protein.

Dr. Girard: One problem with GLUT-3 is to have good antibodies to measure the protein concentration. This is a very important aspect and probably the reason why there is such discrepancy between one group and another.

Dr. Herrera: I would like to ask you whether GLUT-3 expression is also modified by giving a metabolic inhibitor of glucose utilization.

Dr. Girard: We have not done that *in vivo*. What we expect to do is to use a rat cell line for experiments on the regulation of glucose transporter. The next step will be to see to what extent glucose is capable of increasing GLUT-3 expression in syncytiotrophoblast cells *in vitro*, and if these cells are responsive to glucose, to try to identify the region of the promoter that is capable of responding to glucose concentration. That is the next step. We have not done it yet.

Dr. Soares: With regard to the effects of fatty acid on liver gene expression, do you think that this is probably acting through some type of nuclear receptor, an orphan receptor of some sort?

Dr. Girard: We think that it is not acting through a PPAR (peroxisome proliferator-activated protein), which is expected by most people to be the protein that allows fatty acids to activate transcription. This PPAR is very similar to the hormone-activated receptors, retinoic acid receptors, or thyroid hormone receptors. We have one experiment I have not discussed in which we have exposed our fetal hepatocytes to clofibrate. Clofibrate is a stimulator of PPAR. In this experiment we showed that clofibrate is a strong stimulator of CPT-2 gene expression, but fatty acids are not. So there is a dissociation between the effects of fatty acids and clofibrate. So we think that the fatty acids are probably not acting on the gene through PPAR but through a protein that could be an acyl-CoA binding protein. PPAR is a very good substrate for fatty acids but not for fatty acyl-CoA. So we have to identify a protein that will be a specific fatty acyl-CoA binding protein.

Dr. Battaglia: What was the evidence that it is not the fatty acid but the fatty acyl-CoA that is the inducer?

Dr. Girard: What we have done is to use an inhibitor of long-chain fatty acid oxidation, a drug that doesn't allow activated acyl-CoA to enter the mitochondria and be oxidized. This is known as *tetradecylglycidic acid*. With this agent we have a marked potentiation of the effect of fatty acids, which is much increased, whereas tetradecylglycidic acid by itself has no effect.

Dr. Battaglia: You mean that when you use this inhibitor, the intracellular fatty acid concentration does not increase, only the fatty acyl-CoA?

Dr. Girard: Yes, exactly.

Dr. Nicolaides: Can you please speculate on the possible differences between your rat diabetic model and human diabetes in relation to fetal growth?

Dr. Girard: What is clear in the rat is that when you induce severe diabetes, such as in our experiments, there is increased placental weight and decreased fetal weight. But if you induce diabetes with a much smaller degree of hyperglycemia, you get a fetus with a higher weight and a placenta that is also higher in weight. So the effects depend on the severity of the diabetes. A very important question we asked when we had seen our results was, What is the physiologic meaning of increased GLUT-3 expression? Is it to increase glucose utilization by the placenta, or to increase glucose transport to the fetus? We think that increased GLUT-3 expression in the diabetic pregnancy could be a means of protecting the fetus, because these transporters facilitate glucose transport in the direction of the glucose gradient. So this may be a means of avoiding having too severe fetal growth retardation.

Dr. Battaglia: You studied hyperinsulinemia, but in fact the streptozotocin animals get hypoinsulinemic, so that would be the advantage of doing some fasting or starvation studies. You increased the insulin, but you don't yet know the impact if you have a low insulin level.

Dr. Girard: I think the experiments with phlorizin answer this question, because when you compare streptozotocin diabetes and streptozotocin diabetes plus phlorizin, you have one case in which the mother is hyperglycemic and hypoinsulinemic, and another case in which she is normoglycemic and hypoinsulinemic. Phlorizin doesn't correct the low plasma insulin concentration but only the hyperglycemia, so our conclusion was that the overexpression was caused by an increased glucose concentration and not by the lack of insulin.

Dr. Battaglia: These are old inhibitors that are not terribly specific. That is the problem.

Dr. Godfrey: I was wondering if you have looked to see whether maternal hyperglycemia during pregnancy had any persistent effects on postnatal intermediary metabolism in the liver. The reason for asking is that Nick Hales in Cambridge has shown that a low-protein diet in the mother just during pregnancy has long-term effects on the ratio of PEPCK to glucokinase in the liver of the offspring, and hence may alter the balance of gluconeogenesis and glycogen metabolism (2).

Dr. Girard: We have not done this, but Van Assche and Ktorza have shown clearly that by inducing moderate diabetes in pregnant rats or by inducing hyperglycemia during the last week of pregnancy, you can induce a diabetic type of metabolism at a later stage in life (3–6).

Dr. Williams: Your data in relation to CPT-1 in fetal hepatocytes suggest that the lack of the enzyme *in utero* is caused by a lack of exposure to substrate. Do you have any data on hepatocytes removed earlier in pregnancy and whether or not they are able to respond to fatty acid supply? And would you expect that in the human there would be less of a transition in the induction of the enzyme at birth?

Dr. Girard: We have not done that experiment, but the situation in the human is very similar to that in the rat. The only exception is that the human placenta is much more permeable to fatty acids, so there is a transfer of free fatty acids to the fetus. But the capacity for fetal tissue to oxidize fatty acids is also very low. So the fatty acids transferred to the fetus are stored as fat and are not oxidized as a fuel in other tissues. I think that the neonatal transition is very similar. We have a change of nutrition from a high-carbohydrate to a high-fat diet after delivery, both in human and in rat. Fetal tissue in the human does not have the capacity to oxidize fatty acids to a large extent.

Dr. Battaglia: But it is an interesting point she is making. They may not have the capacity to oxidize fatty acids, but why not, if they are coming across the placenta? That is an interesting question.

Dr. Girard: I don't know whether it may be possible in the human to induce the capacity for fatty acid oxidation prematurely by loading the mother with fat. These experiments have not been done. It is not possible to do such experiments in the rat, because in the rat the fatty acids do not cross the placenta. But in the human, when free fatty acids are provided to the fetus, perhaps the gene is unable to respond before delivery. There are other situations in which a gene is completely silent because the chromatin structure doesn't allow the protein that binds fatty acyl-CoA to go to the promoter and to stimulate gene transcription. We don't know exactly what the structure of the CPT-1 promoter is during fetal life.

Dr. Marini: In your *in vitro* study, do you try to expose the culture to different oxygen concentrations?

Dr. Girard: No, we have not done that. But it is a very interesting question, because there are many genes that are sensitive to oxygen (7,8), and there is an oxygen-sensitive regulatory element on the DNA that is capable of responding (9,10). We are very interested in that question in relation to GLUT-3, because during fetal growth retardation there is not only a shortage of substrate but sometimes of oxygen, and GLUT-3 can be perhaps regulated by oxygen concentration.

Dr. Battaglia: From the point of view of nutrition, the idea that nutrients regulate gene expression is an old one and very well established in adult biochemistry. The postprandial rise in concentration of many nutrients, amino acids among them, induces the expression of the enzymes involved in their catabolism within the liver. And that is a very fast time curve. It has been intriguing for workers in that area to look at how you can get this quick turn-on and turn-off around the postprandial cycle. So certainly the concept is well established that nutrient concentrations can regulate gene expression. What they do in organs other than the liver isn't, I think, well studied, even in the adult.

Dr. Girard: We have done very similar experiments using adipose tissue. If adipose tissue from suckling rat, for example, which is not able to express the lipogenic enzyme, is put into culture and only glucose is added, glucose alone is capable of turning on the gene within 3 to 6 hours. When you look at textbooks of biochemistry, you see that lipogenic enzymes are supposed to be under the control of insulin. But it is not insulin that turns on the gene, it is glucose, and what insulin is doing is to increase glucose utilization by the cell. So there are many more genes that are carbohydrate-sensitive than that are only insulin-sensitive. Of the latter, the only one I know is glucokinase. Glucokinase in the liver is sensitive to insulin and is not affected by carbohydrate concentration.

Dr. Herrera: I would like to know whether the effect of hyperglycemia on GLUT-3 expression is specific for the placenta. Did you test this in other tissues?

Dr. Girard: We have not done this in other tissues. But GLUT-3 is a transporter in neurons and is specifically expressed in the brain and not in other tissues—not in skeletal muscle, liver, or adipose tissue, for example, although it is in the testis to some extent.

REFERENCES

1. Devaskar SU, Devaskar UP, Schroeder RE, *et al.* Expression of genes involved in placental glucose uptake and transport in the nonobese diabetic mouse pregnancy. *Am J Obstet Gynecol* 1994;171: 1316–1323.
2. Desai M, Crowther NJ, Ozanne SE, *et al.* Adult glucose and lipid metabolism may be programmed during fetal life. *Biochem Soc Trans* 1995;23:331–335.
3. Aerts L, Holemans K, Van Assche FA. Maternal diabetes during pregnancy—consequences for the offspring. *Diabetes Metab Rev* 1990;6:147–167.
4. Van Assche FA, Aerts L, Holemans K. Metabolic alterations in adulthood after intrauterine development in mothers with mild diabetes. *Diabetes* 1991;40(Suppl 2):106–108.
5. Bihoreau MT, Ktorza A, Kinebanyan MF, Picon L. Impaired glucose homeostatis in adult rats from hyperglycemic mothers. *Diabetes* 1986;35:979–984.
6. Gauguier D, Bihoreau MT, Ktorza A, Berthault MF, Picon L. Inheritance of diabetes mellitus as consequence of gestational hyperglycemia in rats. *Diabetes* 1990;39:734–739.
7. Semenza GL, Roth PH, Fang HM, Wang GL. Transcriptional regulation of genes encoding glycolytic enzymes by hypoxia-inducible factor 1. *J Biol Chem* 1994;269:23757–23763.
8. Eckardt KU, Pugh CW, Ratcliffe PJ, Kurtz A. Oxygen-dependent expression of the erythropoietin gene in rat hepatocytes *in vitro. Pflugers Arch* 1993;423:356–364.
9. Kietzmann T, Immenschuh S, Katz N, Jungermann K, Muller-Eberhard U. Modulation of hemopexin gene expression by physiological oxygen tensions in primary rat hepatocyte cultures. *Biochem Biophys Res Comm* 1995;213:397–403.
10. Kietzmann T, Schmidt H, Unthanfechner K, Probst I, Jungermann K. A ferro-heme protein senses oxygen levels, which modulate the glucagon-dependent activation of the phosphoenolpyruvate carboxykinase gene in rat hepatocyte cultures. *Biochem Biophys Res Comm* 1993;195:792–798.

Oxygenation *In Utero*: Placental Determinants and Fetal Requirements

Julie A. Owens, *Karen L. Kind, and #Jeffrey S. Robinson

*Department of Physiology, University of Adelaide, Adelaide; *CSIRO Division of Human Nutrition, Gouger St., Adelaide; #Department of Obstetrics and Gynaecology, University of Adelaide, Adelaide, South Australia, Australia*

Oxygen is an essential substrate for life before birth; it is required to produce energy, maintain tissues already laid down, and support accretion of new tissues. Fetal oxygen requirements are therefore ultimately determined by the rate of fetal growth and the factors that regulate this process. These needs clearly vary with body size, composition, and metabolic activity, and therefore with stage of development (1). In addition, fetal oxygen requirements can vary in the short term, at least during the second half of gestation, when substantial changes in fetal oxygen consumption occur with sleep state and physical movement; at the same time, changes in oxygen delivery can occur with uterine activity (2). Wide variations in oxygenation can exist *in utero*, and in the human fetus hypoxemia is associated with altered growth and with increased morbidity and mortality, both during the perinatal period and in later postnatal life (2).

In mammalian species, the placenta is the organ responsible for the transfer of oxygen from the mother to the fetus (3). The placenta is therefore a major--although not the sole—influence on fetal oxygenation (4). The aim of this brief review is to outline current understanding of placental influences on oxygen supply to the fetus, the nature of fetal oxygen requirements, and the consequences for fetal development of limiting oxygen delivery to the conceptus. In particular, the mechanisms by which oxygen supply influences fetal growth are discussed. The focus of this review is primarily on experimental studies in the sheep, with the relevance to human physiology and pathophysiology indicated when possible.

OXYGENATION *IN UTERO*: PLACENTAL DETERMINANTS

Following implantation, a sequence of events, in part common to all species and in part species-specific, results in the formation of the placenta, an organ in which fetal tissues are closely associated with maternal blood and tissues, to enable controlled transfer of essential substrates from maternal to fetal blood. In addition, as described elsewhere in this volume, the placenta has other important functions; it acts to modulate immune interactions between the mother and fetus and, through the production of steroid and polypeptide hormones, to regulate and coordinate maternal adaptation to pregnancy and fetal growth and development.

The external environment and maternal factors—such as respiratory and cardiovascular adaptations to pregnancy, hemoglobin concentration, and affinity for oxygen—influence the availability of oxygen in maternal blood, the rate of uterine blood flow, and hence the rate of oxygen delivery to the placenta for subsequent transfer to the fetus (3,4) (Table 1). The characteristics of the placenta that influence the rate at which oxygen is transferred from mother to fetus are physiologic and structural in nature (Table 1). The rates of placental perfusion or of maternal and fetal blood flows and their matching, together with the high rate of placental oxygen consumption, are key determinants of placental oxygen transfer (3,4). Within the fetal villi, the close proximity of the arterioles and venules of the umbilical circulation allows direct exchange of highly diffusible substances to occur. This diffusional "shunting" bypasses the area of maternal-fetal exchange and reduces the efficiency of the process. Placental diffusing capacity for oxygen is an important influence on the rate of oxygen transfer and is determined by structural characteristics of the placenta, as well as by physicochemical processes such as oxygen reaction rates with hemoglobin and diffusion rates through plasma and tissues (5). The structural characteristics of the placenta that determine placental diffusing capacity for oxygen

TABLE 1. *Factors influencing oxygenation* in utero

External environment of mother
   Atmospheric pO_2
Maternal factors
   Hemoglobin type (affinity for oxygen) and concentration
   Cardiovascular and respiratory adaptation to pregnancy
   Vascular (uterine) adaptation to pregnancy
Placental factors
Physiologic
   Rates of umbilical and uterine blood flow (perfusion)
   Matching and direction of maternal and fetal blood flows
   Rate of oxygen consumption
   Diffusional shunts
Structural
   Diffusion distance between maternal and fetal blood ("villous membrane")
   Surface area of exchange epithelia and fetal capillaries (and of maternal capillaries in some species)
   Volume of fetal villi and fetal capillaries (and of maternal capillaries in some species)
   Spatial arrangement of vasculature
   Anatomic shunts
Fetal factors
   Hemoglobin type and concentration
   Cardiac output and distribution

include the thickness of the placental barrier (the diffusion distance between maternal and fetal blood) and the surface areas of exchange epithelia and of fetal capillaries. In general terms, these physiologic and structural characteristics are common to the placentae of different mammalian species, although great diversity exists *between* species in the quantitative and qualitative nature of these placental characteristics and in their relative importance in influencing oxygen transfer by the placenta (3). The fetus also influences placental oxygen transfer through characteristics such as hemoglobin concentration and affinity for oxygen and cardiac output and its distribution.

The importance of these various factors for oxygen supply to the fetus under different circumstances in several species has been reviewed recently (3,4). In sheep, the effects on oxygen transfer by the placenta of experimental variations in maternal oxygenation, of maternal and fetal hemoglobin concentration and affinity for oxygen, and of rates of fetal and maternal placental blood flows have been extensively studied (3,4). In this species, placental oxygen transfer to the fetus is determined by both placental oxygen diffusing capacity and placental perfusion, and the former is small relative to fetal and placental oxygen demand (3). Placental oxygen transport in the human is less well understood, with conflicting views on the pattern of exchange and on the main determinants of transfer. The human placental diffusing capacity for oxygen has been estimated morphometrically from quantitative analysis of placental structure and mathematical modeling of the various physicochemical processes involved (5). Morphometric estimates of diffusing capacity are higher than the available physiologic estimates for the human placenta, probably because of a variety of factors that include "shunting," placental oxygen consumption, and the technical and biologic difficulties in obtaining accurate physiologic estimates. The morphometric modeling of diffusion across the human placenta suggests that the major contributor to placental diffusional resistance is the thickness of the villous membrane, followed by the surface areas of the fetal villi and capillaries (6). The relative importance of placental diffusing capacity for oxygen compared with the rates of placental blood flows—or indeed with other factors—in influencing oxygen transfer across the human placenta remains to be determined.

Ontogenic Changes in Placental Oxygen Transfer and Characteristics

Placental growth in terms of mass occurs largely in the first half of gestation (7). In the latter part of pregnancy, fetal size increases exponentially and rapidly exceeds that of the placenta. To meet the ever-increasing substrate demands of the fetus, the functional characteristics of the placenta undergo substantial changes throughout pregnancy, resulting in increases in placental transfer capacity—including that for oxygen—approximately in parallel with fetal growth (1,8). Thus, ontogenic increases in maternal and fetal placental blood flows, villous surface area, vascularity, and placental diffusing capacity for carbon monoxide, and reductions in the thickness of the placenta barrier or the diffusion distance between maternal and fetal blood, have been variously demonstrated in several species, including the human, sheep, cow, and guinea pig (1,8). These physiologic and structural changes increase the placental transfer capacity for oxygen. We currently understand little of the factors that regulate or modulate these processes, although, as discussed later, they can undergo modification in response to various perturbations, including hypoxemia *in utero*.

Relation Between Placental Growth and Oxygen Delivery to the Fetus

In late gestation and at term, much of the variation in fetal or birth weight can be accounted for by variations in placental weight in the human, sheep, and other mammalian species (2,7). Experimental restriction of placental growth has shown that this is a causative relation and that restricting growth reduces placental function in terms of substrate transfer capacity and so limits fetal growth (9–13). In sheep, surgical reduction of the number of implantation sites in the uterus before pregnancy results in a placenta with reduced numbers of placentomes and reduced total weight by late gestation. As the extent of restriction of placental growth increases, the rates of uterine and umbilical blood flow and of flow-determined antipyrine clearance decrease, as does the surface area of the exchange epithelia (10–14) (Fig. 1). Consequently, the rates of delivery of oxygen to the pregnant uterus and to the fetus

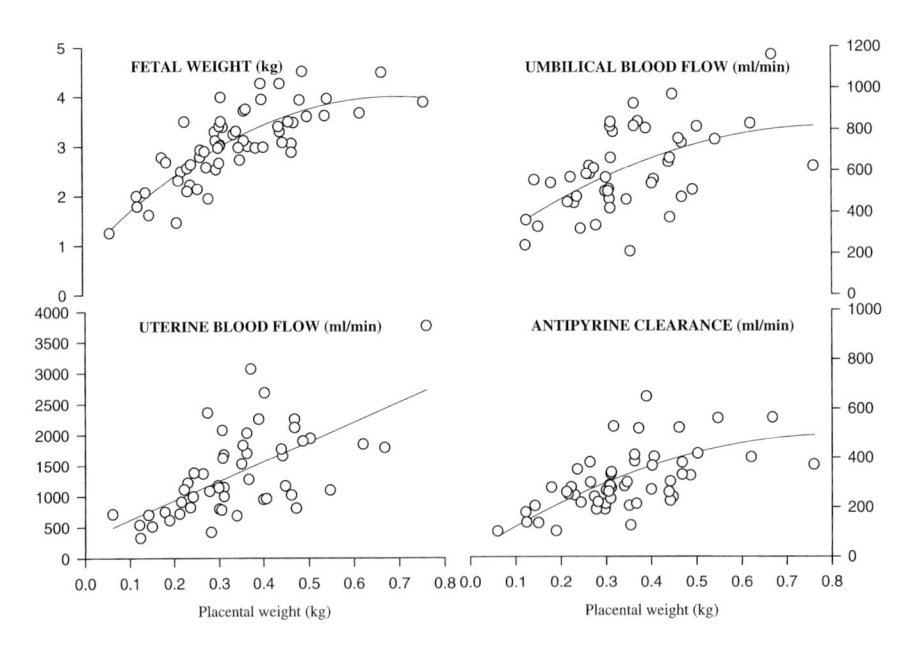

FIG. 1. Relation between placental growth and function in the sheep in late gestation. Some sheep were subjected to restriction of implantation by surgical removal of most placental implantation sites from the uterus before pregnancy (10–13).

RATES OF OXYGEN DELIVERY OR CONSUMPTION
(mmol/min)

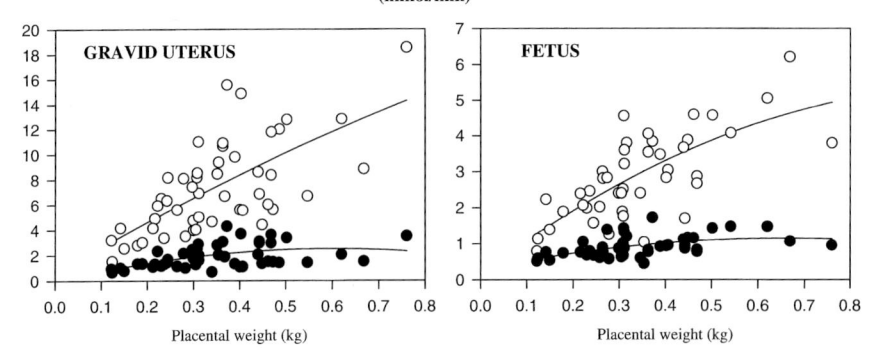

FIG. 2. Relation between placental growth and oxygen delivery to (*empty circles*) and consumption by (*filled circles*) the gravid uterus and fetus in sheep in late gestation. Placental growth was restricted in some sheep as described in Fig. 1.

decrease with decreasing placental weight (Fig. 2). This occurs despite concomitant compensatory changes in the placenta, which should help to maintain the oxygen supply to the fetus. Restriction of placental growth in sheep reduces the connective tissue content of fetal villi, which form part of the barrier to diffusion between maternal and fetal blood, and increases the surface density of the epithelial cell layers responsible for exchange, which should also help to maintain transfer (14). In addition, the rate of oxygen uptake by uteroplacental tissues decreases (Fig. 3), which would further help to maintain oxygen delivery to the fetus by reducing placental competition for this substrate.

In sheep, the consequences of restricted placental growth for the fetus are hypoxemia, hypoglycemia, and disproportionate growth restriction, with relative maintenance of brain growth, a disproportionate reduction in growth of the liver and gut, and a reduction in the ponderal index (9–13). The growth-restricted human fetus is characterized by similar metabolic and phenotypic stigmata (2,15). Studies in sheep and other animals show that restricting placental growth decreases the rate of delivery of glucose as well as of oxygen to the fetus (10–13). In late gestation, the rates of uptake of oxygen and glucose by the placentally restricted fetus are reduced in absolute terms, but they occur at normal rates relative to body weight (Figs. 2 and 3). This suggests that fetal growth is slowed to an extent commensurate with the rate at which the fetus can obtain these essential substrates. The mechanisms by which reduced substrate supply restricts fetal growth are increasingly defined and appear to involve both direct and indirect actions, mediated in part by endocrine pathways. What is less clear are the respective roles and importance of deficits in particular substrates, such as oxygen *vs.* glucose, in mediating placental control of fetal development.

Figure 3

CONTROL (mmol/min)

Placenta 0.41kg | Fetus 3.25kg

- OXYGEN: 2.31 → 1.31 → 1.00
- GLUCOSE: 0.26 → 0.17 → 0.09
- LACTATE: -0.03 / 0.22 → 0.01 → 0.03 / 0.21
- AMINO ACIDS

RESTRICTED

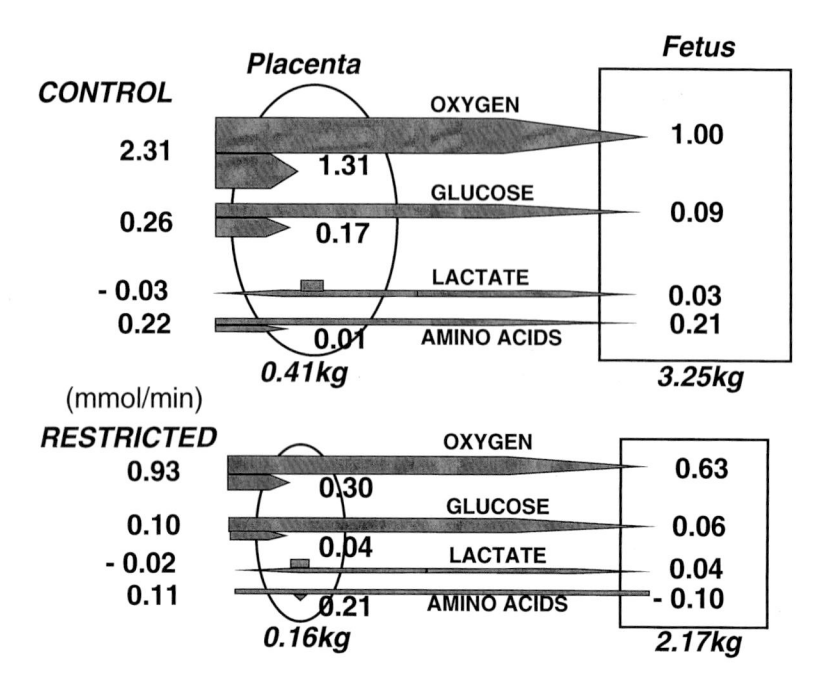

Placenta 0.16kg | Fetus 2.17kg

- OXYGEN: 0.93 → 0.30 → 0.63
- GLUCOSE: 0.10 → 0.04 → 0.06
- LACTATE: -0.02 / 0.11 → 0.21 → 0.04 / -0.10
- AMINO ACIDS

FIG. 3. Partitioning of substrates between placenta and fetus: effect of restricting placental and fetal growth. Rates of flux between mother, placenta, and fetus in control sheep and in sheep with restricted placental and fetal growth in late gestation. Placental growth was restricted as described in Fig. 1. Mean placental and fetal weights are shown in italics.

OXYGENATION *IN UTERO*: FETAL REQUIREMENTS

Acute variations in the rate of oxygen delivery to the fetal sheep generally do not alter fetal oxygen uptake until delivery falls below 0.6 mmol/min/kg, or 60% of the normal rate (4). This is a consequence of the substantial capacity of the fetus to maintain oxygen uptake by increasing extraction. Both the conceptus as a whole and the fetus are capable of increasing oxygen extraction, and maintaining this increased extraction chronically, in response to reduced oxygen availability (12). When placental growth is restricted in sheep, both the gravid uterus and the fetus increase oxygen extraction to help maintain oxygen uptake (Fig. 2). This occurs at the cost of reducing the margin of safety between oxygen delivery and consumption for the placenta and fetus (7,12). Acute variations in fetal oxygen requirements occur with fetal body movements or changes in sleep state, and increased demand may transiently exceed oxygen supply in the growth-restricted fetus, with a reduced margin between delivery and consumption (2). In growth-restricted fetal sheep, acute or chronic episodes of hypoxemia or asphyxia have been observed with onset of uterine contractions. To elucidate the influence of oxygen alone on fetal growth and development and the mechanisms involved, various methods have been adopted specifically to reduce oxygen delivery to the conceptus and fetus, and the consequences have then been determined.

Reduced Oxygen Supply to the Conceptus: Consequences for Growth

In human populations, high altitude is associated with a reduction in birth weight (16). This occurs despite compensatory changes in the human placenta, such as attenuation of the villous membrane and increased vascularization of the fetal villi, which should help to increase the placental diffusing capacity for oxygen (16). Experimental reduction of the supply of oxygen to the fetus has been shown to restrict growth in several species, including the sheep (17–26) (Table 2; Fig. 4). Various direct methods have been used to alter oxygen supply to the fetus, including reduction in the partial pressure of oxygen (PO_2) in maternally inspired air by means of nitrogen gas, increased altitude, or hypobaric conditions, and low-level maternal exposure to carbon monoxide (17–25). Other approaches have been to reduce the rates of uterine or umbilical blood flows by ligation, partial mechanical occlusion, or embolization of the fetal or maternal placental circulations with microspheres. These latter methods have mostly been used in sheep, and they do reduce the delivery of oxygen to the fetus. However, many of these procedures also reduce the rate of delivery or supply of other substrates to the fetus, including glucose, and are therefore not considered here. Although chronic reduction of uterine blood flow reduces the rates of delivery of both oxygen and glucose to the gravid uterus, it appears to reduce the delivery of oxygen to the fetus specifically, and not that of other major substrates,

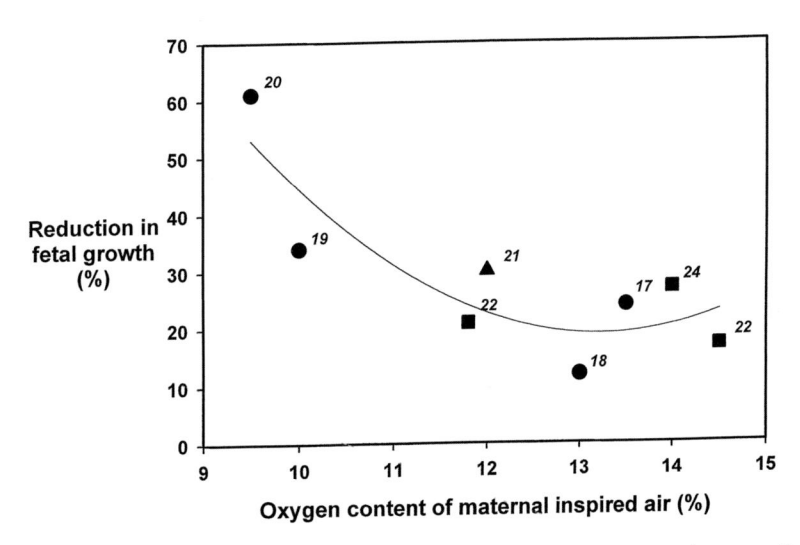

FIG. 4. Relation between fetal growth and prolonged alterations in maternal oxygenation in different species. Data from studies in rat (*circles*), guinea pig (*diamonds*), and sheep (*squares*) as summarized in Table 2. References are indicated by italicized numbers.

TABLE 2. Consequences for fetal growth of restricting oxygen supply

Species	Method	Timing (Fraction of gestation)	Fetal pO$_2$	Fetal O$_2$ content	CRL	Fetus	Placenta	Brain	Liver	Adrenals	Lymphoid tissues
Rat	Normobaric maternal hypoxia[a]										
	13.5% O$_2$[17]	0.67–1.0	na	na	na	−24	−10	na	−20	na	na
	13.0% O$_2$[18]	0.14–0.9	na	na	na	−12	+3	−4	−16	na	na
	13.0% O$_2$[19]	0.67–1.0	na	na	na	−34	na	na	na	na	na
	10.0% O$_2$[19]										
	9.5% O$_2$[20]	0.45–1.0	na	na	na	−61	−15	−23	−44	na	na
Guinea pig	12% O$_2$[21]	0.27–1.0	na	na	na	−30	−5	−17	na	na	na
Sheep	Hypobaric hypoxia[22,23]										
	4572 m	0.2–0.9	na	na	−8	−21	−23	+5	−8	+65	−54
	3048–4572 m	0.8–0.9	−38	−25 (13 days)[b]	−9	−17	−12	−4	−5	+40	−49
	Normobaric maternal hypoxia ∼3860 m[24]	0.83–0.92	−31	−30 (14 days)[b]	na	−27	na	na	na	na	na
	12.5% O$_2$[25]	0.73–0.92	−36	−34 (4 days)[b]	na	+5	na	na	na	na	na
	Reduced uterine blood flow[26]	0.86–0.91	−27	−50 (7 days)[b]	−1	−8	−20	0	−5	na	na

CRL, crown rump length; na, data not available.
[a] Superscripted numbers refer to references.
[b] Duration of reduction in O$_2$ content of fetal blood.

glucose or lactate (26). The consequences for fetal growth of specifically restricting the supply of oxygen to the fetus are summarized in Table 2, in which studies have been ranked in order of increasing degree and duration of treatment.

From these studies, it is evident that restricting oxygen supply to the fetus reduces the fetal growth rate. Moreover, increasing the degree of maternal hypoxia and to a lesser extent the duration of exposure to hypoxia, is broadly associated with a greater reduction in fetal weight in the rat and guinea pig (17–21) (Table 2; Fig. 4). In the sheep, fetal growth is not clearly related to the degree of fetal hypoxia achieved, in terms of fetal PO_2. Rather, fetal growth appears more to reflect the duration of the reduction in fetal oxygen content (22–26) (Table 2). In these studies, oxygen content in fetal blood usually returned to normal before the end of the period of imposed hypoxia, because of a compensatory increase in fetal hematocrit and hemoglobin concentration in the blood (Table 2). When hypobaric hypoxia is imposed on pregnant sheep during late gestation alone (121 to 140 days) or during a longer period of gestation (35 to 135 days), quantitatively similar reductions in fetal growth are observed (22). This suggests either adequate compensation by the fetus during the longer period of hypoxia or developmental changes in sensitivity of fetal growth to limitations of oxygen supply.

In general, restricted oxygen supply is associated with disproportionate fetal growth, with length reduced to a lesser extent than weight and a relative sparing of brain size (17–21) (Table 2). In contrast, growth of the liver is reduced to a similar or lesser extent than fetal body weight. Other changes are disproportionate reductions in the weights of lymphoid tissues and increases in adrenal weight. This suggests that some but not all of the changes in fetal growth following restricted placental growth can be ascribed to hypoxemia (2,7). Chronic fetal hypoxemia caused by hypobaric conditions or reduced uterine blood flow also reduces the weight of skeletal muscle tissues (22), and in the most severely chronically hypoxic fetal sheep, the rate of oxygen consumption by the hindlimb (26). Thus, reduced growth of skeletal muscle tissues as well as of visceral tissues occurs in chronic fetal hypoxemia. Overall, reduced fetal uptake of oxygen could not be demonstrated up to 7 days after the onset of reduction of uterine blood flow and fetal hypoxia, possibly because oxygen consumption was still being largely determined by the size of tissues already laid down, and because there was at least partial maintenance of their oxygen consumption by increased extraction of oxygen (26).

The outcome of chronic restriction of oxygen supply to the conceptus for the placenta varies, with a maintenance of placental weight relative to fetal weight in the rat and guinea pig, which is more marked with earlier onset of restriction of oxygen supply (17–21) (Table 2). This may represent differential sensitivity of the fetus and placenta to oxygen restriction, or a compensatory response by the placenta aimed at maintenance of placental size and function. This does not occur in sheep, particularly when fetal hypoxemia is produced by reducing uterine blood flow (22–26) (Table 2). However, the latter reduces the rate of delivery of glucose as well as of oxygen to the uteroplacental tissues and is accompanied by reductions in uteroplacental uptake of glucose (26). The mechanism by which oxygen deficiency restricts fetal growth may be direct in nature, through inhibition of oxidative metabolism and a reduction in the metabolic rate of sensitive tissues, which in the long term reduces growth. Consistent with this is the observation of reduced hindlimb oxygen uptake in the most severely hypoxic fetal sheep when uterine blood flow is chronically reduced (26). However, reductions in total fetal oxygen uptake are not evident immediately or subsequently when measured *in vivo* during chronic hypoxia (24,26), suggesting that any changes are modest and not detectable by these methods.

Reduced Oxygen Supply to the Conceptus: Consequences for Supply of Other Substrates

Does placental and fetal hypoxia influence growth indirectly by altering the supply of other substrates *in utero*? Chronic maternal hypobaric hypoxia does not alter maternal and fetal arterial concentrations of glucose, confirming that hypoxemia, but not hypoglycemia, is present (23). The concentration of another important fetal nutrient, lactate, increases substantially after 1 day of hypobaric hypoxia, then falls subsequently to a level approximately twice that of the control sheep (23). Similarly, when the rate of uterine blood flow is chronically reduced in sheep, glucose availability is unchanged, and that of lactate increased in the fetus (26). Prolonged reduction in the rate of uterine blood flow reduces oxygen delivery to the uterus and fetus and reduces fetal oxygenation, linear fetal growth, and fetal weight without changes in fetal arterial glucose (26). The rates of fetal uptake of oxygen, glucose, and lactate are not altered by reduced uterine blood flow and consequent fetal hypoxemia for up to 7 days. These findings suggest that reduced oxygen delivery to the fetus and fetal hypoxia do not slow fetal growth by reducing carbohydrate availability (23,26).

The other major class of nutrient used by the fetus for oxidative metabolism and growth is the amino acids. Placental transfer of amino acids from mother to fetus occurs by active transport against a concentration gradient and requires energy (1). In addition, as described elsewhere in this volume, some amino acid requirements of the fetus and placenta may be met by placental and fetal modification and exchange or cycling of certain amino acids (1). To determine if hypoxia *in utero* alters the availability of this class of nutrients, we have examined the consequences of chronic maternal hypobaric hypoxemia on the quantity of 17 individual amino acids in fetal blood in sheep (27). Prolonged hypoxemia does not alter circulating concentrations of individual amino acids in maternal plasma, but it results in substantial reductions in the concentrations of the branched-chain amino acids and phenylalanine, tyrosine, and serine in fetal plasma. Thus, chronic maternal hypoxemia reduces the fetomaternal amino acid gradients for the branched-chain amino acids—and alters the availability of many amino acids in the fetal circulation—by mechanisms not involving altered concentrations in the mother (27). To determine whether the changes in amino acid concentration result from impairment of placental amino acid transfer and exchange with the fetus, the precise consequences of chronic hypoxemia in regard to these processes need to be examined. Equally, it is not known whether reducing the concentrations of particular amino acids in fetal blood alters their uptake and utilization by the fetus for energy production and growth. This question must be addressed and the consequences of chronic hypoxemia for fetal uptake and utilization of amino acids known, to determine whether fetal hypoaminoacidemia contributes to the concomitant reduction in fetal growth. This is particularly important, because similar changes in circulating amino acids and fetomaternal amino acid concentration gradients are frequently observed in the growth-restricted human fetus (15,28), raising the possibility that placental and fetal hypoxemia may impair amino acid supply to the fetus and potentially perturb growth in the human.

Reduced Oxygen Supply to the Conceptus: Endocrine Consequences

Reduced delivery of essential substrates to the fetus may also restrict fetal growth indirectly by endocrine pathways. Experimental and human fetal growth restriction accompanied by fetal hypoxemia and hypoglycemia is typically characterized by a decreased quantity of anabolic hormones and an increased quantity of catabolic hormones in late gestation (2,7). Some of these changes may be specific consequences of fetal hypoxemia and constitute endocrine mechanisms by which oxygen deficit slows and perturbs the pattern of fetal growth. The altered patterns of organ growth in fetal growth restriction resulting from chronic fetal hypoxemia parallel the redistribution of fetal cardiac output to various tissues that occurs in response to acute and chronic fetal hypoxemia (2,29). Normobaric maternal hypoxia increases the concentrations of epinephrine, and transiently those of norepinephrine, in the fetal sheep (25). Therefore, the redistribution of cardiac output appears to be mediated by the sympathoadrenal medullary responses of the fetus to chronic hypoxia, suggesting one mechanism by which the pattern of fetal growth may be perturbed. Hypobaric hypoxia in pregnant sheep does not alter circulating concentrations of insulin or thyroxine in the fetus, but it does delay the rise in concentrations of triiodothyronine in fetal blood that occurs in late gestation (27). The latter normally parallels the ontogenic increase in plasma cortisol near term. The emergence of a reduced quantity of triiodothyronine after prolonged hypoxemia may contribute to fetal growth restriction, as fetal growth is thyroid hormone-dependent (30). With the onset of hypoxia, fetal plasma cortisol increased and underwent a further substantial and accelerated rise late in gestation (27). This is also consistent with the increase in adrenal growth concomitantly observed in response to chronic hypoxemia. Exogenous cortisol inhibits the growth of the fetal sheep in late gestation (30). Therefore, the increased quantity of cortisol in the hypoxic fetal sheep may also contribute to the inhibition of fetal growth by chronic hypoxemia.

Each of these hormonal factors—catecholamines, thyroid hormone, and cortisol--may themselves act in part through another endocrine/paracrine/autocrine axis, that of the insulin-like growth factors, IGF-1 and IGF-2. The IGFs are small, growth-promoting polypeptides that are important mediators of the influence of essential substrates and hormones on fetal and placental growth (7,31). The IGFs have metabolic, mitogenic, and differentiating actions that they exert through cell surface receptors, principally the type 1 IGF receptor (31). Gene deletion studies in mice show that IGF-1 and IGF-2 are both required for normal fetal growth, whereas we have shown that an increased quantity of IGF-1 can promote growth in fetal sheep (32). Recent studies suggest that insulin deficiency and thyroid hormone deficiency are associated with reduced concentrations of IGF-1 in fetal blood in the sheep, whereas cortisol inhibits hepatic IGF-2 gene expression (2). Thus, fetal hypoxia, by inducing thyroid hormone deficiency and increasing cortisol levels, may reduce the amount of IGF-1 and IGF-2 within the conceptus and slow fetal growth. Certainly, acute hypoxia has been shown to reduce the concentrations of IGF-1 rapidly in the blood of fetal sheep (33). In addition, the biologic activities of the IGFs are modulated by up to six IGF binding proteins (IGF-BPs) (31); these sequester the IGFs in blood by slowing their clearance from the vascular space, and usually inhibit the bioactivity of the IGFs by controlling their availability to IGF receptors (31). Postnatally, the levels of the various IGF-BPs are regulated by a range of factors, including various hormones (31). IGF-BP-1 is postulated to have an important acute glucoregulatory role and in its usual highly phosphorylated form is a marked inhibitor of IGF actions (31). The levels of IGF-BP-1 increase rapidly in fetal blood in response to both acute hypoxia and more prolonged hypoxia resulting from either induction of maternal hypoxia or a reduction of uterine blood flow in sheep (33,34). This effect of hypoxia has been shown to be partly caused by an increase in circulating catecholamines, which rapidly induce hepatic IGF-BP-1 synthesis (35). Consistent with this, chronic normobaric hypoxia in the pregnant rat restricts fetal growth and increases the amounts of hepatic IGF-BP-1 and IGF-BP-2 messenger RNA and of circulating IGF-BP-1, -2, and -4 in the fetus (17). Thus, an increase in IGF-BP-1 and other IGF-BPs may reduce the bioactivity of IGFs within the chronically hypoxic fetus and further slow growth.

Reduced Oxygen Supply to the Conceptus: Therapeutic Approaches

As noted earlier, the development of percutaneous sampling of fetal blood has made it possible to show that a significant proportion of human growth-restricted fetuses are hypoxemic (36–38). Can such intrauterine hypoxemia be ameliorated? Experimental studies in rats showed improved survival of fetuses in which growth was restricted by ligation of a single umbilical artery when the mothers were exposed to hyperoxic conditions (39). Similarly, we found that placental restriction and reduced fetal oxygenation in sheep could be overcome by maternal hyperoxia, which increased fetal PO_2 and the margin of safety between delivery of oxygen and its consumption by the growth-restricted fetus. This suggests that placental limitation of oxygen delivery to the conceptus can indeed be ameliorated by increasing maternal oxygenation.

There has recently been controversy about the effectiveness of exposing women to hyperoxic conditions to improve fetal oxygenation. In a randomized trial, maternal hyperoxia in the second stage of labor resulted in a deterioration of cord blood gas values at the time of birth (40). However, during the first stage of labor in women with normal pregnancies, maternal hyperoxia has been shown to increase the concentration of fetal cerebral oxyhemoglobin, with a concomitant reduction in deoxyhemoglobin (41). These changes reversed when the hyperoxia ceased.

Maternal hyperoxia in women significantly increases the umbilical arterial PO_2 in pregnancies complicated by growth restriction (42). A small, randomized trial suggested a benefit from maternal hyperoxia (43). Continuous hyperoxia may be better than bed rest for fetuses of less than 26 weeks' gestation with absent end-diastolic flow in the umbilical artery (44). These are all small studies without sufficient sample size to determine the benefits and hazards of hyperoxia, and larger studies are required before the induction of maternal hyperoxia can be considered as a treatment for growth restriction into clinical practice.

In addition, there are potentially adverse effects of maternal hyperoxia for the fetus that will have to be considered when future trials of maternal hyperoxia are designed. Our studies in sheep show that although maternal hyperoxia increased PO_2 in normal and placentally-restricted fetal sheep, there was no increase in fetal oxygen consumption; however, these were acute studies. After cessation of the hyperoxia, oxygenation of the growth-restricted fetal sheep fell to less than that in the prehyperoxic period. Similar consequences in the human may be inferred by the increase in the number of fetal heart rate decelerations in preterm growth-restricted fetuses after cessation of maternal hyperoxia (45). Furthermore, as maternal hyperoxia improves fetal oxygenation and PO_2, it may result in a redistribution of cardiac output and blood flow to less vital organs in the growth-restricted fetus. Hyperoxia causes an increase in cerebral vascular resistance and a decrease in resistance in the descending aorta of the fetus (46). This may cause a redistribution of essential but scarce nutrients away from vital organs such as the brain and heart, as the supply of several amino acids is marginal in human pregnancy (47). All these considerations have led to a note of caution about adopting apparently simple and effective treatments for fetal growth restriction (48).

SUMMARY

Oxygen is an essential substrate for life before birth, required for the production of energy, the maintenance of tissues already laid down, and the accretion of new tissues. Studies in animals show that that chronic oxygen deficiency restricts and alters the pattern of fetal growth. Reduced oxygen delivery to the fetus does not alter fetal growth by reducing the availability of the carbohydrate substrates glucose and lactate. However, chronic fetal hypoxemia is associated with reduced concentrations of the branched-chain amino acids and of phenylalanine, tyrosine, and serine in fetal plasma and a reduced fetomaternal concentration gradient for the branched-chain amino acids. It remains to be determined whether these changes are a result of hypoxemia inhibiting placental amino acid transport, and if the consequent fetal hypoaminoacidemia limits amino acid utilization for energy production and protein accretion in the fetus and thus restricts growth. In addition, chronic fetal hypoxemia is characterized by reductions in the levels of anabolic hormones, with lowered concentrations of triiodothyronine and possibly lowered concentrations of IGF-1 and IGF-2 in fetal plasma. Concomitantly, the levels of catabolic hormones are increased, with increased concentrations of catecholamines and cortisol, which may limit and alter fetal growth. Increased concentrations of IGF binding protein, particularly IGF-BP-1, in fetal plasma occur in response to fetal hypoxemia, which inhibit the anabolic activities of IGFs within the conceptus. Thus, reduced oxygen delivery to the fetus and placental and fetal hypoxemia may restrict fetal growth directly as well as indirectly—by altering amino acid availability within the fetus and through endocrine mechanisms involving an increase of factors inhibitory to fetal growth and a decrease of other hormonal factors required for normal fetal growth and development. Both experimental animal studies and limited human trials show that maternal hyperoxia can improve oxygenation of the growth-restricted fetus, but that cessation of maternal hyperoxia may be associated with adverse changes in the fetus. Further studies are required to characterize more fully the consequences of maternal oxygen supplementation for the hypoxemic fetus before the adoption of such treatment in clinical practice.

ACKNOWLEDGMENTS

This work was supported by the National Health and Medical Research Council of Australia, and J. A. Owens was the recipient of a National Health and Medical Research Council Research Fellowship.

REFERENCES

1. Hay WW. Energy and substrate requirements of the placenta and fetus. *Proc Nutr Soc* 1991;50: 321–336.
2. Robinson JS, Owens JA, Owens PC. Fetal growth and fetal growth retardation. In: Thorburn GD, Harding R, eds. *Textbook of Fetal Physiology*. Oxford: Oxford University Press; 1994:83–94.
3. Wilkening RB, Meschia G. Current topic: Comparative physiology of placental oxygen transport. *Placenta* 1992;13:1–15.
4. Carter AM. Factors affecting gas transfer across the placenta and the oxygen supply to the fetus. *J Dev Physiol* 1989;12:305–322.
5. Mayhew TM, Joy CF, Haas JD. Structure-function correlation in the human placenta: the morphometric diffusing capacity for oxygen at full term. *J Anat* 1984;139:691–708.
6. Mayhew TM, Jackson MR, Haas JD. Microscopical morphology of the human placenta and its effect on oxygen diffusion: a morphometric model. *Placenta* 1986;7:121–131.
7. Owens JA, Owens PC, Robinson JS. Experimental restriction of fetal growth. In: Hanson MA, Spencer JD, Rodeck CH, eds. *Fetus and the Neonate. Physiology and Clinical Applications*. Cambridge: Cambridge University Press; 1995:139–175 (vol 3).
8. Moll W. Physiological aspects of placental phylogeny. *Placenta* 1985;6:141–154.
9. Robinson JS, Kingston EJ, Jones CT, Thorburn GD. Studies on experimental growth retardation in sheep. The effect of removal of endometrial caruncles on fetal size and metabolism. *J Dev Physiol* 1979;1:379–398.

10. Owens JA, Falconer J, Robinson JS. Effect of restriction of placental growth on umbilical and uterine blood flows. *Am J Physiol* 1986;250:R427–R434.
11. Owens JA, Falconer J, Robinson JS. Effect of restriction of placental growth on fetal and uteroplacental metabolism. *J Dev Physiol* 1987;9:225–238.
12. Owens JA, Falconer J, Robinson JS. Effect of restriction of placental growth on oxygen delivery to and consumption by the pregnant uterus and fetus. *J Dev Physiol* 1987;9:137–150.
13. Owens JA, Falconer J, Robinson JS. Restriction of placental size in sheep enhances the efficiency of placental transfer of antipyrine, 3-O-methyl-D-glucose, but not of urea. *J Dev Physiol* 1987;9: 457–464.
14. Chidzanja S. *Restricted implantation and undernutrition alter development and growth of the ovine placenta* (Thesis). Adelaide: University of Adelaide, 1994.
15. Montemagno R, Soothill P. Human fetal blood gases, glucose, lactate and amino acids. In: Hanson MA, Spencer JD, Rodeck CH, eds. *Fetus and the Neonate. Physiology and Clinical Applications*. Cambridge: Cambridge University Press; 1995:201–221 (vol 3).
16. Mayhew TM, Jackson MR, Haas JD. Oxygen diffusive conductances of human placentae from term pregnancies at low and high altitudes. *Placenta* 1990;11:493–503.
17. Tapanainen PJ, Bang P, Wilson K, Unterman TG, Vreman HJ, Rosenfeld RG. Maternal hypoxia as a model for intrauterine growth retardation: effects on insulin-like growth factors and their binding proteins. *Pediatr Res* 1994;36:152–158.
18. Garvey DJ, Longo LD. Chronic low level maternal carbon monoxide exposure and fetal growth and development. *Biol Reprod* 1978;19:8–14.
19. Larson JE, Thurlbeck WM. The effect of experimental maternal hypoxia on fetal lung growth. *Pediatr Res* 1988;24:156–159.
20. Van Geijn HP, Kaylor WM, Nicola KR, Zuspan FP. Induction of severe intrauterine growth retardation in the Sprague-Dawley rat. *Am J Obstet Gynecol* 1980;137:43–47.
21. Gilbert RD, Cummings LA, Juchua MR, Longo LD. Placental diffusing capacity and fetal development in exercising or hypoxic guinea pigs. *J Appl Physiol* 1979;46:828–834.
22. Jacobs R, Robinson JS, Owens JA, Falconer J, Webster MED. The effect of hypobaric hypoxia on growth of fetal sheep. *J Dev Physiol* 1988;10:97–112.
23. Jacobs R, Owens JA, Falconer J, Webster MED, Robinson JS. Changes in metabolite concentrations in fetal sheep subjected to prolonged hypobaric hypoxia. *J Dev Physiol* 1988;10:113–121.
24. Kamitomo M, Longo LD, Gilbert RD. Cardiac function in fetal sheep during two weeks of hypoxemia. *Am J Physiol* 1994;266:R1778–R1785.
25. Kitanaka T, Alonso JG, Gilbert RD, Siu BL, Clemons GK, Longo LD. Fetal responses to long-term hypoxemia in sheep. *Am J Physiol* 1989;256:R1348–R1354.
26. Boyle DW, Lecklitner S, Liechty EA. Effect of prolonged uterine blood flow reduction on fetal growth in sheep. *Am J Physiol* 1996;270:R246–R253.
27. Owens JA, Kind KL, Robinson JS, Webster MED, Jacobs R. Chronic hypobaric hypoxia alters the ontogeny of circulating amino acids, thyroid hormone and cortisol in the fetal sheep (*unpublished data*).
28. Cetin I, Corbetta C, Sereni LP, Marconi AM, Bozetta P, Pardi G, et al. Umbilical amino acid concentrations in normal and growth-retarded fetuses by cordocentesis. *Am J Obstet Gynecol* 1990; 162:253–261.
29. Kamitomo M, Alonso JG, Okai T, Longo L, Gilbert RD. Effects of long-term, high-altitude hypoxemia on ovine fetal cardiac output and blood flow distribution. *Am J Obstet Gynecol* 1993;169: 701–717.
30. Fowden AL. Endocrine regulation of fetal growth. *Reprod Fertil Dev* 1995;7:49–61.
31. Jones JI, Clemmons DR. Insulin-like growth factors and their binding proteins: biological actions. *Endocr Rev* 1995;16:3–34.
32. Lok F, Owens JA, Mundy L, Robinson JS, Owens PC. Insulin-like growth factor-I promotes growth selectively in fetal sheep in late gestation. *Am J Physiol* 1996;270:R1148–R1155.
33. Iwamoto HS, Murray MA, Chernausek SD. Effects of acute hypoxemia on insulin-like growth factors and their binding proteins in fetal sheep. *Am J Physiol* 1992;263:E1151–E1156.
34. McMellan KC, Hooper SB, Bocking AD, Delhanty PJD, Phillips ID, Hill DJ, et al. Prolonged hypoxia induced by the reduction of maternal uterine blood flow alters insulin-like growth factor-binding protein-1 (IGFBP-1) and IGFBP-2 gene expression in the ovine fetus. *Endocrinology* 1992;131: 1619–1628.
35. Hooper SB, Bocking AD, White SE, Fraher LJ, McDonald TJ, Han VKM. Catecholamines stimulate

the synthesis and release of insulin-like growth factor binding protein-1 (IGFBP-1) by fetal sheep liver in vivo. *Endocrinology* 1994;134:1104–1112.
36. Soothill PW, Nicolaides KH, Rodeck CH, Clewell WH, Lindridge J. Relationship of fetal hemoglobin and oxygen content to lactate concentration in Rh isoimmunized pregnancies. *Obstet Gynecol* 1987; 69:268–271.
37. Economides DL, Nicolaides KH. Metabolic findings in small-for-gestational-age fetuses. *Contemp Rev Obstet Gynaecol* 1990;2:75–79.
38. Pardi G, Marconi AM, Cetin I, Bellotti M, Buscaglia M. Fetal blood sampling during pregnancy—risks and diagnostic advantages. *J Perinat Med* 1994;22:513–516.
39. Vileisis RA. Effect of maternal oxygen inhalation on the fetus with growth retardation. *Pediatr Res* 1985;19:324–327.
40. Thorp JA, Trobough T, Evans R, Hedrick J, Yeast JD. The effect of maternal oxygen administration during the second stage of labor on umbilical cord blood gas values: a randomized controlled prospective trial. *Am J Obstet Gynecol* 1995;172:465–474.
41. Aldrich CJ, Wyatt JS, Spencer JAD, Reynolds EOR, Delpy DT. The effect of maternal oxygen administration on human fetal cerebral oxygenation measured during labour by near infrared spectroscopy. *Br J Obstet Gynaecol* 1994;101:509–513.
42. Nicolaides KH, Campbell S, Bradley RJ, Bilardo CM, Soothill PW, Gibb D. Maternal oxygen therapy for intrauterine growth retardation. *Lancet* 1987;1:942–945.
43. Battaglia FC, Artini PG, Dambrogio G, Galli PA, Segre A, Genazzani AR. Maternal hyperoxygenation in the treatment of intrauterine growth retardation. *Am J Obstet Gynecol* 1992;167:430–435.
44. Johanson R, Lindlow SW, van der Elst C, Jaquire Z, van der Westhuizen S, Tucker A. A prospective randomised comparison of the effect of continuous oxygen therapy and bedrest on fetuses with absent end-diastolic flow on umbilical artery Doppler waveform analysis. *Br J Obstet Gynaecol* 1995;102:662–665.
45. Bekedam DJ, Mulder EJH, Snijders RJM, Visser GHA. The effects of maternal hyperoxia on fetal breathing movements, body movements and heart rate variation in growth retarded fetuses. *Early Hum Dev* 1991;27:223–232.
46. Arduini D, Rizzo G, Mancuso S, Romanini C. Short-term effects of maternal oxygen administration on blood flow velocity waveforms in healthy and growth-retarded fetuses. *Am J Obstet Gynecol* 1988;159:1077–1080.
47. Chien PFW, Smith K, Watt PW, Scrimgeour CM, Taylor DJ, Rennie MJ. Protein turnover in the human fetus studied at term using stable isotope tracer amino acids. *Am J Physiol* 1993;265:E31–E35.
48. Harding JE, Owens JA, Robinson JS. Should we try to supplement the growth retarded fetus? A cautionary tale. *Br J Obstet Gynaecol* 1992;99:707–710.

DISCUSSION

Dr. Rennie: Have you attempted to look at the stoichiometry between the rise of alanine and the fall in the branched-chain amino acids? Because it seems to me that in a situation in which there is an oxygen deficit that is limiting the ability to oxidize fuels, and because protein synthesis is an energy-requiring process, it is unlikely that you are getting an increased disappearance of leucine, valine, and isoleucine into protein, especially as you see an opposite change for lysine, which you would have expected to have gone in the same direction. Is there a connection between the amount of α-amino nitrogen that is disappearing onto alanine and the amount that is coming from the branched chains? If so, have you looked at the ketoacid concentrations, because one would predict that there would be some export of ketoacids back.

Dr. Owens: No, we haven't looked at the relation between, for example, the increase in alanine and the reduction in the branched-chain amino acids, which are the two major quantitative changes, although that would be interesting to do. Like you, intuitively we would suspect it is unlikely that the reductions in concentrations of amino acids that we are seeing are caused by increased utilization. But I think it is very clear that there are many processes that may be determining plasma concentrations, and although we can go a bit farther in doing the sorts of calculations that you have suggested to clarify what may be happening, we really need to set up suitable experiments with catheterized umbilical and uterine circulations, blood flow measurements, and tracers to be able to say conclusively what is happening. I think it is interesting that we see reductions in the branched-chain amino acids, which are transferred from the mother to the fetus intact and in which there is substantial placental deamination. We also see reductions in glycine and serine, and these arrive in fetal blood by such a different route, maternal serine being converted to glycine by the placenta, which then supplies it to the fetal liver, which in turn produces serine. But my view is that there would be quite different pathways and mechanisms involved there.

Dr. Soothill: In your studies of maternal oxygen supplementation, did you find any improvements—increases in glucose or amino acids?

Dr. Owens: We found no change in fetal glucose concentrations or in fetal glucose uptake. It was only 4 hours, so it is quite a short-term experiment. We haven't looked at amino acid concentrations or amino acid exchange in those animals, although we have the samples available.

Dr. Soothill: Why was the experiment only 4 hours? In terms of what is known about induction of some of the transport systems, it would be quite nice to have data for many days, if it is possible.

Dr. Owens: This was really just a first step. What we want to know is whether, when we produce a placenta that is not just small in size but has reduced rates of perfusion, reduced rates of uterine umbilical blood flow, and, as we know now, very much reduced surface exchange area, can we in fact increase oxygenation within the fetus at all—the fetus that is very growth-restricted and with a very small placenta? I agree with you, I think it would be fascinating to go on for longer and perhaps to look at the impact on amino acids.

Dr. Pardi: You reported on the fetal-to-placental weight ratio going from 8 in controls to 12 in severe growth retardation. Could you comment on these data?

Dr. Owens: Yes, when we restrict implantation in the sheep we variably restrict placental growth, and what we consistently find in that perturbation is that there is an increase in the ratio of fetal weight to placental weight in late gestation. This probably reflects compensatory changes on the part of the placenta and the fetus that may help to maintain fetal growth to some extent. The nature of these compensations varies, but within the placenta, for example, we see that although there are reductions in the absolute rates of uterine and umbilical blood flows, umbilical blood flow per gram of placenta seems to increase in the small placenta.

Dr. Pardi: In other words, very roughly and clinically, the placenta loses weight first and then the fetus.

Dr. Owens: We have ontogenic data now in this particular model, and certainly up to early in late gestation the placenta is growing more slowly; in contrast, the fetus up to about day 90, which is late in midgestation in the sheep, is of normal weight, but some tissues such as the gut are starting to show decrements in weight and changes in structure, suggesting that limitation has set in. Thereafter, with cross-sectional data fetal growth rate slows. We don't know whether we actually see placental wasting *per se*, because in the sheep the placental weight normally decreases late in gestation. But there is clearly placental restriction first, and fetal restriction follows subsequent to that.

Dr. Battaglia: I think people are getting misled because you have presented oxygen data in milliliters per minute, and there are good reasons in physiology to express them in milliliters per minute per kilogram. The mouse consumes a lot less oxygen than the elephant, but the oxygen consumption of the mouse is much higher than that of the elephant, and there is certainly no reduction in ATP supply in the mouse. So if you have a small fetus, in which you are studying growth retardation, it seems to me absolutely essential to present the data on a weight-specific basis, because otherwise people are misled. I'm assuming that if you express it per unit weight you will find as we do in growth retardation that you are not getting a reduction in oxygen consumption. So ATP supply is not the problem. I wonder why you are presenting it in absolute terms. The other comment I have is about amino acids. I know of no relation between changes in concentration and uptake. When we are talking about growth and nutrition, we are talking about uptake. So again, I have a problem with your interpretation of concentrations alone.

Dr. Owens: In terms of looking at the impact of these perturbations on fetal oxygen consumption, what I did today was simply to present the data in absolute terms. You can see in our papers that indeed, at least up to 130 days' gestation, the placentally restricted fetal sheep is consuming oxygen at a normal rate on a per kilogram basis. We now have some data showing that eventually oxygen consumption may start to decrease, but it is only very late that you start to get a decrement in oxygen flux when corrections for weight are made. Interestingly, when we look at several of our studies combined, we find that the very small placenta in late gestation is consuming oxygen at a reduced rate per gram. Although there are changes in structure and composition of such placentae, nevertheless it seems that the restricted implantation placenta may be suffering from reduced energy production. On your other point about trying to relate circulating concentrations of amino acids to their utilization, particularly for growth, I think you are absolutely right. All we can say here, for example, where we have a chronically restricted oxygen supply using hypobaric hypoxemia and induced changes in concentrations of amino acids in fetal plasma, is that there is evidence that some perturbation is occurring. We have no idea, however, what is happening to flux, what is happening to transfer, or what is happening to utilization. I think that all these data are telling us is that some of the changes that you see in plasma concentrations in the growth-restricted human fetus can be produced in the sheep by restricting oxygen supply alone, but how that relates to growth and whether it has any relevance to it is another question.

Dr. Doris Campbell: I was interested in the idea that the placenta is restricted from the time of implantation, because in terms of the human work there is a great deal of interest in what is controlling implantation and trophoblast invasion, particularly in the field of hypertension, and what the signal is for trophoblast development. I wonder if you have any information about what the decidual fetal signals might be that control that.

Dr. Owens: We don't have that information from our studies directly. What we see early on in terms of the placentomes that can form at the few sites of implantation that are left, and what we see subsequently up to midgestation at least, is that at those sites there is if anything an overgrowth, or compensatory growth, so in that sense I don't think it is analogous to what you are looking at in the human, where you have impaired or imperfect implantation and impaired subsequent placentation. The signals, of course, would be fascinating to investigate, because treatment such as maternal oxygen supplementation may prove to be valuable when you have identified that you have a problem on your hands, and I would really like to know in addition whether we can intervene very early on in women who we know are likely to go on and have problems with placentation and pregnancy.

Dr. Sibley: There are very interesting data coming from Susan Fischer's lab at the University of California in San Francisco that oxygen might play a key role in the implantation process in inducing various integrins and similar molecules. I would like to know what happens to blood flow in the hypoxic situation, because it strikes me that all your data might be explained by reduced blood flow and a change in vascular resistance. A third point: Everything you said in your model in terms of amino acid concentrations is quite similar to the human studies, except for alanine. As I understand it, in the Milan study and I think in the London study also, alanine, if anything, goes down despite the fact that, as in your study, lactate goes up. So I really have two questions: What happens to blood flow, and is there any explanation for the discrepancy between alanine in the human and sheep model?

Dr. Owens: Taking the first question, in our study in which we imposed hypobaric hypoxemia in the sheep, we don't know what happened to blood flow. There is only one study that I know of, again in sheep but with normobaric hypoxemia, in which uterine blood flow was looked at, and they did not find any chronic changes in uteroplacental flow (1). But these sorts of measurements are extremely difficult to do, so I think it remains an open question. Intuitively, you would expect no change or perhaps even an increase in umbilical blood flow in response to maternal hypoxia, but I don't think we know whether that could be sustained. On your second question in relation to alanine, I should say that in our placentally restricted animals, we don't find increases in lactate until quite late in gestation, so there may be an element of timing in that once metabolic acidosis sets in, that may be when you see a change in alanine.

Dr. Battaglia: Dr. Meschia, would you like to comment? You did high-altitude studies at about 14,000 feet. What was the uterine flow? Was there a consistent change in flow?

Dr. Meschia: At that time we could not establish any increase in blood flow, but that was many years ago.

Dr. Battaglia: But you were looking for an increase. At least there was no reduction in flow.

Dr. Meschia: No. In acute hypoxia there can be some reduction, but it is very modest. What amazes me is how modest all the changes are with changes in oxygenation; even in growth retardation the effects are relatively small compared with what you get with heat stress.

Dr. Battaglia: Just on the alanine and lactate, I don't think it is going to end up being a species difference. In sheep with acute hypoxia, alanine and lactate concentrations are directly correlated because they are freely exchangeable. The transaminase reaction is readily reversible, so alanine, pyruvate, and lactate are really interchangeable. With chronic hypoxia that relationship breaks down, so something else is going on, but over 4 to 6 hours you would expect a tight correlation. If lactate is increased threefold or fourfold, it is almost impossible to visualize why you wouldn't have an increase in alanine.

Dr. Milliez: Is there any evidence in humans that hyperoxygenation improves fetal growth?

Dr. Owens: There is no evidence that it improves fetal growth. However, Battaglia *et al.* carried out a randomized controlled trial of maternal hyperoxia in human fetal growth restriction in a small, but I think sufficient, cohort and halved the mortality rate (2). They did not find a restoration of fetal growth rate, but they did improve fetal survival. I certainly agree with Professor Meschia about the limited effect of chronic hypoxemia on fetal growth. It is surprising, particularly when you look at the human growth-restricted fetuses, among which there certainly seems to be a large category that are hypoxemic but not hyperglycemic, yet very growth-restricted. So there may be species differences there, and there may be questions of timing of onset and of magnitude as well.

REFERENCES

1. Kitanaka T, Gilbert RD, Longo LD. Maternal and fetal responses to long-term hypoxemia in sheep. In: Kunzel W, Jensen A, eds. *The Endocrine Control of the Fetus.* Berlin-Heidelberg: Springer-Verlag; 1988:38–63.
2. Battaglia FC, Artini PG, D'Ambrogio G, Galli PA, Segre A, Genazzani AR. Maternal hyperoxygenation in the treatment of intrauterine growth retardation. *Am J Obstet Gynecol* 1992;167:430–435.

Placental Function and Fetal Nutrition,
edited by Frederick C. Battaglia,
Nestlé Nutrition Workshop Series, Vol. 39.
Nestec Ltd., Vevey/Lippincott-Raven Publishers,
Philadelphia, © 1997.

Placental Transport in Fetal Growth Retardation

Edward S. Ogata, Robert H. Lane, Rebecca A. Simmons, and Gregory J. Reid

Division of Neonatology and Departments of Pediatrics and Obstetrics and Gynecology, Children's Memorial Institute for Education and Research, Children's Memorial Hospital/ Northwestern University Medical School, Chicago, Illinois 60614, USA

The factors responsible for retarding fetal growth are numerous and not completely understood. Although it is reasonable to assume that altered placental handling and transport of metabolic fuels can affect fetal growth, little is known about the precise relation between these changes and the numerous aspects of fetal growth (1). Indeed, a comprehensive understanding of the role of the various aspects of placental transport in normal fetal growth remains to be developed. In this review, we present information about alterations in placental transport that are associated with fetal (intrauterine) growth retardation (IUGR). Glucose and amino acid transporters are highlighted, and we present information about the effects of nicotine, alcohol, and cocaine on transport and IUGR.

Among the physiologic factors that influence placental transport of metabolic fuels, acid-base status, and exchange of oxygen and carbon dioxide are maternal (uterine) blood flow and the availability of maternally derived metabolic fuels (2,3). The transport of metabolic substances from either maternal to fetal or fetal to maternal circulations is complex, involving different cell sites and various transporters. For example, in the rat glucose is believed to pass from the maternal circulation through pores in the cytotrophoblast. Glucose transporter-1 (GLUT-l) carries glucose into the cytoplasm of the syncytiotrophoblast-1. Glucose passes through gap junctions into the cytoplasm of syncytiotrophoblast-2, where GLUT-1 on the cell membrane transports it to the fetal endothelium. It then passes through pores on the fetal endothelium into the fetal vasculature. Alterations at any of these sites can affect transfer (Fig. 1). Of course, the placenta is more than a conduit for metabolic fuel provision and gas exchange. It actively participates in fetal metabolism, having metabolic relations with different fetal organs—that is, it supplies, takes up, and modifies specific metabolites from the placental circulation.

Species differences and developmental considerations also complicate our understanding of the relation between fetal growth and placental function. Fetal metabolic requirements differ between species. Anatomic differences between species may also be a factor. The expression and function of the various transporters may change

GLUT 1 LOCALIZATION

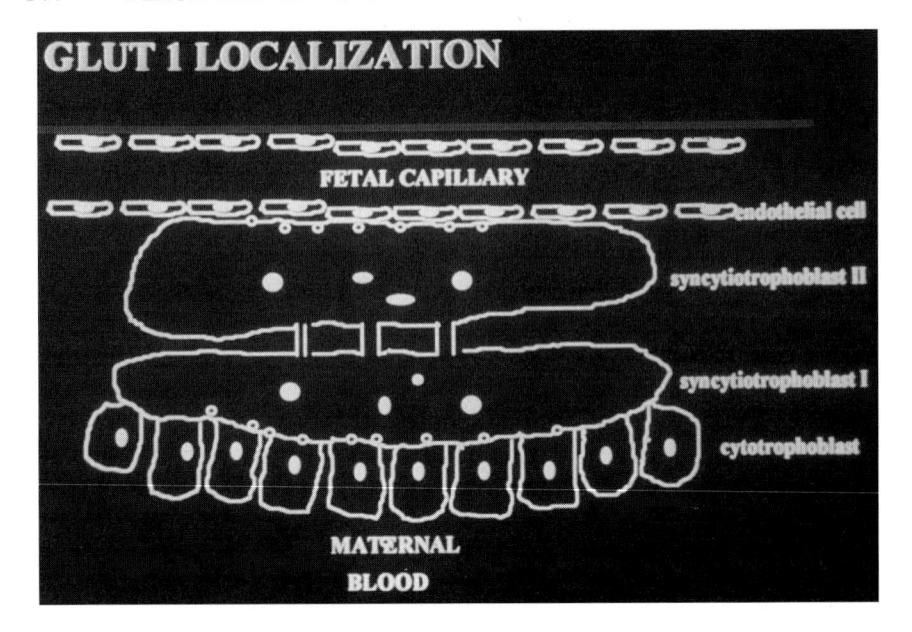

FIG. 1. Schematic representation of glucose transport in the rat placenta. Glucose passes from maternal capillaries into pores located in the cytotrophoblast. GLUT-1 transfers glucose into syncytiotrophoblast-1. Glucose passes through gap junctions from syncytiotrophoblast-1 to syncytiotrophoblast-2. GLUT-1 on the membrane of syncytiotrophoblast-2 transfers glucose into the fetal endothelium.

as gestation progresses. Also, the anatomic and functional relations are complicated in the placenta. For example, the handling of a metabolic substance may differ between the maternal (microvillous) and fetal (basal) facing membranes, cytotrophoblast, and endothelial cells.

Glucose transporters—structurally similar proteins encoded by a family of genes and expressed in a tissue-specific manner (4,5)—have been identified on the syncytiotrophoblast, cytotrophoblast, and endothelial cells of the human placenta and on syncytiotrophoblast-1 and syncytiotrophoblast-2 of the rat placenta. Our understanding of the mechanistic and regulatory role of glucose transporters in facilitating glucose flux between the maternal and the fetal circulations is limited.

Establishing the role of placental amino acid transporters in normal and fetal growth is even more complex. This is because numerous amino acid transporters have been characterized on a functional basis, and each transports more than one amino acid (6,7). More amino acid transporters have been characterized on a functional than on a molecular basis. Indeed, identification of the molecular characteristics of the known amino acid transporters is limited.

GLUCOSE TRANSPORT

Glucose is an important metabolic fuel for the fetus; alterations in its availability directly affect fetal metabolism and thereby potentially affect fetal growth. This concept is complicated by the fact that alterations in other metabolic fuels, such as amino acids, and growth-stimulating factors, such as insulin (8), have cumulative effects on fetal growth. Thus, the precise contribution of glucose in modulating fetal growth under normal and IUGR conditions remains to be defined. In this section, we provide the details of *in vivo* quantitation of glucose flux between mother, placenta, and fetus; of *in vitro* measures of placental function; and of the activity and expression of placental glucose transporters. These data confirm a role for glucose in fetal growth but also show that factors other than glucose contribute to the development of IUGR.

In considering maternal-fetal glucose flux, three glucose pools—maternal, placental, and fetal—must be considered. There is considerable bidirectional flux between the fetal and maternal pools. In the sheep, the uteroplacental mass interposed between the maternal and fetal glucose pools is considerable; it not only transfers glucose in both directions but also rapidly metabolizes glucose (9,10). Indeed, the fetal glucose pool contributes approximately 40% of the glucose metabolized by the placenta. The dynamic interchange between the three pools highlights the complexity of glucose transport and utilization in the sheep.

Several animal models of IUGR have been developed. Heat stress in the maternal ewe from 39 to 124 days of gestation retards fetal growth (11). Heat stress restricts placental growth and decreases fetal plasma glucose concentrations. It is noteworthy that heat stress does not decrease placental perfusion or increase uteroplacental utilization of glucose; rather, it directly limits the ability of the placenta to transport glucose to the fetus. Carunculectomy, which reduces placental mass by 30%, results in a 52% to 59% decrease in fetal glucose turnover in the sheep (12,13). Such a reduction in placental mass reduces umbilical blood flow. Both umbilical and uterine blood flow and placental mass correlate with fetal mass, confirming that diminished blood flow is a major factor in restricting fetal growth. This relationship has also been reported in the rat (14).

Diminished blood flow with concomitant reduction in glucose provision is believed to retard fetal growth in the human. Asymmetric fetal growth retardation is often attributed to "uteroplacental insufficiency," a term suggesting impaired uterine blood flow, compromised gas exchange, and altered metabolic fuel provision to the fetus. Doppler flow studies in human pregnancies with identified IUGR fetuses confirm that uteroplacental blood flow is diminished (15). Such diminished flow may restrict glucose provision.

Studies in smaller mammals show that decreased uteroplacental perfusion contributes to the development of fetal growth retardation. Ligation of the uterine artery in the pregnant guinea pig between 38 and 53 days of gestation restricts placental and fetal growth and decreases fetal plasma glucose and amino acid concentrations (10). In particular, the transfer of labeled aminoisobutyric acid (AIB) remains reduced over a longer period after ligation than the transfer of labeled glucose. This suggests that the availability of amino acids may be more important than the availability of glucose in the development of fetal growth retardation.

Ligation of the uterine artery in the maternal rat also retards fetal growth. This method alters numerous physiologic and metabolic variables; for example, it results in metabolic acidosis, hypoglycemia, and diminished total and branched-chain amino acid availability in the fetus (16,17). It is of interest that these and other metabolic variables (such as energy and redox states) return to normal within 24 to 48 hours after uterine artery ligation; nonetheless, subsequent fetal and postnatal growth is retarded (18). As in the guinea pig, the duration of reduction in supply of branched-chain amino acids is greater than that of glucose.

Although it is not possible to perform long-term kinetic studies in the fetal rat, our laboratory did adapt an isotopic glucose technique for acute quantitation of relative glucose uptake by the placenta and various organs of the IUGR rat fetus. Twenty-four hours after ligation, placental glucose uptake is significantly diminished compared with that of controls; corresponding fetal plasma glucose concentrations are also significantly diminished. By 48 hours, placental glucose uptake and fetal plasma glucose concentrations are similar to control levels. As this method measures the accumulation of a phosphorylated glucose analogue in an organ, these findings cannot be used to determine whether increased placental utilization or diminished transfer of glucose, or both, cause fetal hypoglycemia (19). Although the mechanisms for this are not completely understood, the diminished perfusion and transient acidosis resulting from ligation may limit placental function.

Little information is available concerning placental glucose transport under conditions of IUGR in the human. In a series of studies, Cetin *et al.* (20,21) measured glucose and amino acid concentrations in cord blood from IUGR and normal fetuses at time of cesarean section. They found that umbilical venous-arterial differences (UVAD) in glucose were similar in IUGR and normal fetuses; the glucose-to-oxygen quotient also did not differ. On the other hand, IUGR fetuses had lower UVAD amino acid concentrations than normal fetuses. Branched-chain amino acids were significantly diminished. These observations are consistent with studies in laboratory animals suggesting that alterations in amino acids, particularly the branched-chain amino acids, may be a more important factor than glucose availability in the pathogenesis of IUGR.

Limited information is available concerning the expression and regulation of glucose transporters in the placenta under conditions of either IUGR or normal growth. Recently, Takata *et al.* (22) and Illsley's group (Jansson *et al.*, ref. 23) reported that GLUT-1 is the dominant isoform in human placenta. Jansson *et al.* used several techniques and could not detect GLUT-3. GLUT-1 protein density is greater in the microvillous membrane than in the basal membrane of the syncytiotrophoblast. GLUT-1 appears to be developmentally regulated, as its density increases with gestation.

Although *in vivo* measurement of glucose flux in the human IUGR fetus is not available, studies of membrane vesicles from placentae of IUGR fetuses indicate that D-glucose uptake is probably similar to that of normal fetuses. In addition, GLUT-1 protein densities in the villous and basal membranes of placentae from IUGR fetuses do not differ from those of normal fetuses (23).

Several laboratories have reported the presence of GLUT-1 in the rat placenta

(24,25). Takata *et al.* (25) have pointed out that the proximity of GLUT-1 to gap junctions in microvilli is an important anatomic and functional factor in assuring glucose transport from the syncytiotrophoblast-2 into the fetal vasculature.

Reid *et al.* (26) and Lane *et al.* (27) have confirmed that GLUT-1 messenger RNA and protein are present in the rat placenta. In contrast to the human IUGR placenta, the rat IUGR placenta expresses GLUT-1 messenger RNA and protein to a greater extent than normal. Immunohistocytochemistry confirms that GLUT-1 density is increased in the IUGR syncytiotrophoblast (25–27). The up-regulation of GLUT-1 may represent an attempt to compensate for diminished glucose provision to the IUGR rat fetus. Despite the up-regulation of GLUT-1, fetal plasma glucose is diminished in the IUGR fetus. This suggests that GLUT-l expression is probably not rate-limiting in the transfer of glucose under IUGR conditions in the rat.

Little is known about the control of the expression and function of placental glucose transporters under IUGR conditions. Under normal conditions, insulin up-regulates GLUT-1 in most tissues, including the placenta (28). *In vitro* studies suggest that insulin and the insulin-like growth factors (IGFs) increase glucose transport in cultured placental vesicles (29). Insulin increases trophoblast cell glucose uptake and up-regulates GLUT-1 expression to a greater extent than glucose (28).

Summary

These observations emphasize the complexity of placental glucose transport under normal and IUGR conditions. Glucose flux across the placenta is bidirectional, and the placenta metabolizes glucose as well. Indeed, little is known about fetal utilization of glucose under either normal or IUGR conditions. In the sheep, guinea pig, and rat, various conditions that cause IUGR result in decreased fetal plasma glucose concentrations. The extent to which altered glucose availability causes IUGR in the human is less clear, as data concerning middle and late gestation are limited. The observations that GLUT-1 function and regulation have been reported to be unchanged in human conditions of IUGR suggest that factors other than glucose transport may be more important in restricting growth in the human fetus.

AMINO ACID TRANSPORT

As indicated in the preceding section, the transplacental provision of amino acids is critically important for fetal growth and development. Amino acids are substrates for synthesis and are important fuels for oxidative metabolism. As fetal amino acid concentrations may be altered to a greater extent than glucose under conditions of IUGR, the relative importance of amino acids in influencing fetal growth cannot be underestimated. Unfortunately, understanding of the placental transport of amino acids under conditions of IUGR and normal growth remains rudimentary. This is in part a consequence of the large number of amino acid transporters and their complex biology.

Although amino acid transporters are highly stereospecific, transporting L-amino acids more effectively than D-amino acids, their substrate specificity is low—that is, one transporter may transport a number of different amino acids and different transporters may have overlapping specificities. In addition, microvillous and basal membranes have different populations and densities of the various transporters (30). The regulation of transporter function is not completely understood; the availability of one amino acid may either stimulate or inhibit a transporter's ability to transfer another amino acid. Thus, the biology of amino acid transporter systems is far more complex than that of the glucose transporters.

The microvillus has several transporter systems, including system A, which is sodium-dependent and transports—among other amino acids—alanine, serine, AIB, and proline. System N is also located on the microvillus. It, too, is sodium-dependent and transports histidine and glutamine. The microvillus also has a number of sodium-independent transporters. One system N transporter interacts strongly with leucine, tryptophan, tyrosine, and phenylalanine, and resembles system L. Another sodium-independent transporter transports alanine and serine; it binds weakly with branched-chain and aromatic amino acids (31).

The basal membrane has a sodium-dependent system A, which is similar to the system A transporter found in the microvillus, and it also has a sodium-dependent ASC (alanine-serine-cysteine) system, which can transport alanine, serine, and cysteine, but not AIB. Also on the basal membrane is a sodium-independent L system, which transports leucine and phenylalanine. The basal membrane has a sodium-independent system as well, which transports tyrosine. It is unclear whether the basal membrane has system N (Table 1).

No information is available concerning the coordination of amino acid transporter function between the microvillous and basal membranes. Logically, amino acid transporters on the two membranes must act in concert to achieve a concentrative transfer of amino acids from mother to the fetus. The coordinating mechanisms and signals that coordinate these activities remain to be identified.

TABLE 1. *Amino acid transport systems in the syncytiotrophoblast (microvillous and/or basal membrane)*

System	Substrate	Membrane location
A	Neutral AA, AIB	Both
ASC	Ala, Ser, Cys, anionic AA	Basal
N	His, Gln	Microvillous
B	Tau	Microvillous
X_{AG}	Asp, Glu	Both
l	Leu, BCH	Both
Y^+	Lys, Arg	Both
$b^{o,+}$	Lys, Arg	Basal
Y^{+L}	Lys, Arg	Microvillous

AA, amino acid; AIB, amino isobutyric acid; BCH, 2-aminobicyclo-(2,2,1)-heptane-2-carboxylic acid.

In vitro and *in vivo* physiologic studies have been the primary basis for classification of the amino acid transporters. Unlike the glucose transporters, which primarily transfer glucose (GLUT-5 also transports fructose), each amino acid transporter has the capability of transporting more than one amino acid. The molecular characterization of amino acid transporters remains in its infancy. At present, it is extremely difficult to correlate the few cloned amino acid transporter genes with the physiologically characterized transporters. Thus, it is difficult to identify the specific changes in amino acid transporters that are responsible for retarding fetal growth.

The chronically catheterized fetal sheep model has allowed quantitation of maternal-fetal amino acid flux. Studies using this model have shown unique handling of specific amino acids by the placenta under normal circumstances. For example, in late gestation, the fetal liver converts serine to glycine; the placenta has a significant net uptake of fetal serine. The placenta converts at least 15% of serine to glycine, which is released into the umbilical circulation. Glycine is critical for fetal energy metabolism; for example, the fetal hindlimb takes up considerable glycine for oxidation (32,33).

The placenta also modulates placental-fetal metabolism. For example, interorgan cycling of amino acids occurs between fetal liver and placenta. Glutamate is an important amino acid, because it serves as a key intermediate in amino acid metabolism and ammonia homeostasis, and as a neurotransmitter. In the placenta, glutamate is second only to taurine in abundance. Unlike other amino acids, glutamate is not concentrated in fetal blood by the placenta. On the other hand, the placenta does transport glutamine into the fetal circulation. The fetal liver converts glutamine to glutamate. The placenta takes up considerable glutamate from the fetal circulation to allow for protein synthesis and the generation of NADPH (reduced nicotinamide adenine dinucleotide phosphate). This facilitates placental synthesis of cholesterol and steroids. Clearance of glutamate from the fetal circulation is important for the fetus, as excessively raised plasma glutamate concentrations are neurotoxic. As the fetus approaches term, these relations change. Fetal hepatic glutamate release diminishes as glutamate is shifted to fetal hepatic glycogen synthesis (34,35). Several sodium-dependent transporters that can transport glutamate have been cloned and identified. Placental microvilli have both GLT-1 and GLAST-1 (36–38). Their precise location, activity, and expression and involvement in these processes are unclear.

The few data concerning amino acid transport under conditions of IUGR are not consistent, but they do suggest that changes in transporter function or availability contribute to the development of IUGR. In the fetal rat rendered growth-retarded by maternal uterine artery ligation, AIB transport, a marker of sodium-dependent transport, is greatly diminished (39). Similarly, in the guinea pig, maternal uterine artery ligation reduces fetal plasma AIB concentrations by 30% in early gestation and 18% during late gestation. Sodium-dependent transport to the rat fetus rendered growth-retarded by maternal uterine artery ligation is diminished, as labeled AIB is diminished in most fetal organs (16). As maternal uterine artery ligation alters numerous metabolic and physiologic variables, the mechanisms by which this model of uteroplacental insufficiency limits placental amino acid transport is not clear.

A few investigators have used the isolated microvillus method to study this problem. Dicke et al. (40) have reported that the function of a transporter with system A characteristics is significantly diminished in microvilli of placentae from growth-retarded human fetuses. Sibley's group (41) has also observed a similar limitation in the V_{max} of the system A transporter. Another observation that tends to confirm that system A transporter function may affect fetal growth is that system A amino acid transporters are altered in human diabetic pregnancy, resulting in macrosomic fetuses (42). On the other hand, microvillous system A transporter function has been found to be unaffected in placentae of fetal rats rendered growth-retarded by maternal uterine artery ligation (43).

Quantitation of amino acid flux and fetal plasma concentrations under IUGR and normal conditions is limited. Cetin et al. (20,21,44) have used the cordocentesis method to measure fetal plasma amino acid concentrations during middle and late gestation in the human. Their studies show that total α-amino nitrogen and branched-chain amino acids are diminished in the umbilical venous circulation of growth-retarded fetuses. The maternal-fetal ratio of amino acids confirms that transport is reduced under conditions of IUGR. These differences are similar to those reported in the growth-retarded fetal rat (17).

The fact that branched-chain amino acids and particularly leucine are diminished in the circulations during IUGR in both the human and the rat is intriguing and emphasizes the importance of these essential amino acids for normal fetal growth. The branched-chain amino acids are central to protein synthesis and oxidative metabolism. Indeed, under conditions of maternal fuel deprivation, fetal leucine oxidation increases greatly (44,45). Further support for the importance of the branched-chain amino acids comes from studies of normal pregnancy showing that these amino acids are preferentially transported to the fetal circulation. In the sheep, leucine is transported at a rate 95% greater than that of glycine from the maternal to the fetal circulation (46,47). Maternal heat stress in the ewe retards fetal growth. Placental leucine transport, oxidation, and fetal disposal are all significantly reduced (48). Stable isotope studies using cordocentesis in the human also show that the transfer of leucine is significantly greater than that of glycine in normal pregnancies between 20 and 37 weeks of gestation (49).

The precise manner in which the transport of branched-chain amino acids is altered to contribute to the development of IUGR is unclear. Changes in permeability at the syncytiotrophoblast or endothelial interface may be one mechanism. Altered placental and possibly fetal metabolism may also limit branched-chain amino acid availability. In this regard, our laboratory has performed preliminary studies indicating that the expression of a sodium-independent neutral amino acid transporter originally cloned by Tate et al. (50) is diminished in the placenta of the IUGR rat. Lane et al. (51) have found that the messenger RNA for this transporter (307 base pairs) in the IUGR placenta is 85% of normal. This transporter may be one of a family of transporters responsible for branched-chain amino acid transport. Diminished expression of this transporter may be one mechanism responsible for limiting the supply of these critical amino acids to the fetus. The mechanisms by which the altered physiologic and metabolic relations that cause IUGR actually alter placental amino acid transport are unclear. Oxidative metabolism *per se* may not be a critical factor, as perfused human placenta will transport amino acids and carry out protein synthesis even when gassed in 100% nitrogen (52).

Summary

At present, a comprehensive understanding of the role of amino acid transporters in the growth of the normal and the IUGR fetus is not available. This is in part a consequence of the fact that amino acid transporters are located at numerous placental sites and can carry multiple amino acids. In addition, the placenta has a complex metabolic relation with the fetus, in that it processes various amino acids and exchanges them with fetal organs. Fetal utilization of amino acids also complicates understanding of amino acid availability. The *in vivo* data indicating that the availability of amino acids, particularly the branched-chain amino acids, is more profoundly altered than glucose in IUGR pregnancies suggest an important role for amino acids in fetal growth. At this point, limited observations are available concerning the alterations of amino acid transporters at the molecular level.

MATERNAL SUBSTANCE ABUSE AND PLACENTAL TRANSPORT

Maternal use of illicit drugs and excessive consumption of alcohol are associated with IUGR and fetal anomalies. It is likely that multiple factors are responsible for these complications. A few studies have attempted to address the potential effects of these substances on placental transport. For example, limited data suggest that alcohol may not alter placental glucose transport but to some extent does reduce transport of AIB, leucine, and valine (52–54). Alcohol, particularly with prolonged maternal use, reduces the transport of specific amino acids. Several models using isolated villi from primates and rats chronically exposed to ethanol have shown diminished AIB and valine uptake (55). These changes appear to be a direct effect of ethanol rather than of acetoaldehyde (56).

Cocaine abuse and excessive maternal tobacco use are also associated with IUGR. Both nicotine and cocaine reduce AIB and valine uptake in human placental villous slices. Of note, when placental slices are exposed to both ethanol and nicotine, transport is reduced even more; the effects of nicotine and cocaine in reducing AIB transport appear to be additive rather than synergistic (57).

These observations offer only glimpses into a variety of potential mechanisms responsible for IUGR associated with maternal ethanol, cocaine, and nicotine use.

REFERENCES

1. Battaglia FC. New concepts in fetal and placental amino acid metabolism. *J Anim Sci* 1992;70: 3258–3263.

2. Smith CH, Moe AJ, Ganapathy V. Nutrient transport pathways across the epithelium of the placenta. *Annu Rev Nutr* 1992;12:183–206.
3. Battaglia F. Placental transport and utilization of amino acids and carbohydrates. *Fed Proc* 1986; 45:2508–2512.
4. Bell GI, Kayano T, Buse JB, Burant CF, Takeda J, Lin D, *et al.* Molecular biology of mammalian glucose transporters. *Diabetes Care* 1990;13:198–208.
5. Devaskar S, Mueckler M. The mammalian glucose transporter. *Pediatr Res* 1992;31:1–13.
6. Johnson L, Smith C. Neutral amino acid transport systems of microvillous membrane of human placenta. *Am J Physiol* 1988;254:C773–C780.
7. McGivan J, Pastor-Anglada M. Regulatory and molecular aspects of mammalian amino acid transport. *Biochem J* 1994;299:321–334.
8. Hill DJ, Milner RDG. Insulin as a growth factor. *Pediatr Res* 1985;19:879–886.
9. Hay W, Sparks J, Battaglia F, Meschia G. Maternal fetal glucose exchange: necessity of a three pool model. *Am J Physiol* 1984;246:E528–E534.
10. Hay W, Molina R, DeGiacomma J, Meschia G. Model of placental glucose consumption and glucose transfer. *Am J Physiol* 1990;258:R569–R570.
11. Thureen P, Tremble K, Meschia G, Makowski E, Wilkening R. Placental glucose transport in heat induced fetal growth retardation. *Am J Physiol* 1992;263:R578–R585.
12. Owens J, Falconer J, Robinson J. Effect of restriction of placental growth on umbilical and uterine blood flow. *Am J Physiol* 1986;250:R427–R434.
13. Owens J, Falconer J, Robinson J. Glucose metabolism in pregnant sheep when placental growth is restricted. *Am J Physiol* 1989;1257:R350–R357.
14. Gilbert M, Leturque A. Fetal weight and its relationship to placental blood flow and placental weight in experimental intrauterine growth retardation in the rat. *J Dev Physiol* 1982;4:237–246.
15. Laurin J, Lingman G, Marsal K, Persson PH. Fetal blood flow in pregnancies complicated by intrauterine growth retardation. *Obstet Gynecol* 1987;69:895–902.
16. Jansson T, Persson E. Placental transfer of glucose and amino acids in intrauterine growth retardation: studies with substrate analogs in the awake guinea pig. *Pediatr Res* 1990;28:203–208.
17. Ogata ES, Buesey M, Finley S. Altered gas exchange, limited glucose, branched chain amino acids and hyperinsulinism retard fetal growth in the rat. *Metabolism* 1986;35:950–977.
18. Ogata ES, Swanson SL, Collins JW, Finley SL. Intrauterine growth retardation: altered hepatic energy and redox states in the fetal rat. *Pediatr Res* 1990;27:56–63.
19. Lueder F, Ogata ES. Uterine artery ligation in the maternal rat alters fetal tissue glucose utilization. *Pediatr Res* 1990;28:464–468.
20. Cetin I, Marconi A, Bozzetti P, Sereni L, Corbetta C, Pardi G, *et al.* Umbilical amino acid concentrations in appropriate and small for gestational age infants: a biochemical difference present *in utero*. *Am J Obstet Gynecol* 1988;158:120–126.
21. Cetin I, Marconi AM, Corbetta C, Perugino G, Ronzoni S, Battaglia FC, et al. The relative uptake of amino acid, glucose and oxygen across the umbilical circulation in normal and intrauterine growth retarded (IUGR) pregnancies. *SGI Proceedings*, 1994(abst).
22. Takata K, Kasahara T, Kasahara M, Ezaki D, Hirano H. Localization of erythrocyte/HepG2 type glucose transport (Glut 1) in human placental villi. *Cell Tissue Res* 1992;267:407–412.
23. Jansson T, Wennergren M, Illsley N. Glucose transporter protein expression in human placenta throughout gestation and in intrauterine growth retardation. *J Clin Endocrinol Metab* 1993;77:1554–1562.
24. Zhou J, Bondy C. Placental glucose transporter gene expression and metabolism in the rat. *J Clin Invest* 1993;91:845–852.
25. Takata K, Kasahara T, Kasahara M, Ezaki O, Hirano H. Immunolocalization of glucose transporter Glut 1 in the rat placental barrier: possible role of Glut 1 and the gap junction in the transport of glucose across the placental barrier. *Cell Tissue Res* 1994;276:411–418.
26. Reid GJ, Lane RH, Flozak AS, Simmons RA. Placental expression of glucose transporter protein-1 (Glut 1) in fetal overgrowth. *Pediatr Res* 1996;39:318A(abst).
27. Lane RH, Flozak AS, Simmons RA. Placental Glut 1 and Glut 3 gene expression in normal and growth-retarded fetal rats. *Clin Res* 1994;42:347A(abst).
28. Gordon MC, Zimmerman P, Landon M, Gabbe S, Kniss D. Insulin and glucose modulates glucose transporter messenger ribonucleic and expression and glucose uptake in trophoblasts isolated from first trimester chorionic villi. *Am J Obstet Gynecol* 1995;173:1089–1097.
29. Kniss D, Shubert P, Zimmerman P, Landon M, Gabbe S. Insulin-like growth factors: the regulation

of glucose and amino acid transport in placental trophoblasts isolated from first trimester chorionic villi. *J Reprod Med* 1994;39:249–256.
30. McGiven J, Pastor Angladi A. Regulatory and molecular aspects of mammalian amino acid transport. *Biochem J* 1993;299:321–334.
31. Smith CH, Moe A. Nutrient transport pathway across the epithelium of the placenta. *Annu Rev Nutr* 1992;12:183–206.
32. Moores R, Couter B, Meschia G, Fennessy P, Battaglia F. Placental and fetal serine fluxes at mid-gestation in the fetal lamb. *Am J Physiol* 1994;267:E150–E155.
33. Cetin I, Fennessy P, Sparks J, Meschia G, Battaglia F. Fetal serine fluxes across fetal liver, hindlimb, and placenta in late gestation. *Am J Physiol* 1992;263:E786–E793.
34. Guyton TS, Fennessey F, Battaglia F, Meschia G, Wilkening RB. Plasma lactate disposal, decarboxylation rate, and entry into the tricarboxycylic acid cycle in the fetal lamb. *FASEB J* 1994;8:A918(abst 5320).
35. Broeder J, Smith C, Moe H. Glutamate oxidation by trophoblast *in vitro*. *Am J Physiol* 1994;266: C189–C194.
36. Pines G, Danbolt NC, Bjoras M, Zhang Y, Bendahan A, Eide L, et al. Cloning and expression of a rat brain L-glutamate transporter. *Nature* 1992;360:464–467.
37. Storck T, Schulte S, Hofman K, Stoffel W. Structure, expression, and functional analysis of a Na^+-dependent glutamate/aspartate transporter from rat brain. *Proc Natl Acad Sci U S A* 1994;89: 10955–10959.
38. Kanai Y, Hediger M. Primary structure and functional characterization of a high affinity glutamate transporter. *Nature* 1992;360:467–471.
39. Nitzan M, Orloff S, Schulman J. Placental transfer of analogs of glucose and amino acids in experimental intrauterine growth retardation. *Pediatr Res* 1979;13:100–103.
40. Dicke JM, Henderson GI. Placental amino acid uptake in normal and complicated pregnancies. *Am J Med Sci* 1988;295:223–227.
41. Mahendran D, Donnai P, Glazier JD, D'Souza SW, Boyd RDH, Sibley CP. Amino acid (system A) transporter activity in microvillous membrane vesicles from the placentas of appropriate and small for gestational age babies. *Pediatr Res* 1993;34:661–666.
42. Kuruvilla A, D'Souza S, Glazier J, Mahendian D, Maresh M, Sibley C. Altered activity of system A amino acid transporter in microvillous membrane vesicles from placentas of macrosomic babies born to diabetic women. *J Clin Invest* 1994;94:689–695.
43. Glazier J, Sibley C, Carter M. Effect of fetal growth restriction on system A amino acid transporter activity in the maternal facing plasma membrane of rat syncytiotrophoblast. *Pediatr Res* 1996;40(2): 325–329.
44. Cetin I, Marconi A, Corbetta C, Lanfranchi A, Baggiani AM, Battaglia F, et al. Fetal amino acids in normal pregnancies and in pregnancies complicated by intrauterine growth retardation. *Early Hum Dev* 1992;29:183–186.
45. Marconi AM, Battaglia F, Meschia G, Sparks J. A comparison of amino acid arteriovenous differences across the liver and placenta of the fetal lamb. *Am J Physiol* 1989;257:E909–E915.
46. Liechty E, Denne S, Lemons J, Kien L. Effects of glucose infusion on leucine transamination and oxidation in the ovine fetus. *Pediatr Res* 1991;30:423–429.
47. Geddie S, Quick AN, Meschia G, Wilkening RB, Fennesey PV, Battaglia FC. Study of the transport of amino acids across the sheep placenta during non-steady state conditions. *Pediatr Res* 1992;3: 43A(abst).
48. Ross J, Fennessey R, Wilkening R, Battaglia F, Meschia G. Placental transport and fetal utilization of leucine in a model of fetal growth retardation. *Am J Physiol* 1996;270:E491–E503.
49. Cetin I, Marconi AM, Baggiani AM, Buscaglia M, Pardi G, Fennessey PV, et al. *In vivo* placental transport of glycine and leucine in human pregnancies. *Pediatr Res* 1995;37:571–575.
50. Tate S, Yan N, Udenfriend S. Expression cloning of a Na^+-independent neutral amino acid transporter from rat kidney. *Proc Natl Acad Sci U S A* 1992;89:1–5.
51. Lane RH, Flozak AS, Ogata ES, Simmons RA. Expression of a neutral amino acid transporter is down-regulated in growth-retarded fetal rat placenta. *J Invest Med* 1995;43.
52. Penfold P, Illsley N, Purkiss P, Jenning P. Human placental amino acid transfer and metabolism in oxygenated and anoxic conditions. *Trophoblast Res* 1983;1:27–36.
53. Schenker S, Dicke J, Johnson R, Hay S, Henderson GI. Effect of ethanol on human placental transport of amino acids and glucose. *Alcohol Clin Exp Res* 1989;13:112–119.
54. Patwardhan R, Schenker S, Henderson G, Abor Mourad N, Hoyumpa A. Short-term and long-term

ethanol administration inhibits the placental uptake and transport of valine in rat. *J Lab Clin Med* 1981;98:251–262.
55. Fisher S, Atkins M, Jacobson S, Sehgel L, Burnap J, Holmes E, *et al*. Selective fetal malnutrition: the effect of *in vivo* ethanol exposure upon *in vitro* placental uptake of amino acids in the non-human primate. *Pediatr Res* 1983;17:704–709.
56. Henderson G, Turner D, Patwardhan R, Lumey L, Hoyumpa A, Schenler S. Inhibition of placental valine uptake after acute and chronic maternal ethanol consumption. *J Pharmacol Exp Ther* 1981; 216:465–472.
57. Barnwell S, Ramsastry B. Depression of amino acid uptake in human placental villus by cocaine, morphine, and nicotine. *Trophoblast Res* 1983;1:101–120.

DISCUSSION

Dr. Talamantes: Why do you measure IGF-BP-1 in pregnancy in the rat? Is that the main binding protein?

Dr. Ogata: I did not show BP-3, I didn't want to go off on a tangent on the fetus, but we found that both BP-1 and BP-3 are up in the fetal rat; the whole issue of which is the more important binding protein is, I think, still up in the air.

Dr. Talamantes: I think just as important would be the protease, much more than the binding protein. Do you get an increase or an alteration of the BP protease?

Dr. Ogata: We have no data.

Dr. Talamantes: When you measure protein for glucose transporter and say it is up or down, how do you know that the structure of the receptor itself isn't altered, and how do you account for alterations in the structure of the transporter?

Dr. Ogata: In the placenta we have not done actual glucose transport studies. In our other fetal organs we have done both *in vivo* and *in vitro* studies to look at deoxyglucose uptake. So I think we feel reasonably comfortable that function correlates with what we see with respect to protein and NMR. But I should caution that we have not done any isolated vesicle work in the placenta.

Dr. Rennie: Was that NAT transporter actually the Tates clone?

Dr. Ogata: Yes.

Dr. Rennie: So are you aware that there is a lot of controversy about whether that is indeed a transporter?

Dr. Ogata: In Tates' article, he says it is the system L transporter. I realize it has gone back and forth as to what it is, and I think there was also a suggestion that it may be a co-transporter rather than a system L.

Dr. Rennie: I think there is a lot of evidence that it is an amino acid transport activator, which of course would be very interesting, because it appears that if you inject it into oocytes it causes such a widespread increase in amino acid transport that it is almost inconceivable that a single transporter of protein is responsible for the phenomena observed. Therefore, that is the evidence that it is actually some kind of activator. The other thing is that it has only three membrane-spanning domains, so it doesn't look like a conventional transporter, but it would be very interesting if a single protein regulated a whole lot of other proteins in a coordinated fashion.

Dr. Ogata: This is the whole issue of trying to get at the molecular biology of amino acid transporters. There has been such a tremendous amount of work done to characterize these on a physiologic level, but again this particular transporter was received from complementary DNA from kidney injected into oocytes, and so we are going in the other direction here.

Dr. Rennie: I think that we have to address an important theoretical issue that often seems to get much behind, which is that for amino acid transport in terms of metabolism what is important is the relation between the first-order rate constant for transport—in other words, the ratio between V_{max} and K_m, and the necessary rate of disposal for appropriate growth. I think there is a good possibility that for the branched-chain amino acids and possibly a couple of others, including maybe methionine for other reasons, there is the strong likelihood that a decrease in transporter activity would be important in limiting protein accretion. But I find it very hard to believe that transporters that transport nonessential amino acids, with the possible exception of glycine or serine if collagen synthesis is important, really matter very much at all. I think this is something that people often don't think about—whether there is just such a large capacity there that it doesn't really matter if you halve it or reduce it by 75%, and so far we have not really attempted to match up the numbers here. I think that is something we should be constrained to do—to really see to what extent a fall of 75% would make any difference whatsoever in the capacity of the placenta to deliver sufficient amino acids. It is something we should keep in mind.

Dr. Sibley: We found a decrease in system A activity, and the human data suggest that there is a decreased fetal plasma concentration of amino acids that would be transported by that transporter, so the two do go together, although I accept what you say, that you have to do the calculations. Nevertheless, the data suggest that the two go together. But we must not forget a whole raft of things we don't know about: we know only about the microvillous membrane—we don't know if that's rate-limiting; the basal plasma membrane might be rate-limiting for transports; and we don't know anything about the basal membrane in IUGR. We know that amino acid transporters, particularly system A, are affected by a number of variables, such as the intracellular concentration of amino acids—system A shows *trans* inhibition—and we don't know what the concentrations of amino acids in the syncytiotrophoblast are in IUGR. We also know that system A is affected by pH and we don't know what the pH of the trophoblast is in IUGR; we do know that the IUGR fetus is acidemic. So I absolutely agree with you, we are at a very basic level in understanding this problem, and we should not forget all the complications involved.

Dr. Battaglia: There is another point, though, that maybe got lost. It is not just a matter of how much you need for protein synthesis, because you are oxidizing essential amino acids and you are losing them from the fetal circulation into the placenta. For the only one for which we have really good data, leucine (in the heat stress model), the fetus makes an interesting adjustment. It lowers the concentration, and because oxidation rate is driven by concentration, this leads to a lower oxidation rate. The back flux is also concentration-dependent, so you reduce the loss of leucine to the placenta. So with one simple step, you have adjusted the outflow of leucine and redirected it to protein synthesis. The real question is: what are the endocrine regulators that led to resetting leucine concentration lower? The lowering of leucine concentration should not be interpreted as implying that the placenta is not working. This is a resetting, which has very significant survival value to the fetus, because it is redirecting output towards accretion and away from oxidation and loss into the placenta. So far, we have studied only one amino acid in detail, but there the situation is clear.

Dr. Rennie: I think that one of the fascinating links here might be transport of methionine, because if serine is making mainly glycine, then you have to have some methyl groups to get that reaction to go, so the one-carbon pool is going to be important there.

Dr. Battaglia: You don't need the methyl group for glycine production, you need it for resynthesizing serine, and that goes on in the liver.

Dr. Rennie: But nevertheless there is going to be a requirement for that if that is to happen. Methionine is something we haven't really looked at, and the cysteine-methionine metabolism is likely to be very important.

Dr. Battaglia: I agree with you.

Fetal Lipid Requirements: Implications in Fetal Growth Retardation

Jacqueline Jumpsen, John Van Aerde, and M. Thomas Clandinin

Nutrition and Metabolism Research Group, University of Alberta, Edmonton, Alberta, Canada T6G 2P5, and University of Alberta Hospitals, Edmonton, Alberta T6G 2B7, Canada

The importance of lipid metabolism in intrauterine growth retardation (IUGR) has not been extensively studied. Although little is known of the effect of marginal dietary intakes of essential fatty acids on fetal lipid metabolism, there is evidence that placental lipids of infants that are small for gestational age (SGA) are low in 20:4 n-6 and 22:6 n-3. There also is evidence that the placenta transports long-chain polyunsaturated essential fatty acids from the maternal to the fetal circulation. The degree to which the placenta may modify the essential fatty acid precursors, 18:2 n-6 and 18:3 n-3, to longer-chain homologues utilized in fetal tissue synthesis is unknown and is central to understanding whether or not reduced placental transfer of 20:4 n-6 and 22:6 n-3 limits fetal growth. It is also not clear whether limited transfer of 20:4 n-6 and 22:6 n-3 by the placenta may arise from limitations inherent in the metabolic capability of the placenta, or whether it is caused by marginal or low maternal intake of essential fatty acid precursors. Nutritional status of the mother during gestation has been related to fetal growth. In general, reduced nutritional status with respect to n-6 and n-3 essential fatty acids has been correlated with reduced neonatal growth and head circumference. These observations also associate lower nutritional status with lower scores for some behavioral assessments in infants. During the last trimester of gestation, large amounts of essential and nonessential fatty acids are utilized in the synthesis of fetal tissues. The degree to which reduced accretion of lipid is caused by reduced placental transfer of lipid is not clear, nor are the mechanisms that limit fat accretion in the SGA infant apparent.

INTRAUTERINE/FETAL GROWTH RETARDATION

Intrauterine growth retardation is a common generic clinical term used to describe the perinate with a birth weight at or below a specific weight percentile for sex and gestational age. In North America, the 10th centile for birth weight is used. In Britain and Europe, an infant is considered growth-retarded if the birth weight is at or below the third percentile, or is two standard deviations below normal. As part of the clinical definition, IUGR is a result of pathologic processes inhibiting the normal intrinsic growth potential of the fetus. Comparatively, SGA infants are clinically distinct from intrauterine growth-retarded infants by the absence of pathologic processes. SGA infants are considered normal small fetuses, reflecting the normal but lower distribution of perinatal weight. Much of the current literature, however, does not make this distinction, and in most discussions the two terms appear synonymous. Further research is needed to develop more appropriate definitions of IUGR, focusing more on qualitative aspects of growth than on size (1). Quality or "composition" of growth must also be distinguished from quantity of growth. Determining which tissues grow or fail to grow if nutrition or placental function is compromised may be important to developmental progress of the fetus/infant.

The causes associated with growth retardation are a result of fetal, maternal, and placental disorders working alone or in combination. Nutritional deficiencies affecting fetal growth may result from any of these disorders. In some fetal disorders (e.g., inborn errors of metabolism), nutritional status and growth of the fetus may be affected by the inability to metabolize or utilize certain nutrients. Placental function and nutritional status of the mother during gestation are also related to fetal growth. Inadequate placental vascular development, site of placental development in the uterus, placental function, or maternal nutritional status have been related to the development of intrauterine or fetal growth retardation (1,2). These inadequacies may affect the transport of nutrients from the mother to the fetus. Although the potential impact of disturbed fatty acid transport on the development of fetal growth retardation is unknown, a study comparing the fatty acid composition of placentae from term and preterm human pregnancies has been reported (3). Fatty acids in total triacylglycerol and in phosphatidylcholine and phosphatidylethanolamine phosphoglycerides of placental membrane phospholipids from appropriate-for-gestational-age (AGA) and SGA infants were studied. No differences in the content of triacylglycerol between AGA and SGA placentae was observed. However, a reduction of n-6 fatty acids, particularly 20:3 n-6 and 20:4 n-6, in SGA placental triacylglycerol fatty acids was noted. A reduction in n-3 fatty acids, especially 22:6 n-3 in phosphatidylcholine, was also reported. The investigators suggested that these changes in fatty acid composition in placental membrane phospholipids can affect the transport of important nutrients to the fetus as well as alter the formation of eicosanoids. Although it is not certain how these changes in the placenta affect the fetus, a study by Al *et al.* (4) noted that the placenta is, for the most part, a fetal organ. Thus, it is possible that significant correlations between placental weight and some fetal fatty acid values may be explained by the closer similarity of placental to fetal plasma fatty acid composition than to maternal plasma fatty acid composition (4).

In an assessment of 1560 intrauterine growth-retarded fetuses, it was reported that the risk for perinatal mortality and morbidity progressively increases with decreasing birth weight (5). These infants of low birth weight are at highest risk for brain- and nervous system-related handicaps (6). Because the brain is one of the most lipid-concentrated organs in the body, the lipid requirements and supply during fetal growth are of critical importance.

ROLE OF LIPIDS IN THE DEVELOPING FETUS

Developmental processes in fetal growth occur in a critical sequence over a limited period of time. The significance of lipids during these developmental periods is well established (7–9), and their supply is in high demand. Dietary fat provides the main energy store in pregnancy, is the vehicle for supply of lipid-soluble vitamins, and has functional significance by providing structural components of cell membranes, particularly during the processes of cellular multiplication, differentiation, and cell-to-cell interactions. Furthermore, the 20-carbon polyunsaturated fatty acids are precursors for a group of biologically active compounds. These compounds are the eicosanoids and include thromboxanes, prostaglandins, prostacyclins, leukotrienes, lipoxins, and hydroperoxy and hydroxy fatty acids. The profile of eicosanoids formed can be altered with a change in dietary balance of n-6 and n-3 fatty acids. Eicosanoids are involved in regulation of diverse physiologic processes. This diversity depends on which essential fatty acid precursor is predominant, the site of its release, and the subsequent eicosanoid profile synthesized. The physiologic processes vary from inflammatory and hypersensitivity reactions to control of vasoconstrictive and thrombogenic activities (10). Two such processes relevant to fetal nourishment and parturition are regulation of blood flow and coagulation.

Synthesis of C-20 and C-22 polyunsaturated fatty acids, in particular arachidonic and docosahexaenoic acids, occurs by the desaturation and elongation of the essential fatty acids linoleic (18:2 n-6) and α-linolenic (18:3 n-3) acids, respectively. Both arachidonic acid (20:4 n-6) and docosahexaenoic acid (22:6 n-3) are key components of all membranes but are particularly enriched in neural, mitochondrial, and vascular membranes. These two fatty acids are readily incorporated into the structural lipids of the developing brain (10). As the degree to which the fetus is capable of desaturation and elongation is not clear, the supply of essential fatty acids and long-chain polyunsaturated fatty acids is critical and central to the synthesis of structural lipids and hence to normal development of the fetus (7,11–13). With respect to lipid requirements during development, a large number of changes occur in body composition in the developing fetus during the third trimester of pregnancy. This period encompasses a major change in both body composition of the fetus—involving a rapid increase in adipose tissue development—and growth of the brain, an organ also highly concentrated in complex lipids (14). The rate of incorporation of long-chain polyunsaturated fatty acids is high in growing tissues, particularly in brain structures (15–17). Hence, the third trimester shows the largest quantitative requirement for essential fatty acids and thus for supply of long-chain polyunsaturated fatty acids. It has also been suggested that the last trimester is the time when IUGR is most common and usually most pronounced (18).

SPINAL COLUMN AND LIVER

Accretion rates for fatty acids obtained from fetal and infant spinal cord were quantitatively assessed by Clandinin et al. (16). Sample spinal cord segments from the level of C-1 and L3-4 vertebrae were obtained during autopsy. Accretion of approximately 5.4 mg of fatty acid per gram of tissue in the cervical region occurred during the last trimester of pregnancy. During this period, saturated and n-9 monounsaturated fatty acids are the primary ones deposited (45% and 18% of total tissue fatty acids, respectively). Accretion of fatty acids from the n-6 family was also apparent, representing 16% of fatty acids. Accretion in the lumbar region during the last trimester was lower, but increased during the first 13 weeks of life. An estimated 0.88 mg of n-6 and 0.13 mg of n-3 fatty acids accrue in the cervical region of the spinal cord during the last trimester of fetal development. This accretion of fatty acids parallels increasing neuromotor spinal functions and postnatal development of coordinated motor activity (16).

SOURCES OF LIPIDS IN THE DEVELOPING FETUS

Fetal demands for lipids are met by both placental transfer and endogenous synthesis (14,19). Similar to the adult, the human fetus cannot synthesize the essential fatty acids 18:2 n-6 and 18:3 n-3. Thus, the fetus relies on deriving these fatty acids from the maternal blood across the placenta. Robertson and Sprecher (20) noted that the free fatty acid content of the placenta is different from that of maternal plasma, suggesting that sources other than maternal circulation exist for the derivation of some components of the placental free fatty acid pool. The amount transported and the mechanism by which these fatty acids reach the fetus from the maternal circulation remain to be clarified. Placental transfer of long-chain polyunsaturated fatty acids in mammals is well established. Arachidonic acid and docosahexaenoic acid concentrations increase in the fetus as gestational age increases (20–22). Although the mechanism responsible for this transfer is not clear, it has been suggested that either the fetal or placental capacity to form the longer-chain fatty acids from parent fatty acids is increased, or that a preferential transfer of the longer-chain fatty acids across the placenta from the maternal to fetal circulation occurs (23,24). Both fetal plasma (25) and fetal erythrocytes (26) have been suggested to play a major role in the transport of essential fatty acids into the fetus. Carrier proteins have also been implicated in the uptake of polyunsaturated fatty acids in fetal rat hepatocytes (27). Previous observations suggested that sufficient amounts of long-chain n-6 and n-3 fatty acids for deposition in growing tissues could easily be synthesized from precursor fatty acids in full-term and preterm infants. However, Clandinin et al. (15,16) showed a lag in accretion of brain and liver long-chain polyenoic fatty acids during fetal development. A lag in the mobilization of essential fatty acid deposits in the liver has been demonstrated for a varying period of time following birth (17).

Thus, it is likely that synthesis of chain-elongated and -desaturated fatty acids limits maximum postnatal accretion of these essential fatty acids. In this regard, the concept that intrauterine accretion of long-chain polyenoic fatty acids occurs primarily as a function of mechanisms involving placental transfer is consistent with observations reported by other investigators (4,28).

FETAL LIPID REQUIREMENTS

Although the requirement for lipids in the developing fetus persists throughout gestation, the supply of lipid becomes critically important in the third trimester. This trimester is a period of rapid brain growth and rapid accretion of body fat depots, subject to adequate supply of energy to the fetus. At 28 weeks of gestation, accretion of fat in the normal fetus ranges between 1.2 and 1.8 g/kg/d. By 36 to 40 weeks of gestation, fat accretion is approximately linear, ranging between 1.6 and 3.4 g/kg/d (29). Fatty acid analysis of brain tissue from various species indicates that this complex organ contains large amounts of long-chain polyunsaturated fatty acids, predominantly 20:4 n-6 and 22:6 n-3. These long-chain fatty acids accrue substantially during the last trimester of development in brain (15). Accretion of n-9 and saturated fatty acids also occurs at this time. No significant accretion of 18:2 n-6 and 18:3 n-3 was noted during the last trimester (7). An increase in all long-chain polyunsaturated fatty acids has also been reported in cord blood plasma phospholipids in infants between 24 and 44 weeks of gestation (30).

Analysis of fatty acid accretion in fetal liver enabled assessment of minimal fatty acid requirements for tissue synthesis. The liver contains a significant amount of 20n-6 and 22n-3 fatty acids at the end of the second trimester and during the early period of the third trimester of fetal development. During the progression of the third trimester, liver weight, when expressed in grams per kilogram of body weight, decreases as total body weight increases; thus, the liver represents a declining potential reserve of essential fatty acids for the developing fetus (17).

Beyond 30 weeks of gestation, accumulation of fat considerably exceeds that of nonfat components (29). Fetal requirements (mean ± 2 SD) for essential fatty acids and long-chain fatty acids are estimated to be 1100 mg of n-6 fatty acids per day (400 mg/kg of body weight) and 140 mg of n-3 fatty acids per day (50 mg/kg of body weight) (14), based on analysis of fatty acid accretion and estimates for tissue synthesis in fetal brain, liver, and adipose tissue. Rapid accretion of n-6 and n-3 long-chain polyenoic fatty acids in the fetal brain has been indicated by examination of intrauterine fatty acid accretion (15). During the last trimester, the major fatty acids to accrue in the brain are the chain elongation-desaturation products. It is estimated that the developing brain accumulates approximately 43 mg of n-6 polyenoic and 22 mg of n-3 polyenoic fatty acids per week (14). Examination of accretion of fatty acids in the fetal liver from 22 weeks of gestation to term indicates that 13.5 mg of n-6 and 3.8 mg of n-3 fatty acids accrue per week (17).

RELATIONSHIP BETWEEN FATTY ACIDS AND FETAL GROWTH

As the fetus grows and develops, body mass increases between the end of the first trimester and term. During this period there is less reliance on hyperplasia and more on cellular hypertrophy accompanying tissue maturation. In the third trimester, this increase in body mass represents in part preparation for extrauterine life, as adiposity and glycogen storage increase. An increase in the number of cells and tissue formation require formation of new membranes, most of which are high in arachidonic and docosahexaenoic acids (31). Thus, it is logical that these fatty acids must be related to tissue growth. Dynamic markers of circulating pools providing these essential fatty acids are not clear postnatally, but lipoprotein phospholipid and cholesterol ester fractions are likely candidates (32).

Research by Leaf et al. (12) examined the relation between plasma choline phosphoglyceride long-chain polyunsaturated fatty acid composition and measurements of fetal growth and maturity. Analysis indicated a strong correlation of 22:6 n-3 content in plasma phosphatidylcholine with gestational age as well as with fetal head circumference and birth weight. Arachidonic acid correlated most strongly with weight and head circumference. In a study of infants of low birth weight, a relation was found between the long-chain n-6 and n-3 essential fatty acids, birth weight, and head circumference (28). The authors suggest that this does not necessarily imply that low birth weight is a result of essential fatty acid deficiency, but suggests that the relation of lipids to vascular nutrition may be important in placental and fetal development. Research by Koletzko and Braun (33) also provides evidence for a positive correlation between arachidonic acid, as measured in plasma triglyceride content, and body weight. As plasma triglyceride primarily reflects dietary intake, and protein and energy intakes were not controlled in this study, it is not clear how 20:4 n-6 levels in plasma triglycerides might be related to growth. A recent study (11) examined the relation of long-chain polyunsaturated fatty acid supply with prenatal growth. This study analyzed long-chain polyenoic fatty acids in phospholipids from plasma and erythrocytes from the umbilical artery wall. Fifty-two preterm infants ranging in weight from 650 to 1860 g and with gestational ages between 26 and 36 weeks were investigated. Because plasma phospholipids are affected by relatively short-term dietary influences, measures from umbilical artery walls were used as longer-term indicators of long-chain polyenoic status. Results indicate that the relative amounts of n-6 and n-3 long-chain polyenoic fatty acids in umbilical artery walls and relative amounts of n-3 long-chain polyenes in cord plasma were positively correlated with gestational age. Levels of docosahexaenoic acid measured in the arterial cord vessel walls were significantly correlated with weight, head circumference, and length at birth, independently of gestational age at birth. This study suggests that a striking relation exists between docosahexaenoic acid status and prenatal growth. An earlier experiment (34) also examined the relation of fatty acid composition of umbilical artery and vein wall to normal or retarded fetal growth. SGA infants in this study were identified by an abdominal circumference of less than the 10th centile for gestational age. Levels of docosahexaenoic acid measured in the umbilical venous and arterial wall were positively associated with birth weight and head circumference. Carlson et al. (35) have related plasma phosphatidylcholine 20:4 n-6 concentrations in preterm infants to growth, and 20:5 n-3 levels to reduction in growth.

Ontogeny of the human fetal gastrointestinal tract occurs between the 14th day of gestation and the 12th week of embryonic life, by which time glucose and amino acids are actively transported (36). By 26 weeks of intrauterine life, the fetus has the capacity for limited digestion and absorption. Before this, functional development is limited. The development may be influenced by the intrauterine nutritional state of the fetus. In rats, malnourishment at this stage or postnatally alters normal morphologic and functional maturation of the intestinal tract (A.B.R. Thomson and M.T. Clandinin, *unpublished observations*). In suckling rats, the brush border membrane lipid composition can also be influenced by dietary composition, which can alter enterocyte enzyme activity and transport properties. The effect of maternal diet on the developing intestinal tract *in utero* is unknown, as are changes that may be occurring in fatty acid-containing components of the amniotic fluid. However, it appears that early nutritional uptake has effects on intestinal function in later life.

The effects of lipids on growth of the fetus may also occur indirectly, through hormonal control of various systems. Hormonal effects on development have been shown to exist at the level of the central nervous system. Thyroid hormone in particular has been shown to control at least two very important steps of brain maturation: neurite outgrowth and myelination (37). Deficiency or excess of thyroid hormone can alter the distribution of catecholamine receptors or acquisition of muscarinic receptors. In a recent study (M.T. Clandinin et al., *unpublished observations*), raised levels of thyroid stimulating hormone occurred in developing rat pups fed diets reflecting the composition of a current infant formula containing physiologic amounts of 22:6 n-3. These results suggest that changes in the balance of 20:4 n-6 to 22:6 n-3 during the development of neural-endocrine tissues can affect metabolic controls by endocrine mechanisms.

Hormones also control the regulation of fetal lung surfactant glycerophospholipid. Pulmonary surfactant consists of 90% lipid and is synthesized and assembled by alveolar epithelial cells. The main function of surfactant is to decrease surface tension, protecting the alveoli against collapse. This property is primarily conferred by dipalmitoyl phosphatidylcholine. The other major lipid components include unsaturated phosphatidylcholine and phosphatidylglycerol. Among the hormonal regulators of lung surfactant are glucocorticoids, prolactin, thyroid hormones, estrogens, androgens, growth factors, insulin, catecholamines, and cyclic AMP (38). Prostaglandins have also been identified as mediators of lung growth as well as surfactant secretion (38). The impact of fetal lipid metabolism on development and maturation of this critical functional constituent in the lung is not well known.

REFERENCES

1. Pollack RN, Divon MY. Intrauterine growth retardation: definition, classification and etiology. *Clin Obstet Gynecol* 1992;35:99–107.

2. Zamenhof S, Van Martens E. Nutritional influence on prenatal brain development. In: Gottlieb G, ed. *Early Influences*. New York: Academic Press; 1978:149–186
3. Percy P, Vilbergsson G, Percy A, Månsson J-E, Wennergren M, Svennerholm L. The fatty acid composition of placenta in intrauterine growth retardation. *Biochim Biophys Acta* 1991;1084: 173–177.
4. Al MDM, Van Houwelingen AC, Kester ADM, Hasaart THM, DeJong AEP, Hornstra G. Maternal essential fatty acid patterns and their relationship to the neonatal essential fatty acid status. *Br J Nutr* 1995;74:55–68.
5. Allen MC. Developmental outcome and follow-up of the small for gestational age infant. *Semin Perinatol* 1984;8:102.
6. Usher RH, McLean FH. In: Davis JA, Dobbing J, eds. *Scientific Foundations of Paediatrics*. London: Heinemann; 1964:69.
7. Clandinin MT, Chappell JE, Leong S, Heim T, Swyer PR, Chance GW. Intrauterine fatty acid accretion rates in human brain: implications for fatty acid requirements. *Early Hum Dev* 1980;4: 121–129.
8. Jumpsen J, Clandinin MT. *Brain Development: Relationship to Dietary Lipid and Lipid Metabolism*. Champaign, IL: AOCS Press; 1995.
9. Martinez M. Developmental profiles of polyunsaturated fatty acids in the brain of normal infants and patients with peroxisomal diseases: severe deficiency of docosahexaenoic acid in Zellweger's and pseudo Zellweger's syndromes. *World Rev Nutr Diet* 1991;66:87–102.
10. Crawford MA, Hassam AG, Williams G, Whitehouse WL. Essential fatty acids and fetal brain growth. *Lancet* 1976;1:452–453.
11. Foreman-van Drongelen MMHP, van Houwelingen AC, Kester ADM, Hasaart THM, Blanco CE, Hornstra G. Long-chain polyunsaturated fatty acids in preterm infants: status at birth and its influence on postnatal levels. *J Pediatr* 1995;126:611–618.
12. Leaf AA, Leightfield MJ, Casteloe KL, Crawford MA. Long-chain polyunsaturated fatty acids and fetal growth. *Early Hum Dev* 1992;30:183–191.
13. Neuringer M, Connor WE. Omega-3 fatty acids in the brain and retina: evidence for their essentiality. *Nutr Rev* 1986;44:285–294.
14. Clandinin MT, Chappell JE, Heim T, Swyer PR, Chance GW. Fatty acid utilization in perinatal *de novo* synthesis of tissues. *Early Hum Dev* 1981;5:355–366.
15. Clandinin MT, Chappell JE, Leong S, Heim T, Swyer PR, Chance GW. Intrauterine fatty acid accretion rates in human brain: implications for fatty acid requirements. *Early Hum Dev* 1980;4: 121–129.
16. Clandinin MT, Chappell JE, Heim T, Swyer PR, Chance GW. Fatty acid accretion in the development of human spinal cord. *Early Hum Dev* 1981;5:1–6.
17. Clandinin MT, Chappell JE, Heim T, Swyer PR, Chance GW. Fatty acid accretion in fetal and neonatal liver: implications for fatty acid requirements. *Early Hum Dev* 1981;5:7–14.
18. Vilbergsson G, Samsioe G, Wennergren M, Karlsson K. Essential fatty acids in pregnancies complicated by intrauterine growth retardation. *Int J Gynaecol Obstet* 1991;36:277–286.
19. Warshaw JB. Fatty acid metabolism during development. *Semin Perinatol* 1979;3:131.
20. Robertson AF, Sprecher H. A review of human placental lipid metabolism and transport. *Acta Paediatr Scand* 1968;Suppl 183:2–18.
21. Menon NK, Dhopeshwarkar GA. Essential fatty acid deficiency and brain development. *Prog Lipid Res* 1986;25:355–364.
22. Poissennet CM, Lavelle M, Burdi AR. Growth and development of adipose tissue. *J Pediatr* 1988; 113:1–9.
23. Neuringer M, Connor WE, Van Patten C, Barstad L. Dietary omega-3 fatty acid deficiency and visual loss in infant rhesus monkeys. *J Clin Invest* 1984;73:272–276.
24. Kuhn DC, Crawford M. Placental essential fatty acid transport and prostaglandin synthesis. *Prog Lipid Res* 1986;25:345–353.
25. Matorras R, Perteagudo L, Nieto A, Sanjurjo P. Intrauterine growth retardation and plasma fatty acids in the mother and the fetus. *Eur J Obstet Gynecol Reprod Biol* 1994;57:189–193.
26. Ruyle M, Connor WE, Anderson GJ, Lowensohn RL. Placental transfer of essential fatty acids in humans: venous-arterial difference for docosahexaenoic acid in fetal umbilical erythrocytes. *Proc Natl Acad Sci U S A* 1990;87:7902–7906.
27. Inturralde M, Alva MA, Gonzalez B, Anel A, Pineiro A. Effect of alpha-fetoprotein and albumin

on the uptake of polyunsaturated fatty acids by rat hepatoma and fetal rat hepatocytes. *Biochim Biophys Acta* 1991;1086:81–88.
28. Crawford MA, Doyle W, Drury P, Lennon A, Costeloe K, Leighfield M. n-6 and n-3 fatty acids during early human development. *J Intern Med* 1989;225:159–169.
29. Heim T. Energy and lipid requirements of the fetus and the preterm infant. *J Pediatr Gastroenterol Nutr* 1983;2:1–16.
30. Friedman Z, Danon A, Lamberth EL, Mann WJ. Cord blood fatty acid composition in infants and their mothers during the third trimester. *J Pediatr* 1978;92:461.
31. Clandinin MT. Infant nutrition: effects of lipid on later life. *Curr Opin Lipidol* 1995;6:28–31.
32. Clandinin MT, Zuberbuhler P, Brown NE, Kielo ES, Goh YK. Fatty acid pool size in plasma lipoprotein fractions of cystic fibrosis patients. *Am J Clin Nutr* 1995;62:1268–1275.
33. Koletzko B, Braun M. Arachidonic acid and early human growth: is there a relation? *Ann Nutr Metab* 1991;35:128–131.
34. Felton CV, Chang TC, Crook D, Marsh M, Robson SC, Spencer JAD. Umbilical vessel wall fatty acids after normal and retarded fetal growth. *Arch Dis Child* 1994;70:F36–F37.
35. Carlson SE, Werkman SH, Peeples JM, Cooke RJ, Tolley EA. Arachidonic acid status correlates with first-year growth in preterm infants. *Proc Natl Acad Sci U S A* 1993;90:1073–1077.
36. Thomson ABR, Keelan M. The development of the small intestine. *Can J Physiol Pharmacol* 1986;64:13–29.
37. Nunez J. Effects of thyroid hormones during brain differentiation. *Mol Cell Endocrinol* 1984;7:125–132.
38. Mendelson CR, Boggaram V. Hormonal control of the surfactant system in fetal lung. *Annu Rev Physiol* 1991;53:415–440.

DISCUSSION

Dr. Battaglia: During the last day and half, we have talked about the asymmetric growth-retarded baby. It is certainly true that statistically the brain is closer to normal weight than is body weight or other anthropomorphic measurements, but the question of whether it has developed normally in IUGR fetuses is a big one for me. Looking at your data on the distribution of the many long-chain polyunsaturated fatty acids present in the brain, it almost looks like a way in which you can "fingerprint" a tissue. I wonder whether you have looked at normal infants and IUGR infants with supposed brain sparing who have died for other reasons in terms of brain composition?

Dr. Clandinin: No, but we have perhaps done one half of it. We have characterized the compositional changes in neuronal and glial cells in the rat during development and in response to different diet treatments, and it would be fairly easy for us to begin to compare those data with some of the rat models. It would be a very good thing to do.

Dr. Haschke: Data on DHA (docosahexaenoic acid) and arachidonic acid in infant brains indicate that arachidonic acid is not influenced by diet, whereas the DHA concentration in the brain is much influenced by the diet. It is highest in fish eaters and lowest in vegetarians.

Dr. Clandinin: I have seen those data, and one of the difficulties is the way the analyses are expressed as a relative % fatty acid analysis as opposed to a microgram per gram of total tissue quantitative analysis. So it is an interesting observation, but it's difficult to compare it to this kind of data. I guess what you are alluding to is that if the DHA content or the EPA content of the diet varies a lot, the omega-3 would vary, whereas the arachidonic is relatively constant. My interpretation of that would be that arachidonate is one of the really major components in brain, and what I feared about some of the earlier studies in which infants were fed fish oil was that you would compromise arachidonate status unless you fed arachidonate. I guess what one would need to look at in the Gibson data is whether in specific cases in which the dietary DHA was high, was the arachidonate lower? I don't know the answer to that.

Dr. Haschke: The data for preterm infants who were fed fish oil-supplemented formula (containing 0.2% DHA, 0.3% EPA) without arachidonic acid indicated that arachidonic acid in plasma and red blood cells was suppressed (1). Moreover, in these infants, it was shown that linear growth was also suppressed (2). However, it seems that if formulas with lower levels of DHA are fed, arachidonic acid in plasma and red blood cells is no more suppressed. Gibson has unpublished data for infants who were given DHA and GLA (τ-linolenic acid), who therefore didn't receive arachidonic acid but received a precursor. In those infants, arachidonic acid and DHA in erythrocytes and plasma were very close to the values in breast-fed infants. So it seems to be a matter of balance how much we give to infants. However, it is likely that premature infants deviate from term infants as far as requirements are concerned.

Dr. Clandinin: Your point is a good one in that it is a matter of balance between the two, because basically both use the same pathways. In terms of the Carlson study, probably the early effect on the arachidonate was a result of that the way those infants were supplemented with fish oil also provided a significant amount of EPA, and that probably wasn't a good thing to do. It is now possible, as you know, to develop a feed without the EPA so you can avoid that problem.

Dr. Williams: Your estimated weekly requirements for long-chain n-3 polyunsaturated fatty acids, based on the tissue accretion, are actually fairly close to the mean adult weekly intakes of those fatty acids in the UK. How would you suggest that these requirements are being met?

Dr. Clandinin: Certainly we would expect that on a per kilogram basis the requirement of the infant would be high compared with an adult because of the intensive tissue growth that is going on. If you do the same kind of calculations from intakes of human milk, you come up with similar numbers.

Dr. Williams: But *in utero* how are they being met?

Dr. Clandinin: In utero I think we know that the essential fatty acids cross the placenta. There have been early suggestions, from some of the Crawford work that has not been followed up. There may even be selective transfer of some of the chain-elongated forms of the essential fatty acids, but in terms of essential fatty acid transfer and metabolism by placenta to fetus, this is an unstudied area.

Dr. Williams: But would you suggest that there would have to be selective mobilization of these fatty acids from the maternal adipose tissue stores? If the dietary intakes are equivalent only to the fetal requirements, the mother's requirements and the fetal requirements could not be met.

Dr. Clandinin: There are two aspects in that question. One is that the adipose store of the mother is actually rather large with respect to essential fatty acids, and the other is that what we recommend for an adult as a minimum requirement is vastly below what they normally eat—what they normally eat is an order of magnitude greater than what we recommend as a minimum intake.

Dr. Page: It might be pertinent just to comment on the recent study we have been completing in my laboratory in Aberdeen. We did a perfused placental study in which we were able to demonstrate that there was indeed an enhanced transfer of linoleic and α-linolenic acids compared with oleic, and also of DHA, which was even greater. We were unable to find any evidence of chain elongation in our study, and we could not actually demonstrate any enhanced transfer of arachidonic acid. We are following that up, but we think it is metabolized very quickly in the perfused placenta.

Dr. Godfrey: It is important that we do not overinterpret the Leaf data (3) on head circumference and concentrations. Firstly, it is not adjusted for gestational age, and secondly, head circumference at birth is very strongly tied in with placental size, and reduced placental transfer of fatty acids may underlie the lower concentrations. So I think it is very dangerous to infer cause and effect there. Secondly, in relation to the socioeconomic differences in birth weight, differences in maternal size account for a part of that, and differences in maternal smoking for another part of that gradient. Having said that, the WIC (women-infants-children) Nutritional Supplementation Program in the United States was not associated with consistent increases in birth weight, but it was associated with consistent increases in head circumference at birth. So there is a very complex set of areas to address there. In our data from Southampton, we find relations between the mothers' diet and fetal growth that occur at all levels of maternal social class (4). So I think it is dangerous to point specifically towards essential fatty acids; there is a whole series of issues that needs to be addressed.

Dr. Clandinin: I would agree with you. To come back to the serine and glycine story, I actually don't think that serine in liver goes to glycine; I think its purpose is to make choline.

Dr. Battaglia: I guess what we mean by *essential* is that all those nutrients need to be there in adequate amounts, and you have called attention to one set of structural compounds that are needed. I think it is interesting to start working on the placental delivery of these compounds—we need to know a lot more about them. Every time I hear a discussion of diet and fetal growth, I keep thinking of the marvelous biologic example that I know most of you are aware of—hibernation. Bears that hibernate don't eat and they don't drink water, but they produce very nice baby bears that are not growth-retarded. So you can build a perfectly normal baby without any intake in the mother provided there is a mechanism that stops all nitrogen loss. I guess that what we are trying to find out for human is that when you have a restriction, what are the adaptive mechanisms that are made successfully in one pregnancy and not so successfully in another?

REFERENCES

1. Carlson SE, Cooke RJ, Rhodes PG, *et al.* Long-term feeding of formulas high in linolenic acid and marine oil to very low birth weight infants: phospholipid fatty acids. *Pediatr Res* 1991;30:404–412.
2. Carlson SE, Cooke RJ, Werkman SH, Tolley EA. First year growth of preterm infants fed standard compared to marine oil n-3 supplemented formula. *Lipids* 1992;27:901–907.
3. Leaf AA, Leighfield MJ, Costeloe KL, Crawford MA. Long chain polyunsaturated fatty acids and fetal growth. *Early Hum Dev* 1992;30:183–191.
4. Godfrey KM, Robinson S, Barker DJP, Osmond C, Cox V. Maternal nutrition in early and late pregnancy in relation to placental and fetal growth. *Br Med J* 1996;312:410–414.

Placental Function and Fetal Nutrition,
edited by Frederick C. Battaglia,
Nestlé Nutrition Workshop Series, Vol. 39.
Nestec Ltd., Vevey/Lippincott-Raven Publishers,
Philadelphia, © 1997.

Maternal Lipid Metabolism and Its Implications for Fetal Growth

Emilio Herrera and Maria A. Munilla

Facultad de Ciencias Experimentales y Técnicas, Universidad San Pablo-CEU, Boadilla E-28668, Madrid, Spain

During gestation, the mother has to adapt her own metabolism to support a continuous extraction of nutrients through the placenta to sustain fetal development. Quantitatively, glucose and amino acids are the most abundant of these nutrients crossing the placenta (1,2), and the continuous dependence of the fetus on these compounds is well-known. However, the placenta is practically impermeable to lipids, except for free fatty acids (FFA) and ketone bodies (3). Nevertheless, the marked changes in the maternal lipid metabolism during gestation do have important implications for fetal growth. Two consistent manifestations of altered maternal lipid metabolism occurring during gestation are the accumulation of lipids in maternal tissues (4,5) and the development of maternal hyperlipidemia (6,7). It is known that conditions that restrain or alter any of these manifestations—such as hypothyroidism or overt diabetes during the first half of gestation—will greatly affect fetal growth at late gestation, even if they are compensated for by appropriate hormonal treatment during the second half of gestation (8,9).

In this chapter, we analyze the changes that occur in maternal lipid metabolism during gestation and how they contribute to fetal development.

MATERNAL ADIPOSE TISSUE METABOLISM

The increase in maternal body weight during gestation corresponds both to the growth of the fetal-placental unit and to the increase in the mother's own structures, which is mainly related to lipid accumulation in fat depots. A phenomenon common to humans (5,10) and rats (4,11), it occurs during the first two thirds of gestation, accounts for most of the conceptus-free increase in maternal body weight, and is directly related to maternal hyperphagia, as it disappears with food restriction (12).

The increase in maternal fat depots seems to be mainly a result of enhanced lipogenesis, which has been demonstrated both *in vivo* (13) and in periuterine adipose tissue *in situ* (14); it corresponds to an increase in the synthesis of both fatty acids and glyceride glycerol, indicating that triglyceride synthesis is enhanced.

The tendency to accumulate fat in the mother ceases during the last trimester of gestation (5,10,15), when maternal lipid metabolism switches to a catabolic state because of the coincidence of several changes taking place in her adipose tissue metabolism at this time: (a) The augmented lipogenic activity decreases rapidly (14); (b) lipolytic activity becomes highly enhanced (16) because of increased activity by the key enzyme in the lipolytic cascade, hormone-sensitive lipase (HSL) (17); and (c) tissue uptake of circulating triglycerides decreases (6) because of reduced lipoprotein lipase (LPL) activity (18,19). The adipose tissue HSL-to-LPL messenger RNA and activity ratios appear enhanced during late gestation (17), indicating that net triglyceride breakdown is augmented.

Enhanced adipose tissue lipolytic activity increases the release of both FFA and glycerol into the maternal circulation, where they reach high concentrations in the plasma (16,17). Placental transfer of these two lipolytic products is low (3), and maternal liver is their main receptor (20). As shown in Fig. 1, after being converted in the liver into their respective active forms, FFA to acyl-CoA and glycerol to glycerol-3-phosphate, they may be used for esterification in triglyceride synthesis, or for ketone body production in the case of FFA, or glucose synthesis in the case

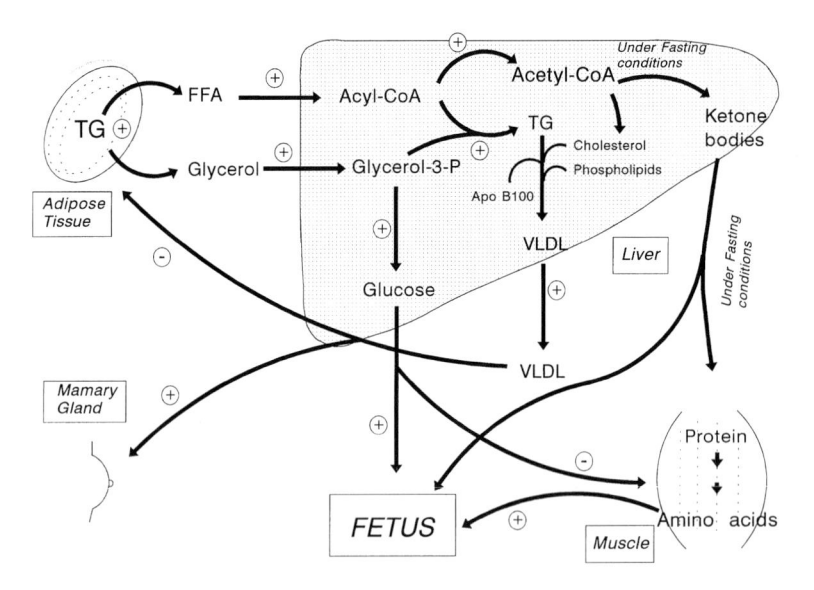

FIG. 1. Major changes in lipid metabolism taking place during late gestation. At this stage, adipose tissue lipolysis becomes a major source of substrates for gluconeogenesis, ketogenesis, and triglyceride synthesis. Glucose and amino acids are essential metabolites for the fetus and continuously cross the placenta, whereas ketone bodies diffuse to the fetus only under maternal fasting conditions, when ketogenesis becomes highly accelerated. +, enhanced pathway; −, inhibited pathway. *TG*, triglyceride; *Apo B-100*, apoprotein B-100; *VLDL*, very-low-density lipoproteins.

of glycerol. All these pathways seem to become enhanced during late gestation. We previously showed that glyceride glycerol synthesis from glycerol is very efficient in the liver of the fed, 21-day pregnant rat (21), and this—together with the increased transfer of FFA and glycerol to the liver from adipose tissue lipolysis—justifies the enhanced esterification and subsequent release in the form of very-low-density lipoprotein (VLDL) triglycerides by the liver, a process that is also known to be enhanced during late pregnancy (22) (Fig. 1). Ketone body synthesis becomes highly enhanced during late pregnancy under fasting conditions (6,18,23), and the use of ketone bodies by certain maternal tissues reduces their consumption of glucose, which is therefore saved for transfer to the fetus. During late gestation, gluconeogenesis from glycerol is highly augmented under both fed and fasting conditions, and this gluconeogenesis is even more efficient than that from other classic gluconeogenic substrates, such as alanine or pyruvate (24,25). It is therefore proposed that the preferential consumption of glycerol for gluconeogenesis spares the use of other possible substrates, such as amino acids, which are more essential for the fetus (Fig. 1).

We may then conclude that besides the availability of essential fatty acids from maternal circulation, the fetus greatly benefits from the end metabolic products of maternal adipose tissue lipolytic activity. Ketone bodies freely cross the placenta (3) and may be used as fetal fuels (26) or even as substrates in brain lipid synthesis (27). The efficient transfer of glucose to the fetus (1,2) and the use of glycerol as a preferential gluconeogenic substrate also benefit the fetus under conditions of reduced availability of other substrates, such as amino acids (1,25,28). Finally, the active adipose tissue lipolytic activity during late gestation also benefits maternal tissues, as at this stage tissue utilization of glucose is greatly decreased because of insulin resistance (29), and the lipolytic products—especially FFA and ketone bodies—can be used as alternative fuels to spare glucose.

MATERNAL HYPERLIPIDEMIA

During normal pregnancy, there is a consistent increase in plasma triglycerides, with smaller rises in phospholipids and cholesterol (7); as shown in Fig. 2, such change corresponds to a specific proportional enrichment of triglycerides in the lipoprotein fractions (30,31), including the low-density lipoproteins (LDL) and high-density lipoproteins (HDL), which normally transport them in very small proportion. Even within the HDL subfractions, there is a specific increment in the proportion of the triglyceride-rich HDL_{2b} subfraction in women during gestation, whereas the proportion of those such as HDL_{2a} or HDL_3, which are poor in triglycerides, is reduced (31). However, the greatest absolute change in plasma triglycerides during gestation corresponds to the VLDL triglycerides (30). These lipoproteins are synthesized in the liver, and the triglycerides that they carry must be derived from the fatty acids and glycerol that are either synthesized within the liver or reach it from

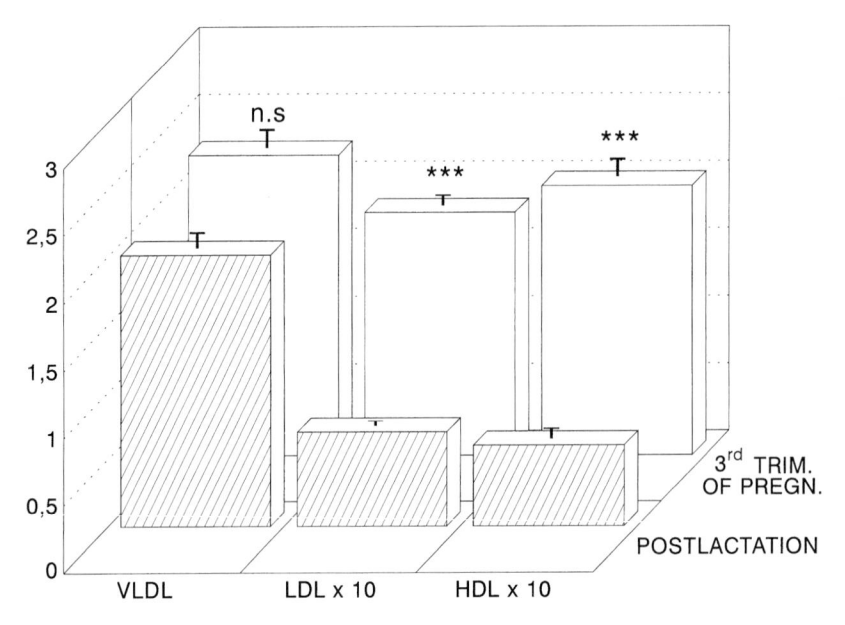

FIG. 2. Plasma lipoprotein triglyceride-to-cholesterol ratio in women during pregnancy and at the end of the lactation period. *Asterisks* correspond to the statistical comparison between values at the third trimester of gestation and at postlactation. $^{***}p < .001$. Adapted from Montelongo et al. (30).

the circulation after being released by adipose tissue lipolysis (Fig. 1), which is highly augmented during late gestation, as described above.

Enhanced liver production of VLDL triglycerides and their decreased removal from the circulation as a result of reduced adipose tissue LPL activity, which is consistently seen during late gestation (17,19,31), seem to be the main factors responsible for the increase in VLDL triglycerides during gestation.

The abundance of VLDL triglycerides in the mother's plasma during gestation, together with other factors summarized in Fig. 3, may contribute to the accumulation of triglycerides in the other lipoproteins. One of these factors is the increase in cholesteryl ester transfer protein (CETP) activity, which was recently found at midgestation (31,32). CETP catalyzes the net mass transfer of triglycerides from VLDL towards triglyceride-poor lipoproteins, LDL and HDL, whereas net mass transfer of cholesteryl ester occurs in the opposite direction, from LDL and HDL towards VLDL; at the same time, LDL and HDL exchange neutral lipid molecules without significant net mass transfer. The increase in the activity of this protein must therefore contribute to the proportional enrichment of triglycerides seen in LDL and HDL during gestation. Another factor contributing to this same effect may be the decrease in the activity of hepatic lipase, which is also seen during late gestation (31). This enzyme controls the conversion of buoyant HDL_2 triglyceride-rich particles into small HDL_3 triglyceride-poor particles, and therefore its decreased activity allows a proportional accumulation in the former, as has been shown during late gestation (31) (Fig. 3).

Among the hormonal factors that are normally modified during gestation, two seem to be responsible for most of these changes. The first is the insulin-resistant condition constantly present during late gestation, which we have recently found contributes to, or is responsible for, both the enhanced adipose tissue lipolytic activity and the decreased LPL activity (29,33). We have seen above that these two changes contribute to both the enhanced availability of substrates for the liver synthesis of triglycerides and the decreased removal from circulation of VLDL triglycerides. The second factor is the progressive increase in plasma estrogen levels during gestation (30,31); this is known to enhance the liver production of VLDL and to decrease hepatic lipase activity, and therefore it actively contributes to several of the changes in lipoprotein metabolism occurring during gestation that end with the development of an exaggerated hypertriglyceridemia (reviewed in ref. 7).

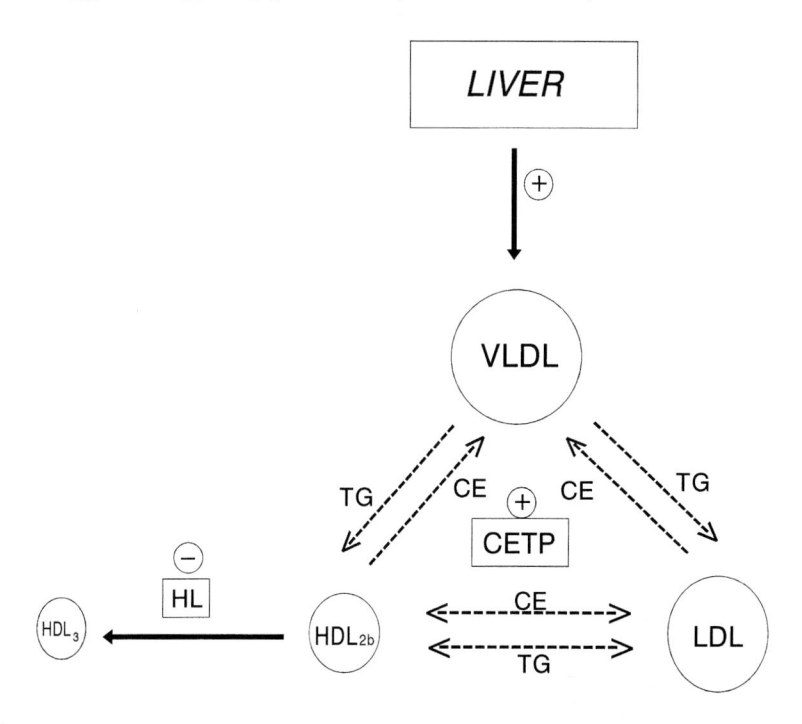

FIG. 3. Proposed factors contributing to the proportional accumulation of triglycerides (TG) in the main circulating lipoproteins during late pregnancy. An enhanced liver production of VLDL seems to be the main factor yielding an increase in plasma VLDL levels. The enhanced CETP activity occurring at midgestation (31,32) facilitates the net mass transfer (*single dotted arrows*) of triglycerides by cholesteryl esters (CE) from VLDL towards lipoproteins of higher density, LDL and HDL, which are poor in TG. Besides this, LDL and HDL can also exchange neutral lipid molecules (*double arrows*) without significant net mass transfer. Because hepatic lipase (HL) activity catalyzes the conversion of triglyceride-rich HDL_{2b} subfractions into HDL_3, which is poor in TG, the decrease of HL seen during gestation (31) would facilitate the accumulation of the former.

BENEFITS OF MATERNAL HYPERTRIGLYCERIDEMIA FOR THE OFFSPRING

Although triglycerides do not cross the placental barrier (3), there are a few mechanisms by which both the fetus and the newborn could benefit from maternal hypertriglyceridemia.

1. Although the liver of the adult rat normally lacks LPL activity, we have consistently seen an intense increase in LPL activity in the liver of the 24-hours fasted, 20-day pregnant rat (18,34,35). This activity may be the result of LPL washout from extrahepatic tissues carried by the triglyceride-rich lipoprotein remnants reaching the liver. Through this mechanism, the liver of the fasted pregnant rat switches from being a triglyceride-exporting organ to being a triglyceride-accepting one, allowing the use of circulating triglycerides as substrates for ketone body synthesis. In this way, ketogenesis in the maternal liver in late gestation becomes highly enhanced under fasting conditions (6,18,23), and this, besides being a mechanism for decreasing glucose use by maternal tissues, directly benefits the fetus by allowing it to obtain ketone bodies through the placenta (see above).

2. Another mechanism by which the fetus may benefit from maternal hypertriglyceridemia is the availability of essential fatty acids from maternal triglycerides. The lipase activities in the placenta hydrolyze maternal triglycerides, and the released FFA can reach the fetus for reconversion into triglycerides.

3. An additional benefit for the offspring of maternal hypertriglyceridemia during gestation is its active contribution to milk synthesis in preparation for lactation (36). Using late-pregnant rats, we showed that there is a rapid appearance of labeled lipids in the mammary gland after an oral load of labeled triglycerides (37), and blocking the increase in mammary gland LPL activity by treatment with progesterone in the late-pregnant rat completely inhibits the decline in plasma triglycerides normally occurring near parturition (38). These findings show that the rapid and intense increase in mammary gland LPL activity that occurs before parturition, at a time when LPL activity in adipose tissue is very low (17,35,38,39), drives circulating triglycerides from the adipose tissue to the mammary gland (Fig. 1) and facilitates the clearance of triglycerides from circulation and their use in milk synthesis. Through this mechanism, essential fatty acids from the mother's diet that circulate in the form of triglycerides become available to the suckling newborn.

EFFECT OF DEVIATIONS IN MATERNAL HYPERLIPIDEMIA TO FETAL GROWTH

The importance of maternal hyperlipidemia to fetal growth may be studied by determining how deviations in this hyperlipidemia affect fetal development.

Treating pregnant rats with fluvastatin, an inhibitor of cholesterol synthesis that does not seem to cross the placental barrier but provokes hypocholesterolemia in the mother, has been shown to reduce fetal weight and even greatly decrease fetal viability (40). Additionally, treating pregnant rats with a nonabsorbable bile acid-binding resin (cholestyramine), which enhances cholesterol synthesis through induction of the key enzyme for this pathway (3-hydroxy-3-methylglutaryl coenzyme A reductase), has also induced the enzyme activity in fetal liver (41). These findings therefore show that fetal growth and metabolism are sensitive to perturbations in maternal lipoprotein metabolism.

Under more physiologic conditions, we have recently found that a sucrose-rich diet in the pregnant rat causes exaggerated hypertriglyceridemia, and this effect is associated with an accumulation of triglycerides in the placenta, an increase in the placental LPL activity, and—what is more important—a significant reduction in fetal weight (42). The possibility then exists that the exaggerated maternal hypertriglyceridemia caused by the sucrose-rich diet--which mainly corresponds to endogenously synthesized fatty acids—has saturated the placental fatty acid transfer process, impeding the adequate transfer of essential fatty acids to the fetus and consequently impairing normal fetal growth.

Although the above reasoning implies that some deviations in maternal hyperlipidemia may cause major alterations in fetal development, there are conditions of maternal hypercholesterolemia that do not seem to affect fetal growth. Pregnant women with pre-existing hypercholesterolemia have been reported not to have problems in the outcome of their pregnancy (43,44).

To study further this apparent protection of fetal development under conditions of maternal hypercholesterolemia, we examined the effects of a cholesterol-rich diet in the pregnant rat. As shown in Fig. 4, plasma cholesterol was greatly enhanced during gestation in rats receiving a standard diet supplemented with 2% cholesterol and 1% cholic acid to facilitate cholesterol absorption, whereas their plasma triglycerides were only mildly, but significantly, augmented in comparison with the values found in pregnant rats fed the standard diet. Regardless of the mechanism responsible for these changes, which is beyond of the scope of this chapter, the outcome of pregnancy in rats receiving the cholesterol-rich diet did not differ from that of the rats under the standard diet, as indicated by an unchanged number of fetuses and the normal weights of both placentae and fetuses (data not shown).

Fetal protection against maternal hypercholesterolemia may be a consequence of the impermeability of the placenta to cholesterol transfer. This has been a question of controversy; early studies have suggested an important contribution of maternal cholesterol to fetal plasma and tissue cholesterol accretion (45), whereas more recent reports have found a minimal transfer of maternal cholesterol (46,47). However, no direct studies investigating this problem have been carried out as yet. In any case, any placental transfer of cholesterol would have to depend on its concentration on the maternal side, and differences such as those caused by a cholesterol-rich maternal diet would have to alter the concentration of lipids in fetal plasma. However, as also shown in Fig. 4, plasma concentrations of cholesterol and triglycerides in fetuses from dams on a cholesterol-rich diet do not differ from those of fetuses from control mothers. The fetal plasma lipoprotein profile is very similar in both groups, whether the mothers received the cholesterol-rich diet or not (data not shown). These findings

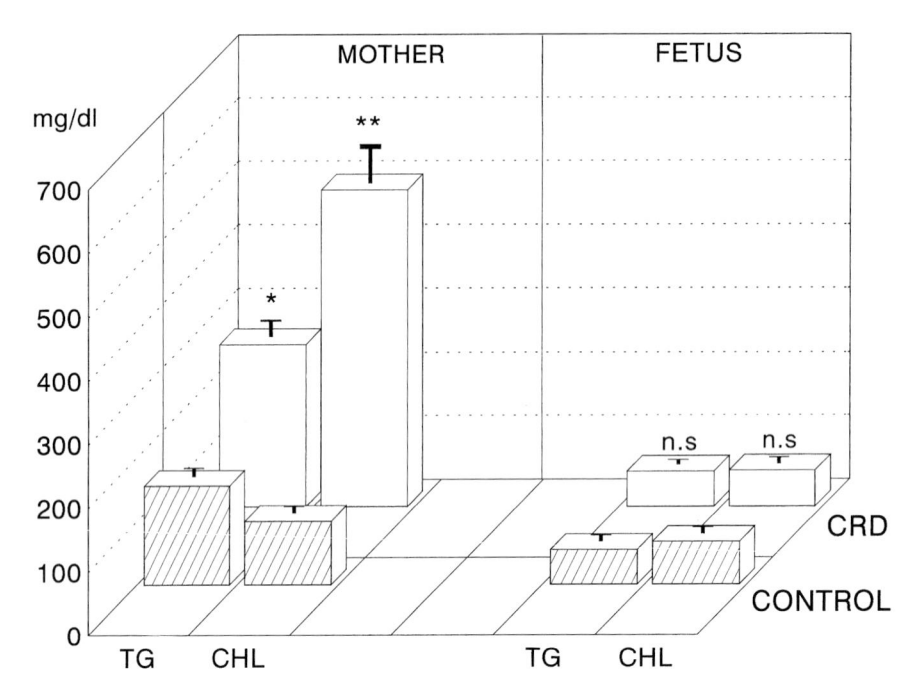

FIG. 4. Effect of feeding pregnant rats with a diet supplemented with 2% cholesterol and 1% cholic acid on plasma lipid concentrations in mothers and fetuses at day 20 of gestation. *Asterisks correspond to the statistical difference between rats receiving or not receiving the cholesterol-rich diet.* $^*p<.05$; $^{**}p<.01$.

therefore support the concept that at least in the rat, cholesterol requirements during fetal life are met by fetal cholesterol synthesis rather than by placental transfer, and maternal hypercholesterolemia affects neither the fetal lipid profile nor fetal development, thanks to the lack of transfer of maternal cholesterol through the placenta. On the basis of the lack of alteration in the gestational outcome of hypercholesterolemic women (43,44), it seems reasonable to assume that such a conclusion is also valid in humans.

We may then conclude that whereas conditions that cause either maternal hypocholesterolemia or exaggerated hypertriglyceridemia greatly affect fetal growth and even viability, conditions of exaggerated hypercholesterolemia do not affect the outcome of pregnancy, probably as the result of the impermeability of the placenta to maternal cholesterol.

SUMMARY AND CONCLUSIONS

During gestation, the increase in the mass of maternal structures mainly corresponds to an accumulation of depot fat, which occurs during the first two thirds of gestation, has a direct relation to maternal hyperphagia, and is a consequence of enhanced adipose tissue lipogenesis. During the last trimester of gestation, maternal lipid metabolism switches to a catabolic condition that leads to a net breakdown of fat depots, thereby increasing the release of FFA and glycerol into the circulation. Placental transfer of these lipolytic products is low and they are dealt with by the maternal liver, where they are either re-esterified for the synthesis of triglycerides, which are released back into the circulation in the form of VLDL, or are oxidized for the synthesis of ketone bodies (FFA) or preferentially transformed into glucose (glycerol). All these pathways are enhanced during late gestation, although ketogenesis is stimulated only under fasting conditions. Enhanced liver production of VLDL triglycerides in the presence of decreased extrahepatic LPL activity, which restrains their removal, causes an exaggerated increase in these lipoproteins. This, together with an increase in CETP activity, facilitates the transfer of triglycerides from VLDL to higher-density lipoproteins, causing a proportional enrichment of triglycerides in all the main circulating lipoproteins.

Despite the impermeability of the placenta to triglycerides, maternal hypertriglyceridemia benefits the offspring in several ways: (a) under fasting conditions, the liver of the mother shows increases in LPL activity, becoming an acceptor organ for circulating triglycerides that are used as substrates for ketone body synthesis, and these compounds easily diffuse through the placenta and are used by the fetus; (b) the presence of lipase activities in the placenta makes essential fatty acids from maternal triglycerides available to the fetus; and (c) the induction of LPL in mammary gland around parturition drives circulating triglycerides to this organ for milk synthesis. Although certain deviations in maternal hyperlipidemia may affect fetal growth, as shown under conditions of hypocholesterolemia or exaggerated hypertriglyceridemia, conditions of hypercholesterolemia do not affect the outcome of pregnancy, probably because of the impermeability of the placenta to maternal cholesterol. It may then be concluded that whereas maternal hyperlipidemia is a constant feature of normal pregnancy and a necessary condition for the continuous availability of substrates to sustain fetal growth, the poor placental transfer of lipids protects the fetus from some—although not all—of the variations in their levels in maternal plasma.

ACKNOWLEDGMENTS

This work has been supported in part by a grant from the Universidad San Pablo-CEU (Grant 6/95). We thank C. F. Warren for her editorial help.

REFERENCES

1. Herrera E, Palacín M, Martín A, Lasunción MA. Relationship between maternal and fetal fuels and placental glucose transfer in rats with maternal diabetes of varying severity. *Diabetes* 1985;34(Suppl 2):42—46.
2. Lasunción MA, Lorenzo J, Palacín M, Herrera E. Maternal factors modulating nutrient transfer to fetus. *Biol Neonate* 1987;51:86—93.

3. Herrera E, Lasunción MA, Asunción M. Placental transport of free fatty acids, glycerol and ketone bodies. In: Polin R, Fox WW, eds. *Fetal and Neonatal Physiology.* Philadelphia: WB Saunders: 1992:291–298.
4. Lopez Luna P, Maier I, Herrera E. Carcass and tissue fat content in the pregnant rat. *Biol Neonate* 1991;60:29–38.
5. Hytten FE, Leitch I. *The Physiology of Human Pregnancy.* Oxford: Blackwell Scientific; 1971.
6. Herrera E, Gomez Coronado D, Lasunción MA. Lipid metabolism in pregnancy. *Biol Neonate* 1987; 51:70–77.
7. Knopp RH, Bonet B, Lasunción MA, Montelongo A, Herrera E. Lipoprotein metabolism in pregnancy. In: Herrera E, Knopp RH, eds. *Perinatal Biochemistry.* Boca Raton: CRC Press; 1992:19–51.
8. Bonet B, Herrera E. Maternal hypothyroidism during the first half of gestation compromises normal catabolic adaptations of late gestation in the rat. *Endocrinology* 1991;129:210—216.
9. Martín A, Herrera E. Different responses to maternal diabetes during the first and second half of gestation in the streptozotocin-treated rat. *Isr J Med Sci* 1991;27:442–448.
10. Villar J, Cogswell M, Kestler E, Castillo P, Menendez R, Repke JT. Effect of fat and fat-free mass deposition during pregnancy on birth weight. *Am J Obstet Gynecol* 1992;167:1344–1352.
11. Moore BJ, Brassel JA. One cycle of reproduction consisting of pregnancy, lactation, and recovery: effects on carcass composition in ad libitum-fed and food-restricted rats. *J Nutr* 1984;114:1548–1559.
12. Lederman SA, Rosso P. Effects of food restriction on maternal weight and body composition in pregnant and non-pregnant rats. *Growth* 1980;44:77–88.
13. Fain JM, Scow RO. Fatty acid synthesis *in vivo* in maternal and fetal tissues in the rat. *Am J Physiol* 1966;210:19–25.
14. Palacín M, Lasunción MA, Asunción M, Herrera E. Circulating metabolite utilization by periuterine adipose tissue *in situ* in the pregnant rat. *Metabolism* 1991;40:534–539.
15. López-Luna P, Muñoz T, Herrera E. Body fat in pregnant rats at mid- and late-gestation. *Life Sci* 1986;39:1389–1393.
16. Knopp RH, Herrera E, Freinkel N. Carbohydrate metabolism in pregnancy. VIII. Metabolism of adipose tissue isolated from fed and fasted pregnant rats during late gestation. *J Clin Invest* 1970; 49:1438–1446.
17. Martin-Hidalgo A, Holm C, Belfrage P, Schotz MC, Herrera E. Lipoprotein lipase and hormone-sensitive lipase activity and mRNA in rat adipose tissue during pregnancy. *Am J Physiol* 1994;266: E930–935.
18. Herrera E, Lasunción MA, Gómez Coronado D, Aranda P, Lopez Luna P, Maier I. Role of lipoprotein lipase activity on lipoprotein metabolism and the fate of circulating triglycerides in pregnancy. *Am J Obstet Gynecol* 1988;158:1575–1583.
19. Otway S, Robinson DS. The significance of changes in tissue clearing-factor lipase activity in relation to the lipaemia of pregnancy. *Biochem J* 1968;106:677–682.
20. Mampel T, Villarroya F, Herrera E. Hepatectomy-nephrectomy effects in the pregnant rat and fetus. *Biochem Biophys Res Commun* 1985;131:1219–1225.
21. Zorzano A, Herrera E. Comparative utilization of glycerol and alanine as liver gluconeogenic substrates in the fed late pregnant rat. *Int J Biochem* 1986;18:583–587.
22. Wasfi I, Weinstein I, Heimberg M. Increased formation of triglyceride from oleate in perfused livers from pregnant rats. *Endocrinology* 1980;107:584–596.
23. Scow RO, Chernick SS, Brinley MS. Hyperlipemia and ketosis in the pregnant rat. *Am J Physiol* 1964;206:796–804.
24. Chaves JM, Herrera E. *In vivo* glycerol metabolism in the pregnant rat. *Biol Neonate* 1980;37: 172–179.
25. Zorzano A, Lasunción MA, Herrera E. Role of the availability of substrates on hepatic and renal gluconeogenesis in the fasted late pregnant rat. *Metabolism* 1986;35:297–303.
26. Shambaugh GE, Metzger BE, Radosevich JA. Nutrient metabolism and fetal brain development. In: Herrera E, Knopp RH, eds. *Perinatal Biochemistry.* Boca Raton: CRC Press; 1992:213–231.
27. Patel MS, Johnson CA, Ratan R, Owen DE. The metabolism of ketone bodies in developing human brain: development of ketone-body utilizing enzymes and ketone bodies as precursors for lipid synthesis. *J Neurochem* 1975;25:905–908.
28. Herrera E, Lasunción MA, Martín A, Zorzano A. Carbohydrate-lipid interactions in pregnancy. In: Herrera E, Knopp RH, eds. *Perinatal Biochemistry.* Boca Raton: CRC Press; 1992:1–18.
29. Ramos P, Herrera E. Reversion of insulin resistance in the rat during late pregnancy by 72-h glucose infusion. *Am J Physiol* 1995;32:E858–E863.

30. Montelongo A, Lasunción MA, Pallardo LF, Herrera E. Longitudinal study of plasma lipoproteins and hormones during pregnancy in normal and diabetic women. *Diabetes* 1992;41:1651–1659.
31. Alvarez JJ, Montelongo A, Iglesias A, Lasunción MA, Herrera E. Longitudinal study on lipoprotein profile, high density lipoprotein subclass and post-heparin lipases during gestation in women. *J Lipid Res* 1996;37:299–308.
32. Iglesias A, Montelongo A, Herrera E, Lasunción MA. Changes in cholesteryl ester transfer protein activity during normal gestation and postpartum. *Clin Biochem* 1994;27:63–68.
33. Herrera E, Ramos P, Martín A. Control by insulin of adipose tissue lipoprotein lipase activity during late pregnancy in the rat. In: Shafrir E, ed. *Frontiers in Diabetes Research. Lessons from Animal Diabetes III.* London: Smith-Gordon; 1990: 551–554.
34. Testar X, Llobera M, Herrera E. Metabolic response to starvation at late gestation in chronically ethanol-treated and pair-fed undernourished rats. *Metabolism* 1988;37:1008–1014.
35. López-Luna P, Olea J, Herrera E. Effect of starvation on lipoprotein lipase activity in different tissues during gestation in the rat. *Biochim Biophys Acta Lipids Lipid Metab* 1994;1215:275–279.
36. Herrera E, Ramos P, López-Luna P, Lasunción MA. Metabolic interactions during pregnancy in preparation for lactation. In: Serrano Ríos M, Sastre A, Perez Juez MA, Entrala A, De Sabesti C, eds. *Dairy Products in Human Health and Nutrition.* Rotterdam: AA Balkema; 1994:189–197.
37. Argiles J, Herrera E. Appearance of circulating and tissue ^{14}C-lipids after oral ^{14}C-tripalmitate administration in the late pregnant rat. *Metabolism* 1989;38:104–108.
38. Ramirez I, Llobera M, Herrera E. Circulating triacylglycerols, lipoproteins, and tissue lipoprotein lipase activities in rat mothers and offspring during the perinatal period: effect of postmaturity. *Metabolism* 1983;32:333–341.
39. Ramos P, Herrera E. Comparative responsiveness to prolonged hyperinsulinemia between adipose tissue and mammary gland lipoprotein lipase activities in pregnant rats. *Early Pregnancy: Biol Med* 1996;2:29–35.
40. Hrab RV, Hartman HA, Cox RH. Prevention of fluvastatin-induced toxicity, mortality, and cardiac myopathy in pregnant rats by mevalonic acid supplementation. *Teratology* 1994;50:19–26.
41. Haave NC, Innis SM. Induction of 3-hydroxy-3-methylglutaryl coenzyme A reductase activity in foetal rats by maternal cholestyramine feeding. *J Dev Physiol* 1988;10:247–255.
42. Soria A, Chicco A, Mocchiutti N, Gutman RA, Lombardo B, Martín-Hidalgo A, Herrera E. A sucrose-rich diet affects triglyceride metabolism differently in pregnant and nonpregnant rats and has negative effects on fetal growth. *J Nutr* 1996;126:2481–2486.
43. Potter JM, Nestel PJ. The hyperlipidemia of pregnancy in normal and complicated pregnancies. *Am J Obstet Gynecol* 1979;133:165–170.
44. Kroon AA, Swinkels DW, Van Dongen PWJ, Stalenhoef AFH. Pregnancy in a patient with homozygous familial hypercholesterolemia treated with long-term low-density lipoprotein apheresis. *Metabolism* 1994;43:1164–1170.
45. Pitkin RM, Connor WE, Lin DS. Cholesterol metabolism and placental transfer in the pregnant rhesus monkey. *J Clin Invest* 1972;51:2584–2592.
46. Parker CR, Deahl T, Drewry P, Hankins G. Analysis of the potential for transfer of lipoprotein-cholesterol across the human placenta. *Early Hum Dev* 1983;8:289–295.
47. Neary RH, Kilby MD, Kumpatula P, et al. Fetal and maternal lipoprotein metabolism in human pregnancy. *Clin Sci* 1995;88:311–318.

DISCUSSION

Dr. Page: Am I right in thinking that placental lipoprotein lipase does not attack chylomicrons?

Dr. Herrera: No, it attacks chylomicrons as well as VLDL triglycerides. Lipoprotein lipase in the placenta does not differentiate between VLDL and chylomicrons.

Dr. Page: Is there any effect of things like estradiol on placental lipoprotein lipase activity?

Dr. Herrera: I don't think so. We have not measured it, but we don't think that there is any effect. We measured lipoprotein lipase activity in adipose tissue of pregnant rats after estradiol administration and found no change.

Dr. Battaglia: If you take a very thin and a very fat pregnant rat, what changes between those two in these adaptations? In other words, how does obesity transform the normal metabolic adaptations to pregnancy?

Dr. Herrera: We did not study obesity, because overfeeding the rats changes the situation too much. With undernutrition in the rats that were kept in a food-restricted condition during pregnancy, there was no increase in liver triglycerides, there was no increase in liver lipoprotein lipase activity, and hyperlipidemia was much more moderate (1). That is why we saw then the possibility of explaining the uptake of triglycerides by the liver of the fasting pregnant rat by the action of the lipoprotein lipase that appears in the liver as a result of the washout of extrahepatic lipoprotein lipase molecules by remnants of triglyceride-rich lipoproteins (2,3).

Dr. Cedard: You explain that the increase of estradiol during pregnancy increases the number of LDL receptors, and this justifies that pregnancy does not enhance the hypercholesterolemic condition of patients having familial hypercholesterolemia. However, another explanation could be the presence in the placenta of a specific receptor for low-density lipoproteins, which are then transformed into progesterone; there are also specific receptors for acetyl lipoprotein, as in macrophages, and also less specific receptors for HDL, although it is possible that the lipoproteins are kept in the placenta and transformed either into steroids or structural components.

Dr. Herrera: The placenta does not affect lipoprotein production. That is modulated by estrogen, but the placenta has lipoprotein receptors, and lipoproteins are taken up from the maternal circulation. This is why I say that one of the physiologic roles of maternal hyperlipidemia is probably to allow enough substrate to be taken up by the placenta for the synthesis of progesterone for steroid hormones.

Dr. Marconi: We know that the second child is usually bigger than the first. Do you think that this could be explained by the fact that insulin resistance increases with further pregnancies?

Dr. Herrera: Maybe. It is true that in the second pregnancy, there is a greater tendency for the mother to be hyperglycemic, so probably there is also a greater amount of glucose crossing the placenta and more possibility for fetal pancreatic β cells to respond to it. Fetal insulin acts as a growth factor, and such a mechanism could contribute to the tendencies of developing fetal macrosomia after several pregnancies.

Dr. K. Taher: I think that as the number of pregnancies increases the insulin sensitivity decreases; that is why maternal diabetes becomes more prevalent with successive pregnancies and why the size of the baby also increases. Have you any comment on that?

Dr. Herrera: Although that is a true fact, we don't know yet its mechanism. Insulin resistance in late pregnancy is caused by several factors, including the presence of counterregulatory hormones and maternal hyperlipidemia, and these factors may be aggravated in successive pregnancies.

Dr. Talamantes: We are doing some studies looking at the effect of placental lactogen on the sensitivity of the mammary gland. With every succeeding pregnancy the mammary gland becomes more sensitive to the actions of prolactin to make casein or fatty acid, so there is an alteration between the first pregnancy and the second and third pregnancies. The mammary gland becomes much more sensitive to the action of hormones, so there is an increased sensitivity that is very interesting. The underlying cause has yet to be determined.

Dr. Herrera: Insulin resistance occurs in many maternal tissues, but it doesn't appear in mammary gland (4,5). Mammary gland responds to insulin in the late-pregnant rat in thesame way as in virgin control animals, and it contributes together with prolactin to the induction of lipoprotein lipase and the other metabolic changes in this specific organ (5,6).

Dr. Nicolaides: We have found that in normal pregnancy there is an exponential decrease in fetal triglyceride levels with gestation, especially after 24 weeks, and that corresponds with increased laying down of fat in the fetus, and in hypoxemia in placental insufficiency the fetal triglyceride levels remain high. We thought the explanation for that was that hypoglycemia mediated hypoinsulinemia, resulting in reduced lipoprotein lipase activity in the fetus, so that was the explanation for fetal hypertriglyceridemia. But I was surprised that on the maternal side the triglyceride levels were normal. And yet you have all these massive efforts for the maternal side to increase triglycerides, but if they are not taken away by the placenta, where do they go?

Dr. Herrera: To the mammary gland, being mediated by the induction of lipoprotein lipase activity occurring in this organ around parturition (7,8).

Dr. Nicolaides: To the mammary gland? So the mothers are producing more milk to feed their growth-retarded babies after birth!

Dr. Herrera: We don't have experience on this specific point.

Dr. Pardi: It is a clinical but important point; perhaps you have data about lactation in growth retardation. In my opinion, the capacity for lactation is decreased in parallel with the degree of placental insufficiency.

Dr. Nicolaides: I haven't any data, but it sounds logical. I have certainly not observed increased lactation in women with growth-retarded babies.

Dr. Herrera: There is also a curious situation concerning hypercholesterolemic pregnant women. Some of these women have familial hypercholesterolemia, which does not worsen during pregnancy. On the contrary, there are some reports saying that plasma cholesterol is decreased because there is induction of LDL receptor caused by the increased estrogen level (9).

Dr. Godfrey: Just to follow on Dr. Marconi's suggestion—it is a nice idea. The epidemiologic data, such as they are, are that if you use maternal fatness—body mass index or perhaps more importantly regional body fat distribution—as a proxy for insulin resistance, the increment in fetal growth associated with increasing parity cannot be explained by maternal fatness.

Dr. Nicolaides: Could you just explain that in a simple way?

Dr. Godfrey: Multiparous women don't have bigger babies simply because they are fatter. And to follow on from that, there are profound changes in regional body fat distribution in human pregnancy, even dating back before the 16 week cutoff in your slide. I was wondering if you had any data from your rat studies, in which I am sure regional body fat distribution is more difficult to study.

Dr. Herrera: No, we did only total carcass analysis (10). An important point is that before the decline of lipoprotein lipase activity in adipose tissue, there is an increase in lipogenesis in adipose tissue (11). Unlike hepatic lipase activity, lipoprotein lipase activity declines only during late gestation (12), when fat is already distributed in the different organs. It seems then that such change plays a role mainly in the preparation of the mother for parturition rather than in the distribution of the accumulation of fat.

Dr. Battaglia: Do we have any long-term data that show differences between women who had no children or one child *vs.* those who have had four children, in terms of later obesity or later complications related to fat metabolism?

Dr. Campbell: The old data from Frank Hytten's group suggested that women did not get fatter with successive pregnancies, looking from para I to II to III, probably up to about para IV, except for a very small number of women who were obese to start with, but they only got fatter with one particular pregnancy, not with each one. So it was not entirely clear from the epidemiologic data what exactly was happening (13).

Dr. Godfrey: From our follow-up studies of 25,000 to 30,000 people whose birth records we have, we found no effects of parity in relation to cardiovascular disease or diabetes in the offspring. In other words, we do not find that men and women who were firstborn or secondborn have any difference in their rates of coronary heart disease or diabetes 50 or 60 years later.

Dr. Van Assche: The adaptation concerning the lipids may not be so important in succeeding pregnancies, but the vascular adaptation is certainly not so good in the first pregnancy, improves in the second and the third, and then maybe deteriorates again in the fourth and fifth. So the change in birth weight is caused by other factors, and the cardiovascular adaptation can be even more important than the metabolic adaptation.

REFERENCES

1. Testar X, Llobera M, Herrera E. Metabolic response to starvation at late gestation in chronically ethanol-treated and pair-fed undernourished rats. *Metabolism* 1988;37:1008–1014.
2. Herrera E, Lasunción MA, Gomez Coronado D, et al. Role of lipoprotein lipase activity on lipoprotein metabolism and the fate of circulating triglycerides in pregnancy. *Am J Obstet Gynecol* 1988;158:1575–1583.
3. Lopez-Luna P, Olea J, Herrera E. Effect of starvation on lipoprotein lipase activity in different tissues during gestation in the rat. *Biochim Biophys Acta* 1994;1215:275–279.
4. Ramos P, Herrera E. Reversion of insulin resistance in the rat during late pregnancy by 72-h glucose infusion. *Am J Physiol Endocrinol Metab* 1995;269:E858–E863.
5. Ramos P, Herrera E. Comparative responsiveness to prolonged hyperinsulinemia between adipose-tissue and mammary-gland lipoprotein lipase activities in pregnant rats. *Early Pregnancy: Biol Med* 1996;2:29–35.
6. Herrera E, Ramos P, Lopez-Luna P, Lasunción MA. Metabolic interactions during pregnancy in preparation for lactation. In: Serrano Rios M, Sastre A, et al, eds. *Dairy Products in Human Health and Nutrition.* Rotterdam: AA Balkema 1994:189–197.
7. Argiles J, Herrera E. Appearance of circulating and tissue ^{14}C-lipids after oral ^{14}C-tripalmitate administration in the late pregnant rat. *Metabolism* 1989;38:104–108.
8. Ramirez I, Llobera M, Herrera E. Circulating triacylglycerols, lipoproteins, and tissue lipoprotein lipase activities in rat mothers and offspring during the perinatal period: effect of postmaturity. *Metabolism* 1983;32:333–341.
9. Mabuchi H, Sakai Y, Watanabe A, et al. Normalization of low-density lipoprotein levels and disappearance of xanthomas during pregnancy in a woman with heterozygous familial hypercholesterolemia. *Metabolism* 1985;34:309–315.
10. Lopez-Luna P, Muñoz T, Herrera E. Body fat in pregnant rats at mid- and late-gestation. *Life Sci* 1986;39:1389–1393.
11. Palacín M, Lasunción MA, Asunción M, Herrera E. Circulating metabolite utilization by periuterine adipose tissue *in situ* in the pregnant rat. *Metabolism* 1991;40:534–539.
12. Alvarez JJ, Montelongo A, Iglesias A, et al. Longitudinal study on lipoprotein profile, high density lipoprotein subclass, and postheparin lipases during gestation in women. *J Lipid Res* 1996;37:299–308.
13. Billewicz WZ, Thomson AM. Body weight in parous women. *Br J Prev Soc Med* 1970;24:97–104.

Oxygen Consumption and Protein Metabolism in the Human Fetus

Michael J. Rennie

Department of Anatomy and Physiology, University of Dundee, Dundee, Scotland, United Kingdom

Much of what we know about placental physiology and biochemistry has come from studies carried out in animals, particularly the guinea pig, rabbit, and sheep. Much less information is available concerning metabolism of the human fetus, for obvious reasons—both ethical and practical. My colleagues and I have attempted to build on what is known from the pioneering work of others (1–4) by using methods that enabled us to apply relatively simple models of fetal metabolism probed by the use of stable isotope tracer techniques.

We have concentrated on fetal amino acid and protein metabolism with the initial aim of simply defining the relative rates of normal fetal and maternal protein turnover and placental transfer. We then began to look at term babies over a large range of body weights and made measurements of fetal oxygen consumption and transport of mannitol and D- and L-amino acids.

METHODOLOGY

We have studied mothers and their babies at the time of elective cesarean delivery (5). We have infused stable isotope-labeled amino acids in the period before delivery and made measurements of umbilical flow and taken samples of umbilical arterial and venous blood while the baby is still attached to the placenta. This has enabled us to make measurements of net exchange of metabolites and oxygen across the placenta and also, when using stable isotope tracers infused into the mother's circulation, to make measurements of unidirectional transfer and back flux from the fetus to the mother as well as estimates of fetal protein turnover, that is, protein synthesis and breakdown.

The conclusions we have reached are very model-dependent, and the assumptions we have made are, in some cases, not easily tested. Nevertheless, the results we obtained appear to us to be coherent and sensible in relation to what is known about fetal growth and metabolism.

OXYGEN CONSUMPTION IN THE HUMAN FETUS

In adult mammals, the rate of oxygen consumption in the resting state, an index of energy expenditure, is not linearly related to body weight but is related to body weight raised to the power 0.75 (6). Thus, the oxygen consumption per kilogram of body weight in an elephant is much less than that in a mouse. However, this allometric relationship between oxygen consumption and body weight does not appear to be shown by fetuses of different species, despite a large range of body size. For example, the guinea pig and the cow have fetuses with a 300-fold difference in body mass, but the rate in fetal oxygen consumption per unit of body weight differs by only 25% (4). Furthermore, physiologic characteristics linked to energy metabolism, such as cardiac output and heart rate, are much less dependent on body weight in mammalian fetuses than in fully grown adults, providing supporting evidence that energy expenditure per body mass is generally less variable in uterine than in postnatal life (4). Information regarding oxygen consumption in the human fetus is sparse, with little published information on fetal oxygen consumption. In one study, fetal oxygen consumption ($\dot{V}O_2$) was determined by observing the differential effect of pregnancy on measured gas exchange in a single woman (7); in another, it was determined in six women by extrapolating from the oxygen left in blood as it drained the uterus and its contents, unfortunately without benefit of measurements of uterine or placental blood flow (8). In each case, the errors were likely to be considerable. Considering the substantial interest in the effects of events during uterine life on human postnatal development and especially on a predisposition to cardiovascular and metabolic disease (9), the lack of accurate information on human fetal energy expenditure constitutes a major gap in our understanding.

We studied oxygen consumption in 40 fetuses about to be delivered by elective cesarean section. The birth weights ranged between 800 and 4300 g. Umbilical blood flow was measured by an ultrasonic transit time flow probe applied to the exteriorized umbilical vein before the baby was delivered (5). Blood samples from the umbilical vein and artery were obtained immediately afterward, and the oxygen saturation and fetal hemoglobin concentration measured using a Radiometer OSM2 hemoximeter. $\dot{V}O_2$ was calculated from the product of the umbilical venous-arterial oxygen concentration difference and the blood flow.

We found that the relation between the whole-body $\dot{V}O_2$ and birth weight (M) was a power function with an exponent significantly greater than unity:

$$\dot{V}O_2 \text{ (ml/min)} = 3.67 \, M^{1.6} \text{ (kg)}$$

Body mass was the best predictor of oxygen consumption; a single equation best described the relationship between the two variables, even for small-for-gestational-age (SGA) and appropriate-for-gestational-age (AGA) fetuses, and sex and gestational age had no significant independent effects. Normalizing birth weight per unit of body length had no effect on the form of the relationship. In addition, the weight-specific oxygen consumption expressed per kilogram of body weight also showed a power relationship with body mass:

$$\dot{V}O_2 \text{ (ml/kg/min)} = 4.17 \, M^{0.53} \text{ (kg)}$$

There is a doubling in the expended energy of the fetus per kilogram of body weight as the body weight increases from 1000 to 3500 g. Fetuses defined as SGA had a mean specific oxygen consumption (6.4 ± 2.6 ml/kg/min; mean ± SD) that was statistically smaller ($p < .05$) than in AGA fetuses (8.4 ± 2.1 ml/kg/min).

One possible explanation for the apparent rise in specific oxygen consumption could have been that the smaller babies lost more heat once the uterus was opened and the cooling effect decreased their oxygen consumption. However, we have measured oxygen consumption in nine babies of birth weights between 1800 and 3000 g in whom central body temperature was also measured, and the small babies had body temperatures that were in the normal range.

The results show clearly that oxygen consumption per kilogram of body weight is not constant in the human fetus but rises with birth weight. What does this mean and how can we explain it?

Differences in growth rate, body composition, and metabolic capacity between babies of different weights (e.g., large for gestational age *vs.* small for gestational age) disappear when the relevant function is plotted against fetal mass (10). Thus, it appears that development is programmed to go hand in hand with fetal mass, and therefore it may be that the results we have obtained provide not only a snapshot of fetal oxygen consumption in babies with different masses but a picture of the developmental changes that occur in all babies.

If it is true, how can we explain the results? As the fetus becomes bigger and more mature, its body composition changes. The proportion that water contributes to the whole-body mass falls considerably as protein is accreted. If we express our results as $\dot{V}O_2$ per kilogram of protein, reflecting the active cell mass of the baby, there is a remarkable constancy throughout the body weight range with $\dot{V}O_2$ of 60 to 64 ml/min/kg protein, suggesting that the metabolic rate of the whole body depends markedly on the mass of active tissue rather than on total mass, which includes water and fat.

What are the implications of our results for the care of premature and SGA babies? This is a difficult question to answer. However, it seems likely that we cannot assume that small, premature babies will have energy requirements like those of larger babies but simply scaled down on a body mass basis.

PROTEIN METABOLISM IN AGA BABIES

We started our studies by investigating the relative rates of fetal uptake and disposal of leucine and phenylalanine in normal, healthy AGA babies (5). We also measured rates of protein synthesis in uterine muscle and placenta, and calculated rates of whole-body protein turnover in the fetus.

The technique we used was to set up a primed constant infusion of the amino acids to achieve a plateau of labeling in the maternal blood some 3 hours before the time of elective cesarean delivery and then exteriorize part of the cord to take blood samples and make umbilical cord blood flow measurements before delivery of the babies. We used L-[^{13}C]leucine and [^{15}N]phenylalanine to make our measurements.

We found that there was a consistent uptake of both tracer-labeled amino acids into the fetus. We were able to use simple steady-state equations to calculate the rates of maternal and fetal appearance of the amino acids and the rates of their disposal by oxidation and by incorporation into protein.

Our results can be summarized as follows: the rates of transfer of amino acids from mother to fetus are only about 5% to 6% of the total rate of maternal appearance of leucine or phenylalanine. In other words, there is no justification whatsoever for the commonly held idea that fetal protein metabolism is a major drain on the resources of maternal metabolism. The needs of the fetus ought to be able to be supplied by very small increases in protein intake (or whole-body protein breakdown) in well-nourished women. We also found that despite the fact that the mothers were in whole-body negative protein balance (they were studied in the postabsorptive state), the fetuses appeared to be in positive balance, with the rate of disappearance of amino acid into protein exceeding that being broken down from protein. The difference between protein synthesis and protein breakdown in the fetus was accounted for by amino acid oxidation. When we compared our values of protein (1.98 ± 0.50 g/kg/d) with those obtained for premature infants studied postnatally (11,12), there was a remarkable concordance, although this was very much better with leucine than with phenylalanine.

Another interesting feature of our results is that when comparison was made between the rates of accretion of protein and the rates of transfer of protein across the placenta, the rates of accretion were a substantial proportion (70% to 80%) of the total delivered across the placenta, suggesting that the safety margin of placental transfer rates is not large.

As a by-product of these studies, we also measured rates of placental protein turnover and the rate of turnover of uterine muscle. We found that protein turnover in the placenta was about 20% per day, whereas in uterine muscle it was about 1% per day (P. Chien, D. J. Taylor, and M. J. Rennie, *unpublished results*). In the term fetus, the rate of protein turnover was about 10% per day. As the placenta weighs about one tenth of the weight of the baby, most of the amino acids being taken out from the uterine arteries are likely to be transferred to the fetus, unless there is a very high degree of intermediary metabolism of amino acids in placenta. The contribution by the uterus to the whole fetomaternal unit is obviously very small.

STUDIES OF PLACENTAL TRANSFER IN AGA AND SGA BABIES

On the basis of previous work, we hypothesized that we ought to be able to distinguish between amino acids that are transported by a facilitated process (with amino acid transporter proteins) and those that are passively transferred by diffusion if we were to investigate the transfer of L- and D-amino acids across the placenta.

Our hypothesis was that L-amino acids would be much more likely to be transferred than D-amino acids. We also hypothesized that it ought to be possible to see to what extent diffusion generally is important in the placenta by measuring the transfer of mannitol, a substance that we believe is transferred passively through pericellular routes. Accordingly, we started to make measurements of transfer of racemic mixtures of stable isotope-labeled amino acids plus mannitol using the kind of protocol we had used earlier but shortening the period of maternal infusion to 1.5 to 2 hours.

Our results threw us into considerable confusion. First of all, it appeared that the transfer of mannitol across the placenta is concentration-dependent, and indeed the form of the relationship very much appeared to be one that is saturable, suggesting that mannitol transfer occurs not by a pure diffusive process but by one that is carrier-mediated.

Even more surprising was that for all the L- and D-amino acid pairs we investigated, there seemed to be a concentrative mechanism of transfer for *both* optical isomers; that is, there was a fetal-maternal concentration gradient for each. This suggested that the stereoselective nature of the amino acid transporters was much less rigid than for transporters observed in mammalian tissues during postnatal life.

Nevertheless, we believe that our results remain of considerable interest. For example, for leucine we can show that the fractional extraction and the net flux into the fetus from the placenta is substantially lower in SGA than in AGA babies, irrespective of whether this is expressed in terms of placental size or birth weight. Furthermore, although umbilical blood flow per kilogram of birth weight is not significantly depressed in SGA babies, it is lower, and given the fact that placental weight is also lower, umbilical blood flow per kilogram of placenta is significantly less for SGA pregnancies. In fact, we find that umbilical blood flow is, at about 200 ml/min/kg placenta, only about half of the normal value in AGA pregnancies. When we calculated unidirectional leucine influx across the placenta in the SGA babies, however, this was also only 50% of the value in AGA babies. Because amino acid transfer ought to be carrier- and not flow-limited, these results suggest to us that there are some defects in the capacity of the placenta to transfer leucine. This, of course, is what has been long suspected after the work of Young (2) and Cetin *et al.* (13,14).

What can we conclude from these results? They tend to confirm suspicions that in babies growing more slowly than normal, there are deficiencies in the ability of the placenta to transfer amino acids. For amino acids such as leucine, and possibly for other essential amino acids, such as phenylalanine, such a decrease in the transfer capacity would have substantial effects in limiting the ability of the fetus to make protein at an adequate rate. We have shown elsewhere that protein synthesis in the human body depends very much on the rate of delivery of amino acids, particularly the essential amino acids (15). However, the results also suggest that the SGA fetus is unable to use all the amino acids presented to it. Thus, it is very hard to identify a crucial process (e.g., at the level of the placenta or at the level of the fetus) that one can consider to be rate-limiting for normal development.

ACKNOWLEDGMENTS

I am grateful to my colleagues Professor David Taylor, Dr. Justin Konje, and Dr. Patrick Chien, who carried out the clinical parts of these studies. The laboratory work was carried out mainly by Dr. Patrick Chien and Dr. Ken Smith, with the help of Mr. Shaun Downie. We are especially grateful to the mothers and babies who participated in these studies, and to Action Research, The Wellcome Trust and the UK Medical Research Council, which provided running costs and the capital equipment without which the studies would have been impossible. Other support was provided by the University of Dundee.

REFERENCES

1. Widdowson EM. Changes in body composition during growth. In: Davis JA, Dobbing J, eds. *Scientific Foundations of Paediatrics.* Baltimore: University Park Press; 1981:330–335.
2. Young M. The materno-fetal nitrogen relationship: further observations. *Acta Paediatr Hung* 1993; 33:131–185.
3. Blaxter K. *Energy Metabolism in Animals and Man.* Cambridge: Cambridge University Press; 1989.
4. Battaglia FC, Meschia G. *An Introduction to Fetal Physiology.* Orlando: Academic Press; 1986.
5. Chien PFW, Smith K, Watt PW, Scrimgeour CM, Taylor DJ, Rennie MJ. Protein turnover in the human fetus studied at term using stable isotope tracer amino acids. *Am J Physiol* 1993;265:E31–E35.
6. Kleber M. *The Fire of Life: an Introduction to Animal Energetics.* Huntington, NY: Robert E Krager; 1975.
7. Sandford I, Wheeler T. The basal metabolism before, during and after pregnancy. *J Biol Chem* 1924; 62:329–350.
8. Romney SI, Reid DE, Metcalfe J, Burwell S. Oxygen utilization by the human fetus *in utero. Am J Obstet Gynecol* 1955;70:791–799.
9. Barker EJP. *Mothers, Babies and Diseases in Later Life.* London: BMJ Publishing Group; 1994.
10. Ziegler EE, O'Donnel AN, Nelson SE, Fomon SJ. Body composition of the reference fetus. *Growth* 1979;40:329–341.
11. Catzeflis C, Schutz Y, Micheli J-Y, Welsch C, Arnaud MJ, Jéquier E. Whole body protein synthesis and energy expenditure in very low birth weight infants. *Pediatr Res* 1993;19:679–687.
12. DeBenoist B, Abdulrazzak Y, Brooke OG, Halliday D, Millward DJ. The measurement of whole body protein turnover in the preterm infant with intragastric infusion of L-[1-^{13}C]leucine and sampling of urinary leucine pool. *Clin Sci* 1984;66:155–164.
13. Cetin I, Corbetta C, Sereni L, Marconi AM, Bozzetti P, Pardi G, *et al.* Umbilical amino acid concentrations in normal and growth retarded fetuses sampled *in utero* by cordocentesis. *Am J Obstet Gynecol* 1990;162:253–261.
14. Cetin I, Marconi AM, Bozzetti P, Sereni LP, Corbetta C, Pardi G, *et al.* Umbilical amino acid concentrations in appropriate and small for gestational age infants: a biochemical difference present *in utero. Am J Obstet Gynecol* 1988;158:120–126.
15. Bennet WM, Connacher AA, Scrimgeour CM, Smith K, Rennie MJ. Increase in anterior tibialis muscle protein synthesis in healthy man during mixed amino acid infusion: studies of incorporation of [1-^{13}C]leucine. *Clin Sci* 1989;76:447–454.

DISCUSSION

Dr. Soothill: Would you mind please just explaining in more detail about the technique of measuring the blood flow in the cord? Presumably you did a cesarean section and the umbilical cord was delivered. Was the fetus left in the uterus?

Dr. Rennie: Yes, the fetus is left in, but the cord is exteriorized and the measurement made.

Dr. Soothill: I think it is an exciting technique, but it would be wonderful to have some way of confirming that the cold exposure and the air exposure haven't led to umbilical artery vasoconstriction, because if they have, then that would clearly affect all the figures.

Dr. Rennie: I don't know any way of really checking that. What I can say is that when my collaborators in Leicester used Doppler and measured the umbilical flow in the same babies, and then later they were delivered, there was a very strong correlation between the two sets of values, but there was certainly a lot of slop in the values.

Dr. Soothill: I think it is a difficult technique, because you have obviously ruptured the membranes, and I can imagine that the incision will tend to squash the cord. It must be difficult.

Dr. Rennie: Yes, I think it is.

Dr. Pardi: We clinicians are very worried, because we all know that just touching the cord causes compression. Are you using a round probe?

Dr. Rennie: It is a probe that has a rounded square profile with a back plate. You put the vessel in surrounded by jelly.

Dr. Pardi: And the value of 76 ml/kg per minute is consistent with the findings *in utero* by Vladimirov and others?

Dr. Rennie: The values that we have per kilogram of baby apparently scale quite well with Doppler ultrasound values, but I don't know to what extent they are acceptable in other terms. But they do appear to be internally consistent; the range of values that we get is not huge—it is not twofold or anything like that. It may be that the values are scaled in some way to the real values even if they are not the actual values, and that is a possibility. I don't know how you would check this out.

Dr. Soothill: The danger is that the intrauterine growth-retarded fetal cord will have less Wharton's jelly and there will be more oligohydramnios, but it would also be interesting to present the data without the blood flow variable, the differences between artery and vein and those sorts of things.

Dr. Jensen: I would like to make a comment on the puzzle that you presented with respect to the oxygen consumption of the fetus. I just think we need a little bit more information on the oxygen content in the umbilical blood of those fetuses that were growth-retarded. The relation established by the Denver group between oxygen delivery and fetal oxygen consumption is curvilinear, so in cases where your SGA fetuses were on the steep part of the curve, oxygen delivery to those fetuses would almost linearly determine oxygen consumption. So this could explain why your SGA fetuses would come up with a reduced oxygen consumption per weight. Did you calculate oxygen content and oxygen delivery?

Dr. Rennie: What we did was to use the Radiometer OSM2 hemoximeter, so that we were able to calculate the saturation of fetal hemoglobin, and then we multiplied that by the hemoglobin concentration and the flow to get the answer. I think these values very much depend on flow, but I don't really think that the relationship per kilogram would necessarily have been affected by that.

Dr. Battaglia: We have many concerns about blood flows measured in this manner, and I don't think it is very useful to go into it in a lot of detail. But the observations you made with the D-amino acids and mannitol of a pumping-up gradient has nothing to do with flow. For this reason, I just wanted to get clear whether you think these compounds are going by transporters.

Dr. Rennie: For the mannitol there isn't any uphill gradient, but it is saturable. Therefore, there appears to be a facilitated mechanism, if you believe that saturability is a robust criterion of a transporter. But the D-amino acids appear at a higher concentration, and you have to assume therefore that there is some energy-dependent process that is pushing them across, and the only energy-dependent processes I know are sodium-dependent transport. So it was really a very great shock to get these data and to be sure that it was happening.

Dr. Meschia: You reached a steady state in each experiment?

Dr. Rennie: Yes, we reached steady state remarkably quickly as far as we could tell.

Dr. Meschia: I was wondering how long it took.

Dr. Rennie: What we would have liked to have done would have been to infuse for different periods of time, but we have never done that because of the variability between mothers and babies, and anyway that might have been difficult. In the event, we usually chose a period of about 90 minutes. When we looked at women between about 80 minutes and 2 1/2 hours, there was no suggestion that we hadn't reached a steady state. If you think about the pool sizes involved and the turnover rates, you ought to be able to get the steady state quite quickly.

Dr. Schneider: We have always noticed that in the *in vitro* preparation the difference between D- and L-amino acids, for leucine and lysine, is rather small, much smaller than for D- and L-glucose. With D- and L-glucose you get a two to three times difference in the *in vitro* preparation, whereas for amino acids this preferential transfer of L-amino acids is quite small *in vitro*. When we compared the flux of D- and L-leucine, mother (M) to fetus (F) and F to M, and then normalized that for creatinine, which we considered a passive diffusion indicator, then there was an increased flux for D-leucine from M to F and also from F to M, although clearly lower than for L-leucine. That puzzled us at the time, but we didn't pursue it.

Dr. Rennie: This would be rather hard to check out with radioactive tracers because there haven't traditionally been any D-tracers.

Dr. Pardi: If I understand your slides correctly, the growth-retarded fetuses were all mildly growth-retarded. In those fetuses the transfer of leucine was reduced. Does this indicate that this derangement is one of the first steps of the disease?

Dr. Rennie: I don't know. Is it suck or is it blow? That is the problem. In other words, does the fetus not suck enough? Or does the mother not blow enough? That's what it comes down to. If a defect, for example, in oxygen delivery to the fetus causes increased glycolysis, so that pyruvate production goes up and the pyruvate—because of the equilibrium nature of alanine aminotransferase—essentially steals nitrogen from branched-chain amino acids, it would mean that those branched-chain amino acids weren't available to be put into protein. So you can construct a scenario in which the primary defect is not necessarily transport. I was quite impressed with Dr. Owens' data; it is possible to think of a way in which oxygen consumption or delivery has this effect. However, if there are some specific defects of the transporter system in the placenta, that would certainly tend to lower the availability of branched-chain amino acids in the fetal circulation. And as I said, a lot of experiments we have done in liver and muscle suggest that protein synthesis is to a large extent driven by the availability of the amino acids, so accretion could be less because there are less amino acids there, and I don't know which of those two is correct.

Placental Function and Fetal Nutrition,
edited by Frederick C. Battaglia,
Nestlé Nutrition Workshop Series, Vol. 39.
Nestec Ltd., Vevey/Lippincott-Raven Publishers,
Philadelphia, © 1997.

Nutrient Supply in Human Fetal Growth Retardation

Anna Maria Marconi

Department of Obstetrics and Gynecology, San Paolo Institute of Biomedical Sciences, University of Milan, Milan, Italy

Our ability to understand the physiology of the fetus *in utero* and the metabolic changes associated with pregnancy has increased in the last 10 years because of the development of fetal blood sampling techniques and the application of stable isotope methods.

The availability of techniques for sampling fetal cord blood *in utero* under ultrasonic guidance has made it possible to investigate the intrauterine environment of the human fetus under relatively undisturbed conditions (1). Several investigators have evaluated the respiratory gases and acid-base balance, the concentration and fetal-maternal relationships of nutrients, the endocrinology, and the hematology of the human fetus through gestation (1). Subsequently, fetal blood sampling has been extensively used in cases of intrauterine growth retardation (IUGR) for the assessment of fetal well-being (2,3). The results of fetal blood analysis have been compared with those of other noninvasive biophysical procedures to obtain a better understanding of the intrauterine conditions of fetuses with IUGR (4,5). We have recently proposed a classification of the clinical severity of fetal growth retardation that is based on the analysis of noninvasive biophysical indices, such as Doppler velocimetry of the umbilical artery and fetal heart rate pattern (6). According to this classification, fetuses are placed in group 1 if they have a normal pulsatility index of the umbilical artery and a normal fetal heart rate; group 2 fetuses have an increased pulsatility index of the umbilical artery and a normal fetal heart rate; fetuses in group 3 have an increased pulsatility index of the umbilical artery and an abnormal fetal heart rate. The evaluation of fetal respiratory gases and lactate concentration performed *in utero* at the time of fetal blood sampling has revealed significant differences in oxygenation and acid-base balance within the three groups, according to clinical severity. All fetuses in group 1 have normal oxygenation and blood lactate concentration. In group 2, fetal hypoxia and acidosis are uncommon, whereas most fetuses in group 3 have hypoxia and lactic acidemia (6).

At the same time, the use of stable isotopes, which is safe in human pregnancies, allows investigation of the maternal disposal rate of nutrients (7–9). In addition, comparison of fetal and maternal enrichments of labeled compounds at the time of fetal blood sampling or cesarean delivery provides information on the transplacental passage of nutrients (10) as well as on fetal and placental nutrient metabolism (11,12).

Some of the results of the studies on nutrient supply in human fetal growth retardation are presented below.

GLUCOSE

Evaluation of maternal and fetal glucose concentrations in normal pregnancies at the time of fetal blood sampling has shown that umbilical venous glucose concentration decreases significantly with increasing gestational age (13). As maternal glucose concentration is fairly constant and independent of gestational age, the maternal-fetal glucose concentration difference increases significantly during human pregnancy (13). These results suggest that one of the mechanisms by which an increased placental transport of glucose is achieved in human pregnancies is by the development of an increasing maternal-fetal glucose gradient as gestation advances.

As in normal pregnancies, a significant linear relationship between fetal and maternal glucose concentrations is present in IUGR pregnancies (13,14) (Fig. 1). However, the evaluation of the maternal-fetal gradient shows that although there is no difference between the normal fetuses and the IUGR fetuses of group 1, there is a significant and progressive increase of the gradient in IUGR fetuses of groups 2 and 3

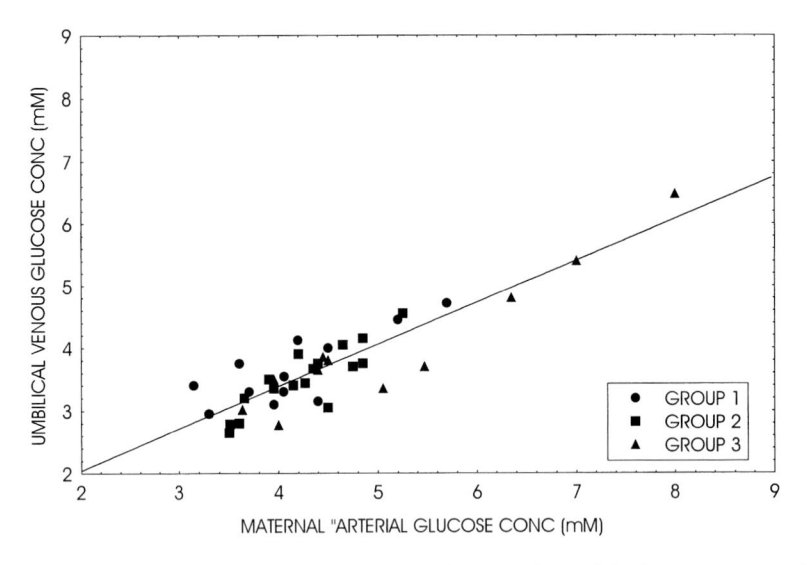

FIG. 1. Relationship between umbilical venous and maternal "arterial" glucose concentrations in growth-retarded fetuses. Fetal glucose concentration (mM) = 0.7 + 0.67 maternal concentration (mM); $r^2 = .77$; $p < .001$.

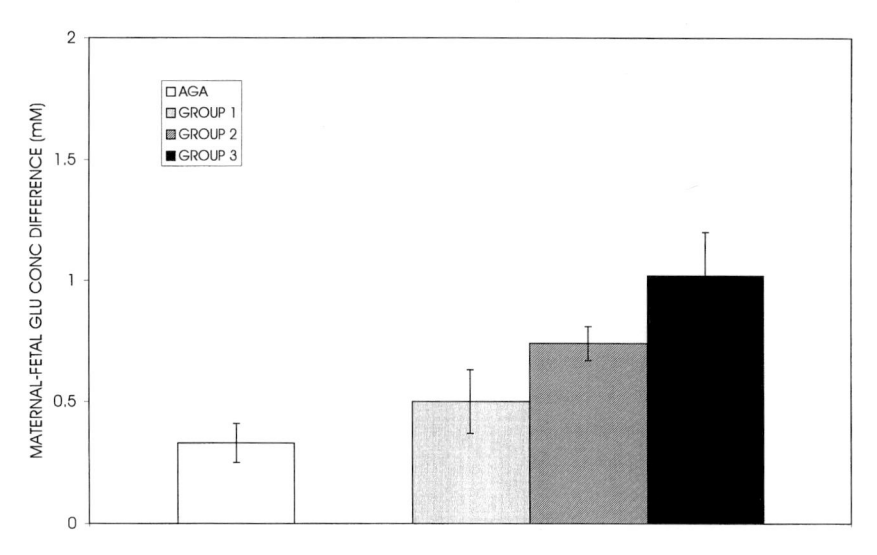

FIG. 2. Maternal-fetal glucose concentration difference in normal and growth-retarded pregnancies divided according to clinical severity (see text). AGA vs. group 1, NS; AGA vs. group 2, $p < .01$; AGA vs. group 3, $p < .001$.

(Fig. 2). Thus, as a consequence of the reduction in placental size, there is a significant reduction of fetal glucose concentration, which increases the transplacental glucose gradient. Figure 3 shows that in IUGR fetuses at the time of elective cesarean delivery, as the transplacental glucose gradient increases the umbilical uptake of glucose also increases. Thus, it is likely that this increase in gradient represents an adaptive mechanism by which the human fetus faces the restriction of placental size, thereby maintaining the glucose uptake. This hypothesis is further supported by experimental studies performed in the heat-exposed model of growth-retarded fetal lambs, where as a compensatory response to the decreased placental capacity for glucose transport, there is a decrease in fetal glucose concentration and a consequent increase in the transplacental glucose concentration difference, which increases the net flux of glucose from placenta to fetus by approximately 50% (15).

The importance of maintaining an adequate supply of glucose to the fetal compartment is further supported by a study performed with D-[U^{13}C]glucose infused in patients with pregnancies complicated by IUGR at the time of fetal blood sampling (11). No significant differences were detected between fetal and maternal glucose enrichments (0.47% ± 0.04 vs. 0.47% ± 0.03), with a mean fetal-maternal MPE (molar percent enrichment) ratio of 0.99 ± 0.01, not significantly different from 1. This implies that there is little if any glucogenesis within the fetus. Thus, transplacental transport represents the most important source of glucose for the growth-retarded fetus.

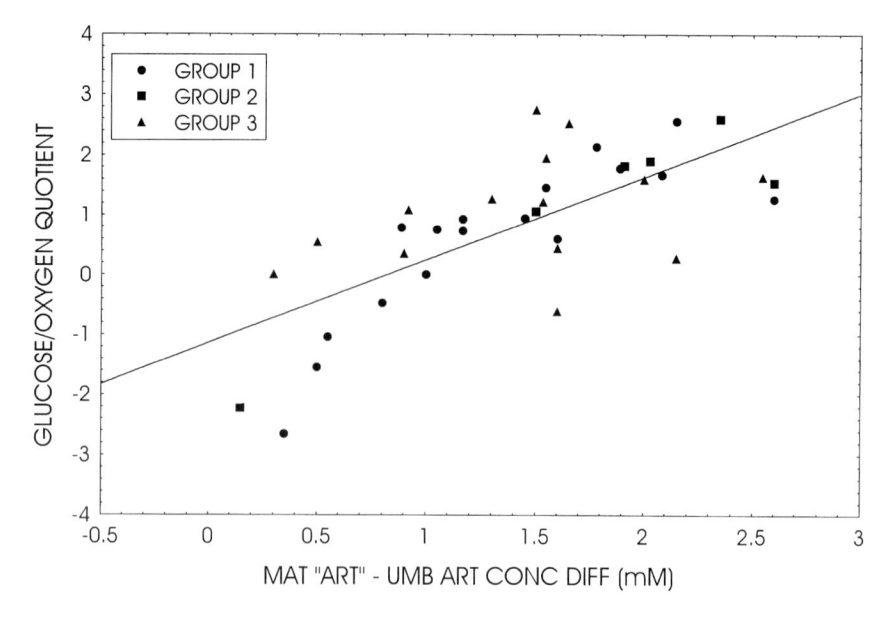

FIG. 3. Relationship between umbilical glucose/oxygen quotient and transplacental glucose gradient in growth-retarded pregnancies at the time of elective cesarean delivery. $G/O_2 = -1.12 + 1.38$ M"A" $-$ UA (mM); $r^2 = .52$; $p < .001$.

AMINO ACIDS

Many studies have shown that the concentration of fetal amino acids is significantly decreased in IUGR pregnancies, both at the time of fetal blood sampling (16,17) and at delivery (18,19). At cesarean delivery, the umbilical venoarterial difference of α-amino nitrogen is significantly reduced in IUGR fetuses when compared with appropriate-for-gestational-age (AGA) fetuses (18). Given that umbilical blood flow is often reduced in these pregnancies, this would imply that the umbilical uptake of amino acids is also reduced.

In IUGR fetuses sampled *in utero* as early as 26 weeks, the umbilical venous plasma concentration of the three branched-chain amino acids—leucine, valine, and isoleucine—is significantly reduced. This reduction is independent of the clinical severity of IUGR and might reflect the presence of an early alteration in the placental transport of amino acids (6). Studies on the system A amino acid transporter in the microvillous membrane of placentae of growth-retarded babies have shown that the activity is reduced compared with the placentae of AGA babies (20).

In a recent investigation in which 23 IUGR pregnancies were studied at the time of fetal blood sampling, we have shown that the fetomaternal concentration difference of most amino acids and of total α-amino nitrogen is significantly reduced in IUGR (21) (Fig. 4). This difference is caused by a decrease in fetal and an increase in maternal amino acid concentrations. In IUGR mothers, the concentration of lysine,

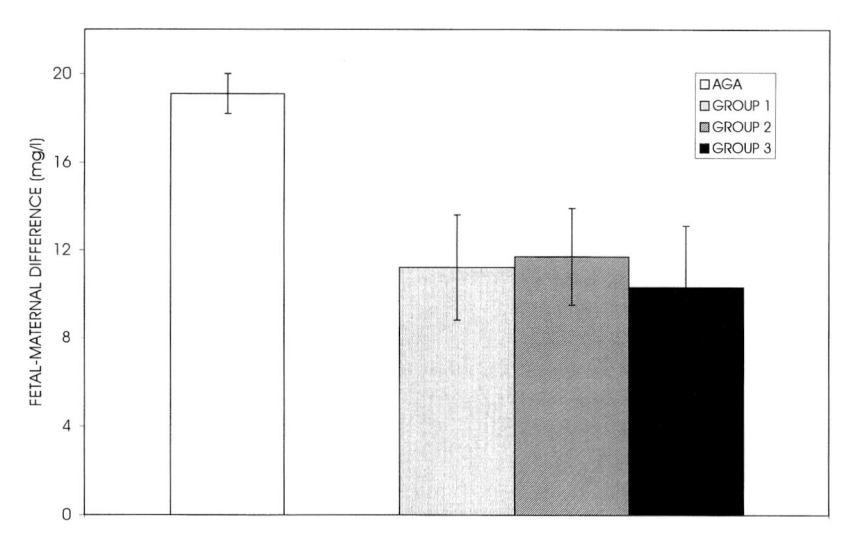

FIG. 4. Umbilical venous-maternal "arterial" plasma concentration difference of total α-amino nitrogen in AGA and IUGR pregnancies divided according to clinical severity (see text). AGA vs. each IUGR group, $p < .01$.

histidine, valine, isoleucine, leucine, phenylalanine, arginine, alanine, and tyrosine is significantly increased when compared with AGA mothers. Total α-amino nitrogen is also significantly increased. In addition, for most amino acids there is a significant relationship between fetal and maternal concentrations, both in AGA and IUGR pregnancies. However, even though the plasma umbilical venous concentration of the individual amino acids does not differ significantly between AGA and IUGR, the relationship between fetal and maternal concentrations is significantly different in IUGR; the relationship between umbilical venous and maternal leucine concentrations is shown, as an example, in Fig. 5. No significant differences are present among the three groups of IUGR pregnancies as far as the maternal-fetal amino acid relationships are concerned. Thus, the decrease in fetal concentrations and in the fetomaternal concentration difference is independent of subgroups and therefore—within these limits—of fetal oxygenation and perfusion.

SUMMARY

IUGR complicates approximately 4% to 10% of deliveries and represents an important cause of perinatal morbidity and mortality (22). At present, no intrauterine treatment is available, and the clinical management relies on the choice of the best timing of delivery. However, in growth-retarded pregnancies there are fetal as well as maternal metabolic differences in comparison with normal pregnancies. It is possible to speculate that the intrauterine detection of such derangements might be used

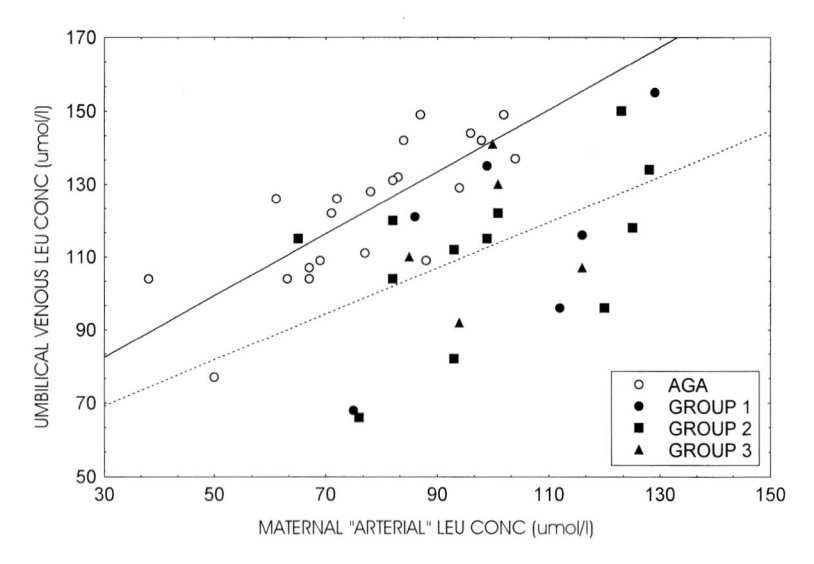

FIG. 5. Relationship between umbilical venous and maternal "arterial" plasma concentrations of leucine in AGA (y = 57 + 0.8x; r^2 = .60; p <.001) and IUGR (y = 50.4 + 0.6x; r^2 = .25; p <.01) pregnancies.

in defining new nutritional therapeutic strategies in these pregnancies, according to clinical severity.

REFERENCES

1. Marconi AM, Cetin I, Buscaglia M, Pardi G. Midgestation cord sampling: what have we learned. *Placenta* 1992;13:115–122.
2. Nicolaides KH, Economides DL, Soothill PW. Blood gases, pH and lactate in appropriate and small-for-gestational-age fetuses. *Am J Obstet Gynecol* 1989;161:996–1001.
3. Pardi G, Buscaglia M, Ferrazzi E, Bozzetti P, Marconi AM, Cetin I, et al. Cord sampling for the evaluation of oxygenation and acid-base balance in growth-retarded human fetuses. *Am J Obstet Gynecol* 1987;157:1221–1228.
4. Visser GHA, Sadovsky G, Nicolaides KH. Antepartum heart rate patterns in small-for-gestational-age third-trimester fetuses: correlations with blood gas values obtained at cordocentesis. *Am J Obstet Gynecol* 1990;162:698–703.
5. Ferrazzi E, Pardi G, Buscaglia M, Marconi AM, Gementi P, Bellotti M, et al. The correlation of biochemical monitoring *versus* umbilical flow velocity measurements of the human fetus. *Am J Obstet Gynecol* 1988;159:1081–1087.
6. Pardi G, Cetin I, Marconi AM, Lanfranchi A, Bozzetti P, Ferrazzi E, et al. Diagnostic value of blood sampling in fetuses with growth retardation. *N Engl J Med* 1993;328:692–696.
7. Marconi AM, Davoli E, Cetin I, Lanfranchi A, Zerbe G, Fanelli R, et al. Impact of conceptus mass on glucose disposal rate in pregnant women. *Am J Physiol* 1993;264(*Endocrinol Metab* 27): E514–E518.
8. Denne SC, Patel D, Kalhan SC. Leucine kinetics and fuel utilization during a brief fast in human pregnancy. *Metabolism* 1991;40:1249–1256.
9. Thompson GN, Halliday D. Protein turnover in pregnancy. *Eur J Clin Nutr* 1992;46:411–417.
10. Cetin I, Marconi AM, Baggiani AM, Buscaglia AM, Pardi G, Fennessey PV, et al. *In vivo* placental transport of glycine and leucine in human pregnancies. *Pediatr Res* 1995;37:571–575.

11. Marconi AM, Cetin I, Davoli E, Baggiani AM, Fanelli R, Fennessey PV, et al. An evaluation of fetal glucogenesis in intrauterine growth retarded pregnancies. *Metabolism* 1993;42:860–864.
12. Marconi AM, Cetin I, Davoli E, Paolini C, Ronzoni S, Fanelli R, *et al.* An evaluation of fetal/maternal plasma leucine enrichments in normal and intrauterine growth retarded pregnancies. *Am J Obstet Gynecol* 1996;174:378.
13. Marconi AM, Paolini C, Buscaglia M, Zerbe G, Battaglia FC, Pardi G. The impact of gestational age and of intrauterine growth upon the maternal-fetal glucose concentration difference. *Obstet Gynecol* 1996;87:937–942.
14. Bozzetti P, Ferrari MM, Marconi AM, Ferrazzi E, Pardi G, Makowski EL, et al. The relationship of maternal and fetal glucose concentrations in the human from midgestation until term. *Metabolism* 1988;37:358–363.
15. Thureen PJ, Trembler KA, Meschia G, Makowski EL, Wilkening RB. Placental glucose transport in heat-induced fetal growth retardation. *Am J Physiol* 1992;263:R578–R585.
16. Cetin I, Corbetta C, Sereni LP, Marconi AM, Bozzetti P, Pardi G, et al. Umbilical amino acid concentrations in normal and growth-retarded fetuses sampled *in utero* by cordocentesis. *Am J Obstet Gynecol* 1990;162:253–261.
17. Economides DL, Nicolaides KH, Gahl WA, Bernardini I, Evans MI. Plasma amino acids in appropriate- and small-for-gestational-age fetuses. *Am J Obstet Gynecol* 1989;161:1219–1227.
18. Cetin I, Marconi AM, Bozzetti P, Sereni LP, Corbetta C, Pardi G, *et al.* Umbilical amino acid concentrations in appropriate and small for gestational age infants: a biochemical difference present in utero. *Am J Obstet Gynecol* 1988;158:120–126.
19. Young M, Prenton MA. Maternal and fetal plasma amino acid concentrations during gestation and in retarded fetal growth. *J Obstet Gynaecol Br Cwlth* 1969;76:333–334.
20. Mahendran D, Donnai P, Glazier JD, D'Souza SW, Boyd RDH, Sibley CP. Amino acid (system A) transporter activity in microvillous membrane vesicles from the placentas of appropriate and small for gestational age babies. *Pediatr Res* 1993;34:661–665.
21. Cetin I, Ronzoni S, Marconi AM, Perugino G, Corbetta C, Battaglia FC, et al. Maternal concentrations and fetal-maternal concentration differences of plasma amino acids in normal (AGA) and intrauterine growth retarded (IUGR) pregnancies. *Am J Obstet Gynecol* 1996;174:1575–1583.
22. Keirse MJNC. Epidemiology and etiology of the growth retarded baby. *Clin Obstet Gynecol* 1984; 2:415–436.

DISCUSSION

Dr. Soothill: I noticed that some of your babies had an oxygen content less than 2 mmol/l, in fact less than 1 mmol/l in some cases, and that is amazingly hypoxic for a baby with normal Doppler. Could you comment?

Dr. Nicolaides: Those data also included the AGA babies.

Dr. Marconi: Those were data at cesarean section. We think that the reason why we have increased lactate concentration differences in AGA and IUGR of group 1 is that in cesarean section there is an acute stress.

Dr. Battaglia: Statistically, perhaps, some of the analyses from groups 2 and 3 might have been the same, but in fact when you look at the data, it is group 3 that is really different. So it seems that it is for group 2 that we need new ways of assessing those babies, because in group 2 there are a few babies that look as bad as in group 3, but most of them don't. So using this crude classification isn't enough. This is the group in which we need better tools to sort out the infants who in a few days are going to be in group 3. That is where the problem is clinically. I think we need new methods there.

Dr. Herrera: Could NMR (nuclear magnetic resonance) spectrometry be the solution to this question?

Dr. Soothill: In UCL, they are trying to use NMR to assess the oxygen concentration in the fetal brain, but you have to paralyze the fetus because of movement artifact. But this is for the future.

Unidentified questioner: Would you care to speculate on the reason why it appears that the maternal amino acid concentrations are elevated?

Dr. Marconi: I guess it is a maladaptation to pregnancy, probably mediated through some hormonal mechanism. We now have evidence of many differences in these mothers. We have found an increase in triglycerides, amino acids, and lactate, so we can call it a maladaptation to pregnancy, but we don't know yet what the mediator of this situation is.

Dr. Nicolaides: One explanation for the high amino acids in the mother is hemoconcentration because of the reduced maternal blood volume in IUGR.

Dr. Marconi: IUGR mothers are not always hemoconcentrated.

Dr. Nicolaides: Have you any explanations for the high fetal nonessential amino acids? We found that essential amino acids are down in the fetus and the nonessentials are up, except serine, which behaves like an essential amino acid.

Dr. Marconi: In our experience, the concentration of nonessential amino acids is also reduced in the IUGR fetus, even though the concentration only of serine and tyrosine is significantly lower when compared with AGA. This observation is in agreement with *in vitro* studies of placental amino acid uptake in AGA and IUGR pregnancies.

Maternal Vascular Disease and Fetal Growth

Carlo Romanini and Herbert Valensise

Department of Obstetrics and Gynecology, Tor Vergata University of Rome, Policlinico S. Eugenio viale dell'Umanesimo 10, Rome, Italy

Maternal vascular diseases are known to influence fetal growth by reducing the availability of nutrients through the impaired uteroplacental circulation. Intrauterine fetal growth retardation (IUGR) is related to an increased risk for perinatal morbidity and mortality. The etiologic factors that result in IUGR are generally difficult to identify. A distinction can be made between intrinsic and extrinsic factors that cause the restriction of fetal growth potential (Table 1), but in many fetuses IUGR is defined as idiopathic or asymptomatic, as none of the identifying factors can be shown to be responsible for the process. Gestational hypertension and the chronic diseases that affect the maternal placental circulation are the principal factors in IUGR (50% to 60%); chromosomal disorders and congenital anomalies are reported in 5% to 10% of all cases of IUGR, and fewer than 10% may have impaired intrauterine growth secondary to congenital infections (1).

In this chapter, we focus on some findings that seem to open new strategies in the identification and treatment of fetal growth retardation: the possibility of monitoring an increased maternal blood pressure in patients with asymptomatic fetal growth retardation; determination of the relations between maternal hyperinsulinemia and reduced fetal growth; and treatment with intravenous immunoglobulin (IVIG) to reduce the incidence of fetal growth retardation in patients with antiphospholipid antibodies.

ASYMPTOMATIC FETAL GROWTH RETARDATION AND INCREASED MATERNAL BLOOD PRESSURE

The asymptomatic growth-retarded fetus (aIUGR) is one in the left part of the overall birth-weight distribution curve, or whose growth is affected by sex, birth rank, race, or maternal height (2). Recently, the use of portable, noninvasive, 24-hour ambulatory devices to monitor blood pressure has been shown to be harmless and effective in defining maternal pressure parameters (3). As a result, different parameters have been adopted. Our objective was to investigate maternal blood pressure with a portable, automatic 24-hour device after the diagnosis of aIUGR had

TABLE 1. *Etiologic factors in intrauterine growth retardation*

Intrinsic factors
Chromosomal abnormalities
Congenital malformations
Genetic heritage
Extrinsic factors
Fetoplacental infections
Placental disease
Anomalous placentation
Maternal vascular disease
Maternal cardiopulmonary disease
Unknown factors

been made ultrasonographically, and to assess the possible role of an undiagnosed hypertensive status in the etiology of growth retardation.

Singleton pregnancies with a first-trimester ultrasonographic scan to assess correct gestational age were included in the study once ultrasonographic diagnosis of fetal growth retardation had been made. Gestational age was above the 28th week, and fetal abdominal circumference below the 10th centile for gestational age for our growth curves, with evidence of a decline across the growth centiles. Identified or suspected gross fetal anomalies, positive immunologic response to any infectious disease (toxoplasmosis, rubella, cytomegalovirus infection), and any chronic or hypertensive disease of the mother were considered to be exclusion criteria. In the week following the ultrasonography and Doppler evaluation, we recorded maternal blood pressure with two portable automatic devices. SpaceLabs 90207 was programmed by a DOS-PC through specific hardware, SpaceLabs 90209 (SpaceLabs Inc., Redmond, WA, USA). Ambulatory recordings were obtained by oscillometry every 30 minutes from 08.00 to 20.00 and from 20.00 to 08.00 during 24 hours, for a total of 50 recordings. The data obtained were analyzed at the end of the 24-hour recording. To describe the whole maternal blood pressure regimen, we chose the mean 24-hour diastolic blood pressure (DBP). This index was recently used as a specific predictor of pregnancy hypertension and pre-eclampsia (4). Four different groups were formed for comparison with the results obtained in the aIUGR group: (a) gestational hypertension with IUGR. Gestational hypertension was defined, after Davey and MacGillivray (5), as a recording of diastolic blood pressure higher than or equal to 90 mm Hg on two consecutive occasions 4 hours or more apart in previously normotensive nonproteinuric women after 20 weeks' gestation; (b) pre-eclampsia with IUGR. Pre-eclampsia was identified when gestational hypertension and significant proteinuria (>300 mg/24 h) were present; (c) gestational hypertension without proteinuria and without IUGR; (d) normotensive patients with normal fetal growth matched for gestational age (control group).

The results obtained in the evaluation of the mean 24-hour DBP are presented in

DIASTOLIC MESOR (mmHg)

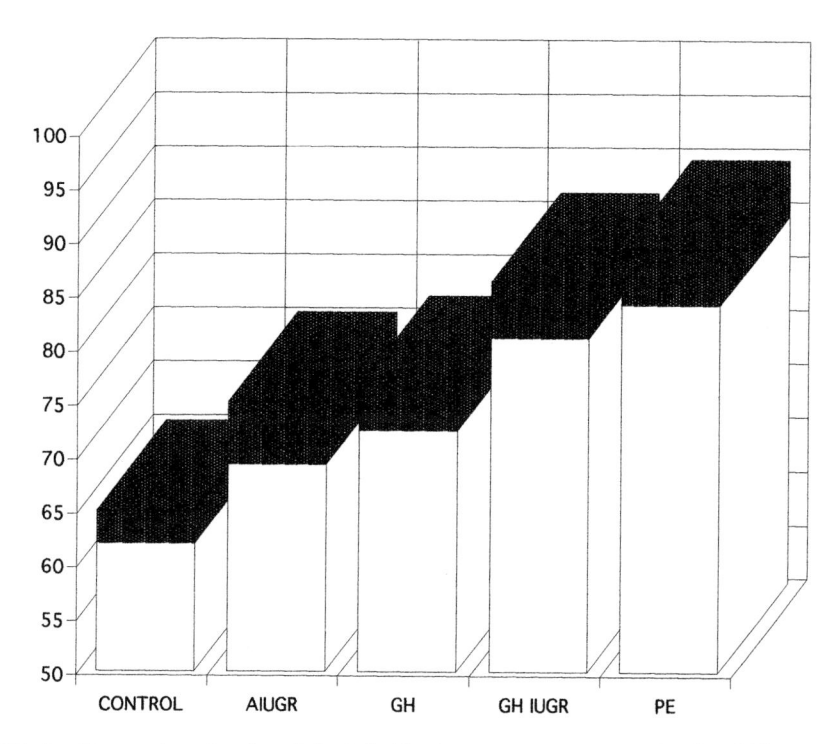

FIG. 1. Mean value of maternal diastolic blood pressure measurements after 24-hour automatic blood pressure monitoring in patients with asymptomatic IUGR (*aIUGR*) compared with controls, patients with gestational hypertension (*GH*), patients with gestational hypertension and IUGR (*GH IUGR*), and patients with pre-eclampsia (*PE*). The value for diastolic blood pressure was higher in patients with aIUGR than in controls ($p < .05$, Student's *t* test) but did not differ from that in patients with GH (NS).

Fig.1, in which the scattered values and median values for each group are given. The highest mean 24-hour DBP value was found in the pre-eclampsia group (84.1 mm Hg). This result does not differ significantly ($p = .38$) from the value obtained in the gestational hypertensive group with IUGR (81.09 mm Hg). The aIUGR group showed a mean 24-hour DBP value of 68.3 mm Hg, which was higher than that in the control normotensive group (61.9; $p < .001$), and lower than that in the gestational hypertensive group without IUGR (75.1 mm Hg; $p < .005$).

Five fetuses had an umbilical S/D (systolic/diastolic) ratio above the S/D cutoff value of 2 for gestational age, whereas PI (pulsatility index) values were all within the normal range. One fetus had a mean cerebral artery PI value above the normal range. Seven patients (38.8%) had an abnormal median uterine resistance index value. A diastolic notch was found in one patient bilaterally and in three patients unilaterally. Our results show that the mean 24-hour DBP value was higher in the aIUGR group than in the control group. Nevertheless, 16 of the 18 patients had a DBP value above the mean value for the normotensive group (61.5 mm Hg), and the two patients who had a normal DBP value had a normal uterine resistance index.

Comment

The condition of an isolated and asymptomatic IUGR fetus is usually defined as idiopathic because of lack of knowledge about the pathophysiologic processes that induce fetal growth retardation. The results obtained in the present series show a significant increase in mean 24-hour DBP in the aIUGR group *vs.* the normotensive control group. Moreover, almost 90% of the patients with an aIUGR fetus showed a mean 24-hour DBP value above the mean of the control group. Hence, in cases of isolated IUGR we recommend a complete evaluation of maternal blood pressure values by 24-hour blood pressure monitoring. The hypothesis that in these patients an incorrect placentation process might lead to a reduction in fetal growth potential rather than to the clinical presentation of maternal hypertension has already been reported by our group (6). The finding that 39% of IUGR fetuses had a high uterine resistance index and an increased mean 24-hour DBP value may provide evidence of an intermediate abnormal implantation process, resulting only in the restriction of fetal growth without the appearance of clinically evident hypertension in the mother. The distribution of abnormal uterine resistance index values in aIUGR infants found in this series overlaps values obtained previously with uterine Doppler resistance index as a screening test for gestational hypertension and IUGR (7). Recent reports (8) have underlined the correlation between abnormal Doppler findings in the uteroplacental circulation and the clinical appearance of hypertension or IUGR. The worst condition of the uterine circulation (bilateral notch and resistance index or PI above the 95th centile for the population studied) is more often linked with pre-eclampsia and IUGR than with isolated IUGR. Ducey *et al.* (9), in their classification of hypertension in pregnancy based on Doppler velocimetry, found only 12 patients among 136 hypertensive women with abnormal uterine and normal umbilical Doppler results. Although differences in peripheral vascular findings in IUGR fetuses have been described using Doppler evaluation both as a screening test and as a diagnostic test (10), no fetuses with absent end-diastolic flow in the umbilical artery were present in this group. This ominous sign in the small-for-gestational-age (SGA) fetus is more commonly detected at earlier gestational ages and in association with pre-eclampsia.

In the presence of fetal growth retardation with normal umbilical Doppler flow measurements, the main advantage in using 24-hour monitoring of maternal blood pressure is to obtain repeated measurements, which are more reliable than the traditional measurements. The use of this technique in patients with aIUGR and normal umbilical PI could then be helpful in the objective quantification of maternal blood pressure. In our series, we found increased maternal blood pressure values in aIUGR pregnancies, equivalent to those of gestational hypertensive patients without IUGR and higher than those of normal patients. Confirmation of our observations by ongoing multicenter clinical trials would allow a new classification of aIUGR fetuses—those suffering from a limitation of growth induced by or complicated by an increase in maternal blood pressure without clinical hypertension. The diagnosis of idiopathic IUGR could then be confined to those fetuses with a reduced rate of growth and normal umbilical and uteroplacental Doppler and mean 24-hour DBP values.

MATERNAL INSULINEMIA AND HYPERTENSION AND FETAL GROWTH RETARDATION

It is well-known that in normal pregnancy insulin secretion increases throughout gestation, whereas peripheral insulin sensitivity decreases (11). Insulin resistance is believed to be the common feature linking hypertension and hyperinsulinemia. The presence of high maternal blood pressure is associated with impaired glucose tolerance and a lower birth weight (12). An increased insulin secretion with insulin resistance and a high insulin-to-glucose ratio may be a predictor of lower birth weight (13). We designed an experimental model to investigate the relation between maternal insulinemia and the glucose-to-insulin ratio in an asymptomatic population, and the subsequent development of gestational hypertension and IUGR. The study was conducted with an asymptomatic population of patients during the second trimester of pregnancy. Patients were submitted to an oral glucose tolerance test, with evaluation of basal and postloading insulinemia. Human placental lactogen was evaluated in the same basal blood sample. Patients were followed using normal procedures until delivery. The longitudinal protocol was based on an ultrasonographic evaluation at 33 to 34 weeks of gestation, and a clinical evaluation of maternal blood pressure and proteinuria every 15 days; 131 patients were then considered for the study. Median maternal age was 30.2 years (SD 3.4; range, 21 to 43). Median gestational age at the time of oral glucose tolerance test was 28.2 weeks (SD 3.1; range, 15 to 39). Median birth weight was 3050 g (SD 345; range, 1800 to 4050). Body mass index (BMI) was calculated as the ratio of weight to the square of the length. Mean BMI was 23.7 (SD 4.7; range, 16 to 41). Patients were divided according to oral glucose tolerance test results into three groups: (a) normal patients (n = 83, 63.3%); (b) patients with gestational diabetes (n = 19, 14.5%); (c) patients with impaired gestational glucose tolerance (IGGT) (n = 29, 22.1%).

IGGT and gestational diabetes patients had values of glycemia at 60 minutes and 120 minutes that were higher than in the control group (p <.001). Basal insulinemia was significantly higher in the IGGT and gestational diabetes group than in the control group. A significant difference in BMI was present (p <.001), with the lowest values in the normal group. Human placental lactogen values did not differ among the three groups of patients, although the IGGT group had the highest values.

INSULINEMIA

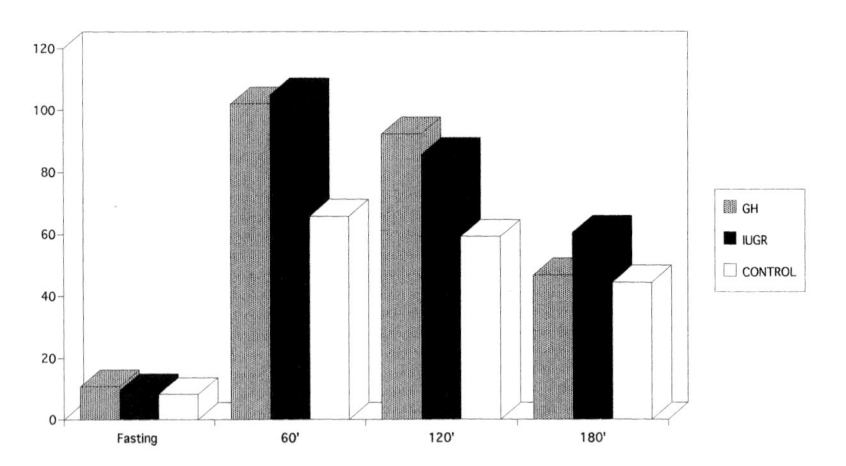

FIG. 2. Mean values of maternal insulinemia after a 100-g oral glucose load in patients in whom gestational hypertension (*GH*) and intrauterine growth retardation (*IUGR*) subsequently developed *vs.* a control group matched for gestational age. An increased level of insulinemia was present in both GH and IUGR patients ($p < .001$) at 60 minutes and 120 minutes after the oral load. The same differences were not apparent with the fasting levels alone.

Birth weight was significantly higher in the IGGT group than in the normal group. In the patients with gestational diabetes, birth weight was not different from that in the normal group.

All the fetuses with isolated IUGR had normal oral glucose tolerance test results. Patients in whom isolated gestational hypertension developed were found in the normal oral glucose tolerance test group (50%) and in the IGGT group (31%). Gestational hypertension and IUGR were present in eleven patients in the normal oral glucose tolerance test group (78.5%) and in three from the gestational diabetes group. Patients with IUGR had 60-minute insulinemia and insulinemic area-under-curve values that were higher than those in controls. The median values of glycemia and insulinemia obtained in the IUGR and gestational hypertension patients with normal responses to the oral glucose load were then compared with those from the normal group: insulinemia at 60 minutes and 120 minutes was significantly increased in the former groups ($p < .05$) (Fig. 2).

Comment

The normal range of maternal plasma insulin in pregnancy is too wide to be useful in identifying hyperinsulinemic patients reliably. Our normal population showed a median level of basal insulinemia of 8.2 mU/l. Patients with gestational diabetes or IGGT showed higher levels of glycemia and insulinemia than did the control group.

Nevertheless, patients with normal responses to the oral glucose load in whom gestational hypertension or IUGR later developed had evidence of increased levels of insulinemia at 60 minutes and 120 minutes after the glucose challenge.

The state of increased insulin resistance, and therefore hyperinsulinemia, could lead to hypertension during pregnancy by several mechanisms, such as retention of sodium and water, activation of the sympathetic nervous system, decreased Na^+/K^+-ATPase activity, increased Na^+/H^+ pump activity, increased cellular accumulation of calcium, and stimulation of growth factor receptors. In nonpregnant women, high blood pressure is prevalent in both obesity and diabetes, conditions associated with insulin resistance; essential hypertension is considered to be an insulin-resistant state (14). Ferranini *et al.* (14) noticed that insulin resistance involves glucose metabolism, is located in peripheral tissues, and is directly correlated with the severity of hypertension. Sowers *et al.* (15) found that women in whom pre-eclampsia developed showed insulin resistance (increased fasting insulin-to-glucose ratios) and abnormal intracellular free calcium metabolism as early as the second trimester of pregnancy. Abnormalities in cellular Ca^{2+} have been observed in women with gestational hypertension (11). These abnormalities include both decreased plasma membrane Ca^{2+}-ATPase activity and abnormal Ca^{2+} responses to vasoactive agonists. Insulin blocks vasoactive receptor and voltage-mediated Ca^{2+} currents in vascular smooth muscle cells, resulting in cell membrane hyperpolarization (15). Insulin also stimulates plasma membrane Ca^{2+}-ATPase and Na^+/K^+-ATPase activity and expression. Insulin-resistant states are associated with decreased plasma membrane Ca^{2+}-ATPase activity, increased Ca^{2+}, and hypertension. The risk for IUGR increases if hypertension and hyperinsulinemia are combined (16). This is probably the result of placental vasculopathy, with reduced or impaired microvascular circulation (16). Solomon *et al.* (17) showed that hypertension in pregnancy occurs in the third trimester, when insulin resistance is greatest. They also noticed that insulin levels measured at the time of oral glucose tolerance test in a subset of women tended to be higher among women in whom hypertension developed during pregnancy. The same results were described with an association between hyperinsulinemia and raised blood pressure during the third trimester of pregnancy (13). Insulin resistance has been related to the development of hypertension, hyperinsulinemia, and increased insulin-to-glucose ratios. The raised blood pressure could be a direct mechanism responsible for the reduced fetal growth. Bevier *et al.* (12) found that within the group of women with gestational diabetes who required insulin, blood pressure and BMI correlated significantly with insulin resistance, quantified by the amount of insulin required to achieve glycemic targets comparable with those achieved in the diet-alone group. In addition, the administration of insulin was accompanied by a significant increase in blood pressure. Patients with normal response to the oral load in whom an IUGR fetus later develops have normal levels of glycemia with increased insulinemia. These two factors might contribute to a chronic state of reduced availability of glucose transferred through the placenta. Decreased availability of maternally derived glucose is responsible for diminished plasma glucose and insulin concentrations in growth-retarded human fetuses (18). Fetal hypoglycemia and hypoinsulinemia are major factors retarding fetal growth; a maternal hyperinsulinemic state can result in maternal and fetal hypoglycemia and hence fetal growth retardation (19). Glucose is a primary fetal metabolic substrate and insulin is a key growth-stimulating hormone that has mitogenic and numerous anabolic effects (18); Breschi et al. (13) found that insulin area under the curve and the ratio of insulin to glucose area were inversely related to birth weight. The inverse correlation was also present in lean mothers, indicating that the link is not forced by obesity. There seems to be an association between maternal hyperinsulinemia and neonatal weight (13). Whether the hyperinsulinemia/insulin resistance is itself a cause of early fetal malnutrition or simply a marker for some underlying mechanism remains to be tested. Moreover, there has been recent interest in the association between intrauterine growth failure and the incidence of hypertension, cardiovascular disease, and syndrome X in adult life (insulin resistance, non-insulin-dependent diabetes, and lipid disorders) (20). It is therefore important to evaluate insulinemia after the oral load to characterize risk factors for the subsequent development of hypertension or retarded fetal growth. We recommend that maternal insulin levels be evaluated both in the fasting state and after a glucose load to characterize patients at risk for hypertension or IUGR.

ANTIPHOSPHOLIPID ANTIBODIES: ROLE OF TREATMENT IN MATERNAL DISEASE AND FETAL GROWTH RETARDATION

Autoimmune factors are recognized to play a role in recurrent pregnancy wastage and obstetric complications (21), even in women with no clinically diagnosed autoimmune disorders. Antiphospholipid antibodies are associated with fetal distress and fetal death. Pre-eclampsia (51%) and severe early-onset pre-eclampsia (27%) have been reported recently in these patients (22). The incidence of fetal growth retardation varies between 30% and 60% of reported cases (23).

Pregnancy complications vary according to the different therapeutic regimens used (corticosteroids, heparin, low-dose aspirin alone or in combination) (22,24,25). The use of high-dose IVIG for preventing recurrent spontaneous abortions and pregnancy complications has been reported in single cases or in small series (26). We have reported normal fetal growth in patients with antiphospholipid syndrome treated with high-dose IVIG (27).

In our series, 14 patients with primary antiphospholipid syndrome received treatment with high-dose IVIG. Ultrasonographic measurements of fetal growth obtained in the group treated with IVIG showed a biparietal diameter below the 10th centile in 23.2% (20/86), but the evaluation of head circumference reduced this to 6.9%. Abdominal circumference below the 10th centile was present in 2.3%, whereas in 90.6% (78/86) the abdominal circumference value was above the 25th centile. The data were assembled for 2-week intervals and compared with the control group. Head circumference was increased in the IVIG group at 36 to 37 weeks ($p < .001$), whereas no significant differences were present at earlier gestational ages. Abdominal circumference was increased in the IVIG group ($p < .05$) in the same weeks of

Abdominal Circumference

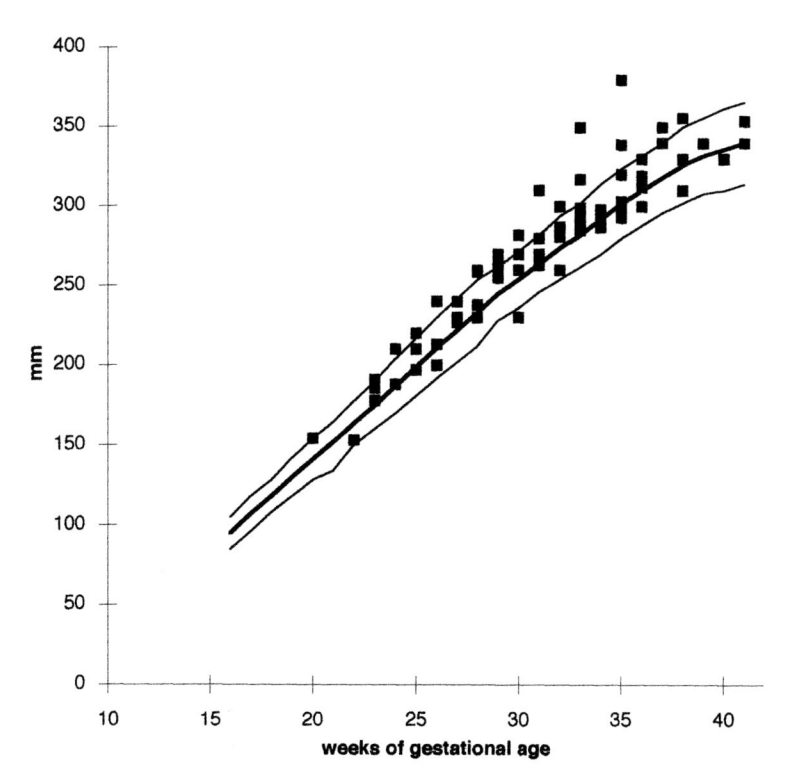

FIG. 3. Scattered reproduction of the values of abdominal circumference observed in the evaluation of fetuses from patients with primary antiphospholipid antibody syndrome treated with IVIG. Normal references are presented as *continuous lines*. No significant reduction in abdominal circumference values was observed in the studied group.

observation (weeks 36 to 37). No significant reduction of fetal abdominal circumference was seen in the treated group compared with the control group (Fig. 3).

Comment

The possibility that immunoglobulin infusions might play a role in the normal evolution of fetal growth should be considered. The type and extension of the placental lesions described in the antiphospholipid-positive patients seem to be of great importance for the availability of fetal nutrients. Placentae from women with adverse pregnancy events in the presence of antiphospholipid show extensive infarction (28), and decidual vasculopathy, placental thrombosis, and infarction are described as major factors in the pathogenesis of fetal growth retardation, intrauterine death, and maternal complications. High titers of antiphospholipid antibodies during pregnancy show greatest sensitivity in predicting placental insufficiency and fetal death, whereas evidence of positive lupus anticoagulant is reported to have the greatest specificity. Moreover, placentae of antiphospholipid-positive patients show an unusual vasculopathy that includes not only histologic evidence of intravascular coagulation, fibrin deposits, and absence of tissue plasminogen activator and thrombomodulin but also endothelial swelling and infiltrates (29). A study of placental abnormalities in women with fetal death showed that those with antiphospholipid antibodies had an increase in placental fibrosis, number of hypovascular villi, and occurrence of thrombosis and infarction, fibrinoid necrosis, and obliterative endoarteritis. There were no signs of inflammation (30). These features were absent in a control group made up of antiphospholipid-negative patients with fetal death. Milder placental histologic abnormalities are found in antiphospholipid-positive patients with liveborn or growth-retarded fetuses. For these reasons, the reduction of fetal growth and of the normal anabolic functions in these patients can be correlated with a direct reduction of placental transfer of nutrients resulting from structural defects induced by the actions of the antiphospholipid antibodies. Several therapeutic regimens have been tried in the past in pregnant women with unexplained autoimmune recurrent fetal loss. These treatments have not always prevented fetal growth retardation or fetal death. Out *et al.* (30) reported IUGR in 24% and intrauterine fetal death in 12% of 59 pregnancies positive for antiphospholipid. Three fetal deaths were present among the 11 pregnancies with persistence of lupus anticoagulant, and treatment with high doses of prednisone could not avoid the reduction in fetal growth observed. Branch *et al.* (22) reported a 43% incidence of fetal growth retardation among 23 patients with antiphospholipid antibodies treated with prednisone and low-dose aspirin; 20% in the group treated with heparin and low-dose aspirin; and 22% in the group treated with prednisone, heparin, and low-dose aspirin. The normal fetal growth reported in our series of antiphospholipid-positive patients treated with IVIG is therefore unusual in the natural history of these patients, and IVIG should not necessarily be considered as the therapeutic solution to this problem. However, we thought it important to present the results obtained on fetal development with IVIG. Although there is the possibility of a "casual" relation, IVIG efficacy is probably a consequence of the presence of anti-idiotypic antibodies in the preparations. It is well-known that these antibodies manipulate the immune system in at least three ways. First, they can neutralize an autoantibody by forming an idiotype/anti-idiotype dimer; then the anti-idiotypic antibodies may bind and down-regulate the B-cell receptor for antigen, decreasing the autoantibody production; finally, regulatory T cells may recognize anti-idiotypic antibody, and a critical concentration of idiotype/anti-idiotype dimers may then be required to activate binding and subsequent suppression through lymphokine production. Furthermore, the beneficial effect of IVIG in patients with autoantibodies might be a result not only of the described mechanism of passive transfer of neutralizing anti-idiotypic antibodies that act against the autoantibodies, but also of the modification of the structure, function, and dynamics of the idiotypic network so that the physiologic control of autoimmunity could be restored and brought to normality. If these are the hypothesized pathways whereby IVIG treatment exerts its positive effects on placental endothelial function and hence on fetal growth, we could in the future regard IVIG therapy as "immunorestoration" of normal function of the network in patients affected by immunologic disorders.

REFERENCES

1. Teberg J, Walther FJ, Pena IC. Mortality, morbidity and outcome of the small for gestational age infant. *Semin Perinatol* 1988;12:84–94.
2. Clapp JF. Etiology and pathophysiology of intrauterine growth retardation. In: Divon M, ed. *Abnormal Fetal Growth*. New York: Elsevier; 1991:83–97.
3. Contard S, Chanundet X, Coisne D, Battistella P, Marichal JF, Pitiot M, et al. Ambulatory monitoring of blood pressure in normal pregnancy. *Am J Hypertens* 1993;6:880–884.
4. Valensise H, Tranquilli AL, Arduini D, Garzetti GG, Romanini C. Screening pregnant women at 22-24 weeks for gestational hypertension or intrauterine growth retardation by Doppler ultrasound followed by 24-hour blood pressure recording. *Hypertension in Pregnancy* 1995;14:351–359.
5. Davey DA, MacGillivray I. The classification and definition of hypertensive disorders of pregnancy. *Am J Obstet Gynecol* 1988;158:892–898.
6. Valensise H, Romanini C. Second trimester uterine artery flow velocity waveform and oral glucose tolerance test as a means of predicting intrauterine growth retardation. *Ultrasound Obstet Gynecol* 1993;3:412–416.
7. Valensise H, Bezzeccheri V, Rizzo G, Tranquilli AL, Garzetti GG, Romanini C. Doppler velocimetry of the uterine artery as a screening test for gestational hypertension. *Ultrasound Obstet Gynecol* 1993;3:18–22.
8. North RA, Ferrier C, Long D, Townsend K, Kincaid-Smith P. Uterine artery Doppler flow velocity waveforms in the second trimester for the prediction of preeclampsia and fetal growth retardation. *Obstet Gynecol* 1994;83:378–386.
9. Ducey J, Schulman H, Farmakides G, Rochelson B, Bracero L, Fleischer A, et al. A classification of hypertension in pregnancy based on Doppler velocimetry. *Am J Obstet Gynecol* 1987;157:680–685.
10. Low JA. The current status of maternal and fetal blood flow velocimetry. *Am J Obstet Gynecol* 1991;164:1049–1063.
11. Reece EA, Homko C, Wiznitzer A. Metabolic changes in diabetic and nondiabetic subjects during pregnancy. *Obstet Gynecol Surv* 1994;49:64–71.
12. Bevier CW, Jovanovic-Peterson L, Burns A, Peterson CM. Blood pressure predicts insulin requirement and exogenous insulin is associated with increased blood pressure in women with gestational diabetes mellitus. *Am J Perinatol* 1994;11:369–373.
13. Breschi MC, Seghieri G, Bartolomei G, Gironi A, Baldi S, Ferrannini E. Relation of birth weight to maternal plasma glucose and insulin concentrations during normal pregnancy. *Diabetologia* 1993; 36:1315–1321.
14. Ferrannini E, Buzzigoli G, Bonadonna R, Giorico MA, Oleggini M, Graziadei L, *et al.* Insulin resistance in essential hypertension. *N Engl J Med* 1987;317:350–357.
15. Sowers JR, Standley PR, Jacober S, Nyogi T, Simpson L. Postpartum abnormalities of carbohydrate and cellular calcium metabolism in pregnancy-induced hypertension. *Am J Hypertens* 1993;6: 302–307.
16. Bauman WA, Maimen M, Langer O. An association between hyperinsulinemia and hypertension during the third trimester of pregnancy. *Am J Obstet Gynecol* 1988;159:446–450.
17. Solomon CG, Graves SW, Greene MF, Seely EW. Glucose intolerance as a predictor of hypertension in pregnancy. *Hypertension* 1994;23:717–721.
18. Frederick LL, Buroker CA, Kim SB, Flozak AS, Ogata ES. Differential effects of short and long durations of insulin-induced maternal hypoglycemia upon fetal rat tissue growth and glucose utilization. *Pediatr Res* 1992;32:436–440.
19. Bagga R, Vasishsta K, Majumdar S, Garg SK. Correlation between human placental lactogen levels and glucose metabolism in pregnant women with intrauterine growth retardation. *Aust N Z J Obstet Gynaecol* 1990;30:310–313.
20. Langford K, Blum W, Nicolaides K, Jones J, McGregor A, Miell J. The pathophysiology of insulin-like growth factor axis in fetal growth failure: a basis for programming by undernutrition? *Eur J Clin Invest* 1994;24:851–856.

21. Rote NS. Pregnancy-associated immunological disorders. *Curr Opin Immunol* 1989;1:1165–1172
22. Branch DW, Silver RM, Blackwell JL, Reading JC, Scott JR. Outcome of treated pregnancies in women with antiphospholipid syndrome: an update of the Utah experience. *Obstet Gynecol* 1992; 80:614–620.
23. Polzin WJ, Kopelman JN, Robinson RD, Read JA, Brady K. The association of antiphospholipid antibodies with pregnancies complicated by fetal growth restriction. *Obstet Gynecol* 1991;78: 1108–1111.
24. Blumenfeld Z, Weiner Z, Lorber M, Sujov P, Thaler I. Anticardiolipin antibodies in patients with recurrent pregnancy wastage: treatment and uterine blood flow. *Obstet Gynecol* 1991;78:584–589.
25. Lockshin MD, Druzin ML, Qamar T. Prednisone does not prevent recurrent fetal death in women with antiphospholipid antibody. *Am J Obstet Gynecol* 1989;160:439–443.
26. Orvieto R, Achirin A, Zion BR, Achiron R. Intravenous immunoglobulin treatment for recurrent abortions caused by antiphospholipid antibodies. *Fertil Steril* 1991;56:1013–1020.
27. Valensise H, Vaquero E, De Crolis C, Stipa E, Perricone R, Arduini D, et al. Normal fetal growth in women with antiphospholipid syndrome treated with high-dose intravenous immunoglobulin (IVIG). *Prenat Diagn* 1995;15:509–517.
28. De Wolf F, Carreras LO, Moerman P, Vermylen J, Van Assche A, Renaer M. Decidual vasculopathy and extensive placental infarction in a patient with repeated thromboembolic accidents, recurrent fetal loss and a lupus anticoagulant. *Am J Obstet Gynecol* 1982;142:829–834.
29. Lockshin MD. Pregnancy and systemic autoimmune disease. *Semin Clin Immunol* 1993;5:5–11.
30. Out HJ, Kooijman CD, Bruinse HW, Derksen RHWM. Histopathological findings in placentae from patients with intrauterine fetal death and antiphospholipid antibodies. *Eur J Obstet Reprod Biol* 1991; 41:179–186.

DISCUSSION

Dr. Soothill: You described your combination of Doppler and 24-hour blood pressure monitoring in predicting outcome, but did your gestational hypertension group have to have proteinuria as well? Because if not, I feel a bit worried about predicting hypertension by blood pressure, because that's self-fulfilling, isn't it?

Dr. Valensise: The problem is that when they had this measurement made at 24 to 25 weeks of gestational age, they did not have evidence of clinical hypertension, so the problem is to find something that could measure what is going on in the mother in a way that could be much more objective than a single measurement. I do agree with your point. If the mother is already hypertensive, there is no need to predict that she will become hypertensive. But the problem is that there may be differences in how the patients will appear in your hands or in my hands on the same day or on two or three different days. That method allows you to have a kind of objective centimeter, as we call it, to which we could refer to categorize a patient and to identify the risk, nothing more than that.

Dr. Soothill: You had a very interesting group—the normal small babies with hyperinsulinemia in the mothers. At what gestational age was that?

Dr. Valensise: The median value is 31.2 weeks, so they are patients who are already in the third trimester. These were very late growth-retarded babies, referred because of suspected growth retardation.

Dr. Battaglia: We keep hearing about normal small babies, and I don't think we should use that term until we know they are normal. Doris Campbell mentioned the other day that we have no follow-up data as to whether these children end up with central nervous system problems later on. I don't know whether they are normal, and I am quite sure no one else knows whether they are normal. Secondly, you said that when you used that term, you were referring to a group of small babies, but did you follow them in the pregnancy, and is it true that they never developed abnormal velocimetry in the fetal vessels?

Dr. Valensise: We could not categorize the babies in exactly the same way as was done by Professor Pardi's group. "Normal small" was a definition to attract attention and nothing more. I still believe that these are babies who need to be followed. In our group a small percentage, about 10%, had an abnormal Doppler. I think that we must include both the umbilical Doppler and the uteroplacental Doppler. I think we should include information from both the maternal side and the fetal side.

Dr. Stuart Campbell: I don't think you could ever call a small fetus "normal small" if there is any abnormal Doppler. And indeed I think you mentioned that many of them had abnormal uterine Doppler, and as soon as you have an abnormal uterine waveform you have to classify that SGA fetus into some sort of category that implies impaired uteroplacental perfusion. So I think "normal small"—if you are ever going to use that expression—means that from all your investigations, you believe that it is a normal, genetically small fetus for normal genetic reasons. I would agree with Professor Battaglia that this is really a retrospective diagnosis.

Dr. Ogata: I am intrigued by your hypothesis about the insulin resistance. There are reports of syndrome X (insulin resistance and hypertension in gestational diabetes), but in that system the insulin resistance results in excess glucose coming across and an increased risk of macrosomia. So if I understand what you are saying, in this particular system you have insulin resistance that overcomes your hyperinsulinemia. Is that right? In one application of this model you can end up with a big baby, and in this application you are reducing glucose availability to the fetus and thus contributing to growth retardation.

Dr. Valensise: This is not my hypothesis, but one that has been presented in the literature. The problem is to try to subdivide the maternal metabolic adaptations, because in gestational diabetes you may find hyperinsulinemia but you may also find normal insulinemia in response to the oral glucose tolerance test. The hypothesis is that maternal hyperinsulinemia could lead to reduced availability of glucose from the maternal side to the fetal side, and this could result in chronically reduced availability of glucose to the fetus, followed by hypoinsulinemia in the fetus and reduced fetal growth. Of course, the pathway can't be that easy, and there must be something else going on—and I refer to all the interactions with the other factors affecting fetal growth. Still, I think it is interesting that some patients who don't show an abnormal response to the oral load and have normal levels of glycemia have levels of insulinemia that are 10-fold those of "normal" patients, and we don't understand why.

Dr. Stuart Campbell: I find it extraordinary that you could have a normal glucose tolerance test and maternal hyperinsulinemia. Could somebody explain that?

Dr. Godfrey: David Phillips from our metabolic programming group in Southampton has done statistical modeling of glucose tolerance tests in individuals in whom insulin resistance and insulin secretion have been specifically measured. My reading of the figure that you showed is that there wasn't fasting hyperinsulinemia but there was an exaggerated insulin response during the glucose tolerance test, and although you would need to apply these statistical models to the data, I would be very surprised, indeed, if those came out showing insulin resistance as opposed to exaggerated insulin secretion. I think there is a further danger in all this, in that we and others have shown profound intergenerational effects on fetal growth and further that men and women who had low birth weights may have a 10-fold increase in syndrome X as adults. So I think we have to be very careful about whether we are looking at intergenerational effects or specific effects relating to placental lactogen or whatever.

Dr. Valensise: I agree with you. Still, when we were looking for hyperinsulinemic patients for the first part of our studies on the receptor, we could find a cutoff value, and the fasting values of insulinemia in literature range from 8 to 25 μU/l, which is a really large variation.

I don't want to say that this is related to insulin resistance, because you need to do something more to measure insulin resistance. You should use a clamp technique, and this was not done. I am not saying that these differences are necessarily significant, but if they are real, they have implications for what has been said in the literature about the chronic action of insulin on the maternal vessels and on the electrolyte content of the vessels. I think we should be aware of that.

Dr. Doris Campbell: We ought to be careful about extrapolating from the results of glucose tolerance testing done at an isolated time in pregnancy to what might be a longitudinal happening, because pregnant women don't drink 100 g of glucose with regularity; they eat food, and the endocrine response in pregnancy is such that it keeps plasma glucose in a very tight band. We must be careful about extrapolating from high levels in response to very high, unphysiologic glucose loading.

Dr. Battaglia: I don't put much credence in the idea that development of any kind of reduction in glucose supply to the pregnant uterus is going to produce growth retardation, because Bill Hay in our department has been producing profound hypoglycemia in pregnant sheep for weeks, and the effect on fetal growth is really minimal—he is getting a 15% reduction in fetal weight, in a species in which you can produce striking growth retardation by other techniques. So I think a limitation of glucose supply alone in large mammals is very unlikely to be a cause of the growth retardation.

Dr. Campbell: I thought it had been shown reasonably conclusively that maternal undernutrition in third-world countries is associated with SGA fetuses.

Dr. Battaglia: We come back to Doris Campbell's point; with undernutrition you are reducing amino acid intake. I am talking about glucose alone. If you restrict glucose, I doubt whether it is going to produce growth retardation in any large mammal.

Dr. Pardi: How did you select the patients followed longitudinally starting from 20 to 24 weeks?

Dr. Valensise: With Doppler evaluation. These patients came from a group of patients referred to our clinic, and they underwent Doppler only when they were in the first pregnancy or they had a previous pathology in their pregnancy that could be related to uteroplacental insufficiency: previous fetal death, previous intrauterine death, previous growth retardation, previous small baby. Those were the selection criteria.

Dr. Boyd: Would it make any difference at all if you used systolic blood pressure from your recordings rather than diastolic? They seem to be extraordinarily parallel.

Dr. Valensise: The slide that you saw was only a graphic reconstruction. When we use systolic blood pressure, we don't have the same results—they are much less significant. The diastolic value is much more useful in this sort of evaluation in the absence of clinical hypertension.

Dr. Boyd: So the slide you showed was atypical, where they were very parallel?

Dr. Valensise: Yes, it was just a representation.

Dr. Fournie: Did you try to link the difference between diurnal and nocturnal pressure measurements?

Dr. Valensise: When these machines first appeared in our department, there was great enthusiasm about the possibility of circadian variation, and people were eagerly awaiting the results to see if there might be differences between patients who retained the normal rhythm and those who had lost it, trying to see whether treatment at a certain time of day could be directed toward restoring the normal rhythm. However, in the patients with a confirmed diagnosis of pre-eclampsia or nonproteinuric pre-eclampsia with growth retardation, the incidence of loss of circadian rhythm was very low, somewhere around 20% to 25%.

Dr. Stuart Campbell: You showed maternal endothelial damage. Could you elaborate on that? What causes this endothelial damage, especially as the endothelium is replaced in the spiral arteries by trophoblast? It always seemed to me to be one of the great mysteries as to why the endothelium is replaced by the placenta. There must be a physiologic reason for that.

Dr. Valensise: It is said that what causes the endothelial damage is a multifactorial process that starts with a reduction in the hemodilution and the presence of hemoconcentration that would increase the sheer stress on the endothelium, and the macrophages or neutrophils would deposit part of their content of aggregating molecules, which will lead to problems.

Dr. Stuart Campbell: You found sustained increased blood pressure in your normal IUGR group. Why?

Dr. Valensise: It was not sustained, but it was certainly different from the median values of the control group. In a scatter diagram, these are in the lowest part, nearer the normal than the abnormal, but they are similar to values in patients who have gestational hypertension without proteinuria. I don't know why. Redman has described normotensive pre-eclampsia, in which the damage to the implantation is not directed toward the maternal organism but toward the fetus (1,2). I don't know whether this is true, and I don't know why this happens.

Dr. Herrera: I would like to comment on damage to the endothelium in this condition. I don't know anything about pre-eclampsia, but it seems to me, at least from the literature, that in this condition there is a large increase in oxidative stress and an increased production of free radicals. These free radicals are taken up by the endothelial cells and maybe could contribute to the damage.

REFERENCES

1. Redman CWG. Current topic: Preeclampsia and the placenta. *Placenta* 1991;2:301–308.
2. Valensise H, Liu YY, Federici M, *et al.* Increased expression of low affinity insulin receptor isoform and insulin/insulin-like growth factor-I hybrid receptors in term placenta from insulin resistant women with gestational hypertension. *Diabetologia* 1996;39:952–960.

Fetal Growth and Long-Term Consequences in Animal Models of Growth Retardation

Kathleen Holemans, Leona Aerts, and F. André Van Assche

Department of Obstetrics and Gynecology, Katholieke Universiteit Leuven, Leuven, Belgium

Fetal growth and development are primarily determined by genetic information in the fetus, but the genetic regulation of fetal growth is influenced by various factors that can exert a stimulatory or inhibitory effect. On the one hand, fetal growth is determined by the capacity of the mother to supply nutrients and by the capacity of the placenta to transport these nutrients to the fetus. On the other hand, the fetus has its own factors that influence its growth and differentiation: the fetal growth factors.

Normal growth demands an equilibrium in the interaction between these different compartments and between the stimulatory and inhibitory factors affecting each of these steps. Disturbance of this equilibrium at any stage can result in intrauterine growth retardation (IUGR) and microsomia or in fetal overgrowth and macrosomia.

The mother's metabolic condition is the first important determinant of fetal growth. Adequate maternal and fetal blood flow is important for placental function, and therefore also for an efficient nutrient supply to the fetus. Malnutrition, as well as diabetes, results in a decreased uteroplacental blood flow during gestation (1,2) and a decreased total milk volume during lactation (3), which hamper normal fetal and neonatal growth. These two conditions can thus provide insight into the adaptations of fetal development in an abnormal intrauterine milieu and thereby into the mechanisms that regulate such development in normal pregnancies as well.

PLACENTAL NUTRIENT TRANSPORT

Normal Pregnancy

Normal fetal growth and development depend on nutrients derived from maternal fuels.

Glucose is the major substrate for the fetus, because—at least in the rat fetus—it cannot be synthesized from placentally transferred substrates. Maternal glucose is therefore retained for transplacental transport and traverses the placenta freely by facilitated diffusion, mediated by glucose transporters. In the rat, GLUT-1 and GLUT-3 have been demonstrated in the placenta within different placental layers (4), but only GLUT-3 is exclusively expressed within the labyrinth, which is the zone of physiologic exchange between the maternal and fetal circulations. It has been suggested, therefore, that GLUT-1 is responsible for supplying glucose as a placental fuel and that GLUT-3 is important for glucose transfer to the fetus. In the human, GLUT-1 is abundant in both syncytiotrophoblast and cytotrophoblast and in fetal endothelial cells in placental villi at term. There is controversy as to whether GLUT-3 is also expressed in human placentae (5). So far as possible regulatory factors are concerned, it has been found that insulin has no effect on glucose uptake and metabolism in a perfused *in vitro* system; only maternal glucose concentration has been shown to direct its uptake.

Amino acids are concentrated in the fetus against a transplacental gradient; the levels of amino acids are higher in the fetus than in the pregnant mother (ratio ≈ 1.5 and 2.0). A similar relation has also been reported in the rhesus monkey and the rat. The transport of amino acids through the placenta is active, with a variety of transport systems for individual amino acids (6). Essential branched-chain amino acids are transported rapidly through the placenta, whereas the transfer of straight-chain amino acids is rather slow.

The transport of *lipids* across the placenta depends on the maternal plasma lipid concentration and the species; placentae of different species have very different permeabilities and transport capacities for fatty acids. As a result, the fat content of the fetuses varies markedly among species in direct relation to placental lipid transport (e.g., the human infant at term has about 18% body fat, whereas the rat fetus has only 1% to 2%). The net flux of lipids across the placenta can occur by at least three mechanisms: (a) direct transfer of fatty acids by specific transport proteins, (b) synthesis of complex lipids from fatty acids within the placenta and subsequent release into the umbilical circulation, and (c) hydrolysis of triglycerides, lipoproteins, and phospholipids and subsequent release into the fetal circulation (7,8).

Diabetic Pregnancy

In diabetic pregnancy, the fuel supply to the fetus is abundant, owing to the accentuated catabolism in the mother. Fetal *glucose* levels are increased relative to the mother's glycemia. GLUT-3 messenger RNA and protein in diabetic rat placentae increase up to fivefold, whereas the expression of GLUT-1 remains unaltered. The same effect could be obtained in pregnant rats during hyperglycemia, but not during euglycemic hyperinsulinemia (4). The transport of *amino acids* depends on an adequate uteroplacental blood flow. The transplacental transport of α-aminoisobutyric acid correlates with the placental blood flow and fetal weight in guinea pigs (9). In diabetic rat pregnancy, the influx of amino acids from the maternal side is largely increased in macrosomic fetuses, whereas amino acid transport to their underweight littermates is significantly reduced (10). Amino acid levels in growth-retarded fetuses of rats with streptozotocin-induced diabetes are decreased (11,12). In human pregnancies, amino acid concentrations are also decreased in small-for-gestational-age (SGA) fetuses (13) and newborns (14). The passage of *lipids* to the fetus in a diabetic pregnancy is promoted by high levels of very-low-density lipoprotein (VLDL) triglycerides and nonesterified fatty acids in maternal plasma (15).

FETAL ENDOCRINE PANCREAS

In the fetal rat pancreas, "islet-like" formations, composed mainly of insulin-containing cells, are clearly present from day 18 of gestation; these cells already co-express GLUT-2, the glucose transporter of the β cell (16). By day 20, the endocrine cells accumulate in clusters, appearing organized into real "mantle-islets" with a core of insulin-producing β cells (17). At the ultrastructural level, the β cells appear as mature synthesizing and secreting cells. Granulation of β cells increases with fetal age, parallel to the increase in pancreatic insulin content (18). With the appearance of small islets of Langerhans (day 20 of gestation), glucose-stimulated insulin release can be triggered *in vivo*. The transition from a fetal to an adult type of insulin release in response to glucose occurs during the last days of gestation and parallels quantitative rather than qualitative changes within the β cells (19). In fetuses of streptozotocin-induced diabetic rats, an evolution similar to that in control fetuses is observed, but the development of the endocrine pancreas is enhanced by the raised blood glucose concentrations, which results in hypertrophy and hyperplasia of the islets from day 20 of gestation until birth (17). When maternal hyperglycemia is severe, fetal pancreatic islets are overstimulated by the excessive glucose concentration. The fetal β cells become degranulated, disorganized, and incapable of reacting to any stimulus (19). Indeed, glucose-stimulated insulin release was absent from pancreases of severely hyperglycemic (15.09 mM) fetuses (19). Incubation of fetal islets with other secretagogues also results in the absence of an insulin response in the fetuses of highly hyperglycemic rats. Only arginine induced a sustained monophasic insulin release, suggesting that the defect may concern stimulus-secretion coupling (20,21). Severe diabetes is associated with fetal growth retardation as a result of fetal malnutrition. Similar findings have also been reported in the fetuses of very poorly controlled diabetic women (22).

Poor nutrition of the mother during pregnancy obviously leads to IUGR. The decreased availability of nutrients for transplacental transport and a decreased placental blood flow result in a decreased nutrient supply to the fetus (1). An inadequate stimulation of the fetal pancreas leads to hypoplasia of the pancreatic endocrine tissue, owing to a smaller size of the islets of Langerhans; pancreatic insulin content is decreased and insulin response to stimuli is altered (23,24), resulting in fetal hypoinsulinemia. The effect was similar whether the maternal rats were restricted in their total food intake or only the protein component of the food was diminished, with or without complementing the diet up to isocaloric levels (23–25).

INSULIN ACTION

In the rat, insulin receptors are present from day 17 of gestation in fetal liver, lung, gastrointestinal tract, and heart. Internalization of the hormone in the hepatocytes occurs as early as insulin receptors are detected, and the rate at which this mechanism proceeds increases with the degree of liver maturation (26).

Fetal hypoinsulinemia and a reduced number of insulin receptors on target cells (27) in fetuses of severely diabetic rats may lead to a reduction in fetal glucose uptake; a reduced fetal glucose uptake has been shown in hypoinsulinemic streptozotocin-injected fetal lambs (28). The growth of the fetal protein mass is suppressed; fetal protein synthesis is consistently lower than control rates, whereas protein degradation increases sharply toward the end of gestation (29).

With maternal malnutrition, the combination of fetal hypoinsulinemia and low substrate availability decreases fetal whole-body glucose utilization rates in sheep (30) and rat (31), mainly through a decrease in glucose uptake by the fetal skeletal muscles and heart; glucose uptake by liver and brain is unaffected (31). A decrease in glucose transporter activity, protein, and messenger RNA has been reported in the lung of SGA fetuses in the rat (32). Also, lipid deposition and protein breakdown are decreased, retarding the growth of muscle and adipose tissue (33).

Malnutrition of the maternal rat prematurely induces gluconeogenesis through a decreased insulin-to-glucagon ratio in the fetus. An increased activity of phosphoenolpyruvate carboxykinase (PEPCK), a key enzyme of gluconeogenesis, was shown in fetal liver after maternal malnutrition (34) and after administration of streptozotocin (35) or anti-insulin serum (34) to fetuses. Moreover, PEPCK activity is increased in neonatal and adult rat liver after perinatal protein deprivation. Glucose-6-phosphatase plays a crucial role in the regulation of hepatic glucose production through either glycogenolysis or gluconeogenesis. Glucose-6-phosphatase activity in fetal liver can be induced by administration of glucagon, cyclic AMP, or epinephrine to the fetus, whereas administration of glucose to the maternal rat prevents an increase in glucose-6-phosphatase activity (36). Insulin injection in the newborn rat also prevents an increase in glucose-6-phosphatase activity (36). Messenger RNA expression of glucokinase, an enzyme of glycolysis, is stimulated by insulin and inhibited by glucagon/cyclic AMP (37). A premature induction of glucokinase messenger RNA expression can also be induced by glucose (38). Glucokinase enzyme activity is decreased in neonatal and adult rats after perinatal protein deprivation. The messenger RNA expression of GLUT-2 seems also to be regulated by glucose (39).

With respect to the peripheral tissues, the perinatal period is also very important for the regulation of the glucose transporters (GLUT-1 and GLUT-4). During fetal life, the glucose transporter GLUT-1 dominates in peripheral tissues. GLUT-1 seems to be negatively regulated by glucose.

After birth, the glucose diet of the fetus changes into the high-fat diet of the suckling rat. The amount of endocrine tissue does not further increase, whereas the pancreatic insulin content exceeds adult values. Plasma insulin concentration decreases and remains low until weaning (11). At weaning, the high-fat diet of the suckling rat is changed into a high-carbohydrate diet. The mass of endocrine tissue and the plasma insulin concentrations increase while pancreatic insulin content decreases (11). The suckling-weaning transition in rats is associated with an increase in insulin sensitivity of the peripheral tissues (40), which may be conferred by an enhanced expression of the GLUT-4 glucose transporter (41). During the neonatal period, GLUT-1 expression decreases while GLUT-4 expression increases. The regulation of GLUT-4 expression depends on the composition of the diet; the suckling-weaning transition in rats is associated with a shift from a high-fat (milk) to a high-carbohydrate diet (rat chow). An increase in GLUT-4 messenger RNA expression can be partly prevented by weaning on a high-fat diet. The expression and translocation of GLUT-4 are also regulated by circulating insulin concentrations (41).

ADULT OFFSPRING

Female offspring of severely diabetic rats have a lower body weight from fetal life onward (Table 1). At adult age (3 months), these offspring appear to have recovered from the influences of a perinatal diabetic environment. They have a morphologically normal endocrine pancreas and normal plasma glucose concentrations (11). Plasma insulin concentrations are normal (Table 1) or increased. During

TABLE 1. *Body weight, plasma glucose and insulin concentrations in the offspring of control, diabetic, and food-restricted rats at various ages*

Group	Body weight, g[a]	Glucose, mmol/l[a]	Insulin, nmol/l[a]
Day 22 of fetal life			
Control	5.11 ± 0.05 (33)	3.68 ± 0.12 (27)	1.59 ± 0.12 (27)
Diabetic	4.23 ± 0.04* (57)	20.4 ± 0.5*** (51)	0.87 ± 0.03* (51)
Food-restricted	4.07 ± 0.05** (35)	2.77 ± 0.08** (30)	0.77 ± 0.07* (30)
Day 20 after birth			
Control	36 ± 0.3 (71)	NM	NM
Diabetic	NM	NM	NM
Food-restricted A	41 ± 0.7* (61)	NM	NM
Food-restricted B	15 ± 0.6* (64)	NM	NM
Day 100 after birth			
Control	202 ± 2 (32)	5.06 ± 0.11 (32)	0.26 ± 0.03 (25)
Diabetic	179 ± 2** (25)	5.11 ± 0.17 (23)	0.26 ± 0.01 (23)
Food-restricted A	218 ± 3* (25)	5.22 ± 0.11 (21)	0.15 ± 0.07* (22)
Food-restricted B	185 ± 4* (21)	5.55 ± 0.17* (21)	0.15 ± 0.01* (25)

NM, not measured; food-restricted A, rats food-restricted during pregnancy; food-restricted B, rats food-restricted during pregnancy and lactation.
[a] Data are presented as means ± SEM. Number of animals is given in parentheses.
* $p < .05$ *vs.* control rats; ** $p < .01$ *vs.* control rats; *** $p < .001$ *vs.* control rats.

a 3-hour glucose infusion, however, these offspring have a raised insulin-to-glucose ratio, suggesting insulin resistance (42). Euglycemic hyperinsulinemic clamp studies combined with isotopic measurement of glucose turnover using [3-^{3}H]-glucose have clearly demonstrated the existence of an insulin resistance in liver and peripheral tissues of adult offspring of severely diabetic rats (43).

The peripheral tissues of offspring of severely diabetic rats are less sensitive to insulin (half-maximal effect), but they display a normal responsiveness to insulin (maximal effect), confirming previous results of the ^{123}I-insulin captation experiments (44). Because in the clamp studies all rats were in the postabsorptive state, the glucose production rate in these studies equals the actual glucose production rate. Endogenous glucose production in offspring of severely diabetic rats is both less sensitive and less responsive to insulin (43).

With the exception of the liver, the hyperinsulinemic clamp does not allow identification of the tissues contributing to the peripheral insulin resistance. To determine the peripheral tissues contributing to the decreased glucose disposal, we used the 2-deoxy-[1-^{3}H]-D-glucose technique in basal conditions and during a clamp at physiologic hyperinsulinemia. We thus determined the *glucose metabolic index* in five skeletal muscles, the diaphragm muscle, white adipose tissue, and two control tissues (brain and duodenum) (Fig. 1). As could be expected, skeletal muscles are primarily responsible for the peripheral insulin resistance that characterizes the adult offspring of severely streptozotocin-induced diabetic rats (45). Indeed, the glucose metabolic index in the skeletal muscles of adult offspring of severely streptozotocin-induced diabetic rats was 9% to 29% lower under basal conditions and 25% to 70% lower at physiologic hyperinsulinemia than that of control rats. Muscles are the main reservoir of insulin-sensitive tissues within the mammalian body, representing 36% to 40% of the body weight. Their contribution to the whole glucose turnover is about 36% in postabsorptive control rats and 50% during euglycemic hyperinsulinemia (46).

Female offspring of rats that are food-restricted (50% of normal food intake) during pregnancy and lactation have a lower body weight from fetal life onward; by contrast, the offspring of rats food-restricted only during pregnancy increased their body weight above control values (Table 1). Nonfasting plasma glucose levels were increased in offspring with malnutrition during both the fetal and neonatal periods (Table 1), indicating that glucose tolerance had deteriorated in this group (25).

With the euglycemic-hyperinsulinemic clamp technique, we have shown that adult female rats subjected during the perinatal period to malnutrition, caused by impaired uteroplacental and mammary transfer of nutrients, are resistant to the action of insulin, as evidenced by the decreased infusion rate of glucose to maintain euglycemia (Fig. 2).

This resistance to insulin was found to be the result of a decreased responsiveness of the liver—that is, a dampened suppression of glucose production during hyperinsulinemia (47). Insulin action at the peripheral tissues, however, remained normal (25).

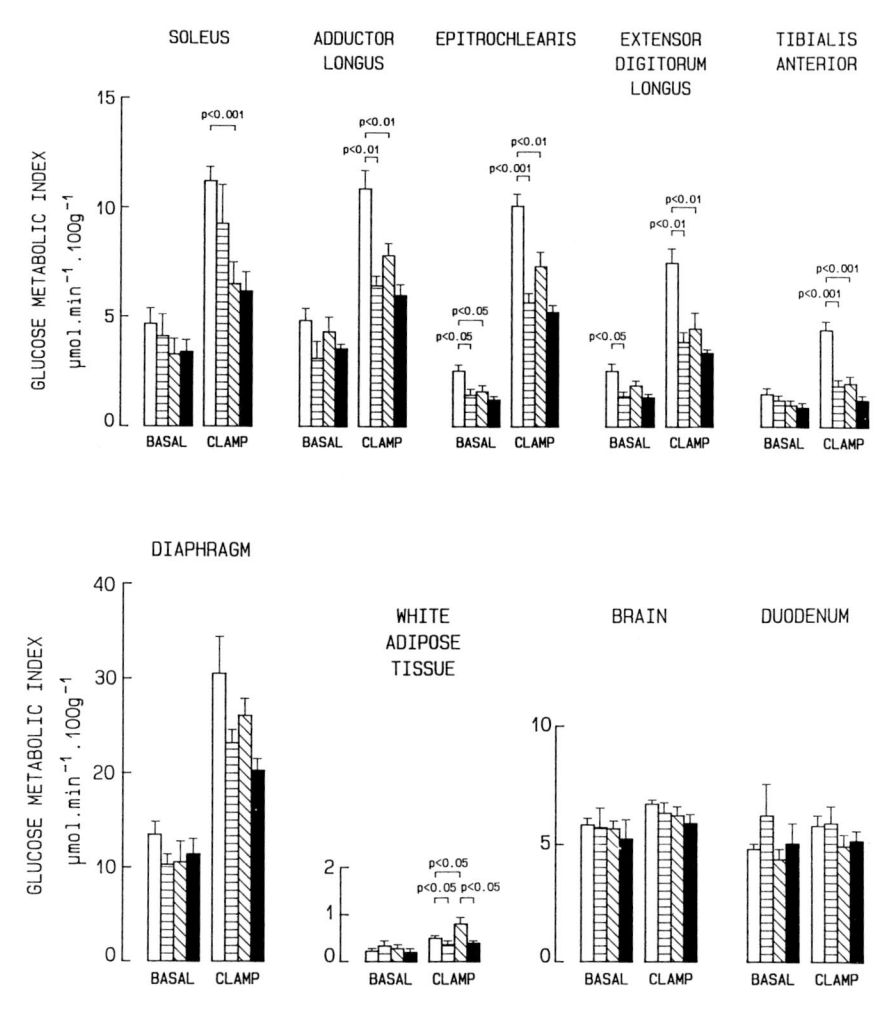

FIG. 1. *In vivo* glucose metabolic index in soleus, adductor longus, epitrochlearis, extensor digitorum longus, and tibialis anterior muscle; and in diaphragm, white adipose tissue, brain, and duodenum of nonpregnant (*empty squares*) and pregnant (*horizontally striped squares*) control rats and of nonpregnant (*diagonally striped squares*) and pregnant (*filled squares*) offspring of rats made diabetic with streptozotocin under basal conditions and at physiologic hyperinsulinemia. Data are means ± SEM of five to ten experiments. From Holemans et al. (45).

Apart from the slight difference in plasma glucose concentrations and a clear difference in body weight (growth retardation at the time of the clamp only in rats undernourished during fetal life), there were no significant differences in the plasma insulin levels or tissue insulin sensitivity of rats subjected to food restriction during the fetal period alone or the fetal and neonatal periods combined. This suggests that fetal malnutrition is the main determinant of hepatic insulin resistance in the rat. By

GLUCOSE INFUSION RATE (μmol.min⁻¹.kg⁻¹)

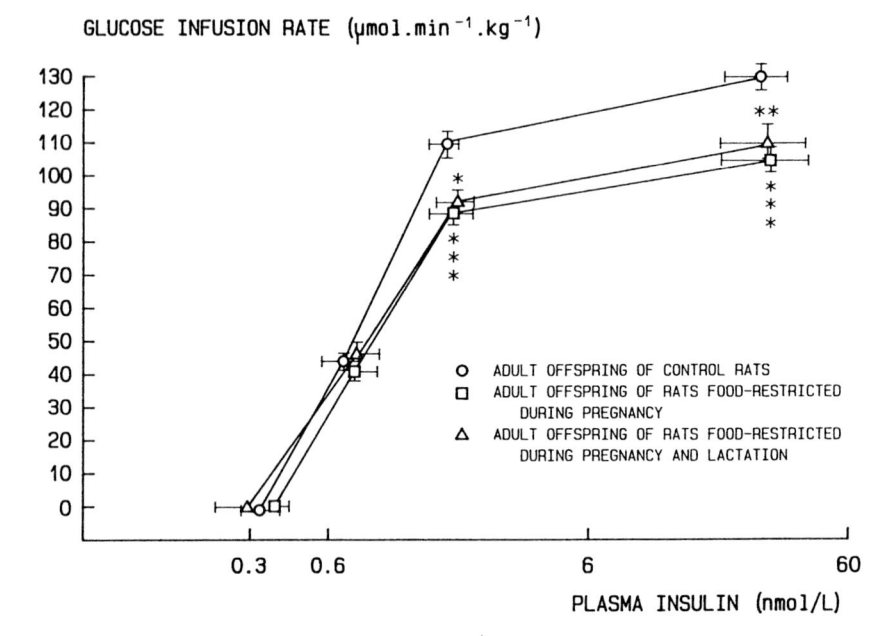

FIG. 2. Insulin dose-response curves for steady-state glucose infusion rate in adult offspring of rats food-restricted during pregnancy (group A; *squares*) or during both pregnancy and lactation (group B; *triangles*) and in rats fed *ad libitum* (group C; *circles*). Data are means ± SEM of five to 10 experiments. $^*p$ <.05; $^{**}p$ <.01; $^{***}p$ <.001 *vs.* control values. From Holemans *et al.* (25).

contrast, although fetal muscle glucose utilization was found to be suppressed by maternal fasting, this did not affect peripheral glucose utilization at adult age. Thus, there is no long-term ''imprinting'' of perinatal malnutrition on muscle glucose utilization.

The growth retardation in adult rats induced by malnutrition during gestation and lactation has different implications for glucose homeostasis than the growth retardation induced by severe diabetes in the maternal rat. We found that the adult offspring of severely diabetic rats had normal nonfasting glucose concentrations and normal or increased nonfasting insulin concentrations. The insulin resistance in these rats was characterized by a decreased sensitivity of the peripheral tissues—that is, the skeletal muscles—and by a decreased sensitivity and responsiveness of the liver (43,45). The insulin secretion in response to glucose *in vitro* was greater in the offspring of diabetic rats than in control rats (44), whereas the inverse seems to be the case in the offspring of food-restricted or protein-restricted rats (25). Thus, the long-term imprinting caused by maternal diabetes on insulin secretion and tissue insulin sensitivity of the adult offspring is very different from that caused by malnutrition.

When the second-generation offspring of severely streptozotocin-induced diabetic rats become pregnant, they exhibit signs of glucose intolerance; they have higher

TABLE 2. *Body weight, plasma glucose and plasma insulin concentrations of pregnant offspring of diabetic rats and their third-generation fetuses*

Group	Body weight, g[a]	Glucose, mmol/l[a]	Insulin, nmol/l[a]
Pregnant offspring			
Control	293 ± 3 (35)	4.3 ± 0.1 (49)	0.40 ± 0.02 (34)
Diabetic	270 ± 3*** (37)	4.7 ± 0.1** (45)	0.34 ± 0.01* (40)
Fetuses			
Control	2.10 ± 0.03 (65)	2.3 ± 0.1 (21)	0.72 ± 0.05 (10)
Diabetic	2.12 ± 0.02 (112)	2.7 ± 0.1** (48)	0.96 ± 0.05** (44)

[a] The measurements were made on day 20 of gestation in pregnant animals and in their fetuses. Values are means ± SEM for the number of rats in parentheses.
* $p < .05$ vs. control rats; ** $p < .01$ vs. control rats; *** $p < .001$ vs. control rats.

glucose levels than normal pregnant rats (Table 2), and the number of granulated β cells in the endocrine pancreas does not increase as in normal rat gestation (11). These data would suggest that a defect is present in offspring of diabetic rats in the pregnancy-induced response of the β cells to glucose. As normal pregnancy is a state of severe physiologic insulin resistance, we wanted to investigate whether the insulin resistance present in the offspring of diabetic rats is further aggravated during gestation. For this purpose, again we used the euglycemic-hyperinsulinemic clamp technique combined with isotopic measurement of glucose turnover (48). The insulin dose-response curve for the increase of glucose metabolic clearance rate over basal values and for inhibition of endogenous glucose production obviously shows that the pregnancy-induced insulin resistance is not found in the offspring of diabetic rats. There is no further decrease in the peripheral tissue sensitivity to insulin, and there is only a small decrease in the hepatic insulin sensitivity. Overall, there are no differences in insulin sensitivity between pregnant control rats and pregnant offspring of diabetic rats. This is also apparent from the glucose metabolic indices determined in various peripheral tissues of both pregnant control rats and pregnant offspring of diabetic rats (Fig. 1). Although the insulin resistance was not markedly aggravated during pregnancy in offspring of diabetic rats, a syndrome of "gestational diabetes" evolved in these rats. The pregnancy-associated increase in circulating insulin concentrations was blunted in offspring of diabetic rats; as a consequence, pregnant offspring of diabetic rats had lower insulin concentrations than pregnant control rats. Their nonfasting glucose levels were also increased, and levels of nonessential fatty acids were markedly elevated (48).

Their fetuses, the third generation offspring, also develop in an abnormal intrauterine milieu. They display islet hyperplasia, β-cell degranulation (11), hyperinsulinemia, and hyperglycemia (48) (Table 2). At adult age, the third generation offspring of streptozotocin-induced diabetic pregnant rats have impaired glucose tolerance with high glucose levels (42). These data clearly show that a diabetogenic tendency is transmitted from the pregnant streptozotocin-induced diabetic rat to her fetuses, with consequences persisting into adulthood and into the next generation. The transmission of diabetes through the maternal line has been confirmed in offspring of rats made hyperglycemic by a continuous glucose infusion during the last week of pregnancy (49).

The inducing factor of the insulin resistance that characterizes the adult offspring of severely streptozotocin-induced diabetic rats must be the abnormal perinatal milieu of the diabetic maternal rat, to which the developing fetus has to adapt. Indeed, normalization of the maternal glycemia from day 15 of gestation by islet transplantation prevents the occurrence of a disturbed glucose tolerance in the offspring (50). The studies of Grill *et al.* (51) and Ktorza *et al.* (49) strongly suggest that the diabetic or hyperglycemic intrauterine milieu must be responsible for the metabolic alterations observed in the offspring, as in both studies the offspring were reared by nondiabetic or normoglycemic foster mothers.

SUMMARY

Perturbations of the maternal environment create an abnormal intrauterine milieu for the developing fetus. The altered fuel supply (depending on substrate availability, placental transport of nutrients, and uteroplacental blood flow) from mother to fetus induces alterations in the development of the fetal endocrine pancreas and adaptations of the fetal metabolism to the altered intrauterine environment, resulting in IUGR.

The alterations induced by maternal diabetes or maternal malnutrition (protein energy or protein deprivation) have consequences for the offspring that persist into adulthood and into the next generation.

REFERENCES

1. Rosso P, Kava R. Effects of food restriction on cardiac ouput and blood flow to the uterus and placenta in the pregnant rat. *J Nutr* 1980;110:2350–2354.
2. Lasunción MA, Lorenzo J, Palacin M, Herrera E. Maternal factors modulating nutrient transfer to fetus. *Biol Neonate* 1987;51:86–93.
3. Rasmussen KM, Warman NL. Effect of maternal malnutrition during the reproductive cycle on growth and nutritional status of suckling rat pups. *Am J Clin Nutr* 1983;38:77–83.
4. Boileau P, Mrejen C, Girard J, Hauguel-de Mouzon S. Overexpression of GLUT3 placental glucose transporter in diabetic rats. *J Clin Invest* 1995;96:309–317.
5. Arnott G, Coghill G, McArdle HJ, Hundal HS. Immunolocalization of GLUT1 and GLUT3 glucose transporters in human placenta. *Biochem Soc Trans* 1994;22:272S(abst).
6. Smith CH. Mechanisms and regulation of placental amino acid transport. *Fed Proc* 1986;45:2443–2445.
7. Hay WW. The placenta. Not just a conduit for maternal fuels. *Diabetes* 1991;40(Suppl 2):44–50.
8. Herrera E, Lasunción MA, Palacin M, Zorzano A, Bonet B. Intermediary metabolism in pregnancy. First theme of the Freinkel era. *Diabetes* 1991;40(Suppl 2):83–88.
9. Saintonge J, Rosso P. Placental blood flow and transfer of nutrient analogs in large, average, and small guinea pig littermates. *Pediatr Res* 1981;15:152–156.
10. Kim IS, Yoon Y, Kim Y. New models for infants of diabetic mothers. In: Shafrir E, Renold AE, eds. *Lessons from Animal Diabetes*. London: John Libbey; 1984:676–684.

11. Aerts L, Holemans K, Van Assche FA. Maternal diabetes during pregnancy: consequences for the offspring. *Diabetes Metab Rev* 1990;6:147–167.
12. Herrera E, Palacin M, Martin A, Lasunción MA. Relationship between maternal and fetal fuels and placental glucose transfer in rats with maternal diabetes of varying severity. *Diabetes* 1985;34(Suppl 2):42–46.
13. Cetin I, Corbetta C, Sereni LP, et al. Umbilical amino acid concentrations in normal and growth-retarded fetuses sampled *in utero* by cordocentesis. *Am J Obstet Gynecol* 1990;162:253–261.
14. Vejtorp M, Pedersen J, Klebbe JG, Lund E. Low concentration of plasma amino acids in newborn babies of diabetic mothers. *Acta Paediatr Scand* 1977;66:53–58.
15. Goldstein R, Levy E, Shafrir E. Increased maternal-fetal transport of fat in diabetes assessed by polyunsaturated fatty acid content in fetal lipids. *Biol Neonate* 1985;47:343–349.
16. Pang K, Mukonoweshuro C, Wong GG. Beta cells arise from glucose transporter type 2 (Glut2)-expressing epithelial cells of the developing rat pancreas. *Proc Natl Acad Sci U S A* 1994;91:9559–9563.
17. Aerts L, Van Assche FA. Rat foetal endocrine pancreas in experimental diabetes. *J Endocrinol* 1977;73:339–346.
18. Perrier-Barta H. A morphometric study of the secretory process in the endocrine pancreas of the foetal rat. *Cell Tissue Res* 1983;229:651–671.
19. Kervran A, Randon J, Girard J. Dynamics of glucose-induced plasma insulin increase in the rat fetus at different stages of gestation: effects of maternal hypothermia and fetal decapitation. *Biol Neonate* 1979;35:242–248.
20. Bihoreau MT, Ktorza A, Picon L. Gestational hyperglycaemia and insulin release by the fetal rat pancreas *in vitro*: effect of amino acids and glyceraldehyde. *Diabetologia* 1986;29:434–439.
21. Bihoreau MT, Ktorza A, Kervran A, Picon L. Effect of gestational hyperglycemia on insulin secretion *in vivo* and *in vitro* by fetal rat pancreas. *Am J Physiol* 1986;251:E86–E91.
22. Van Assche FA, Aerts L, De Prins FA. Degranulation of the insulin-producing beta cells in an infant of a diabetic mother. Case report. *Br J Obstet Gynaecol* 1983;90:182–185.
23. Dahri S, Snoeck A, Reusens-Billen B, Remacle C, Hoet JJ. Islet function in offspring of mothers on low-protein diet during gestation. *Diabetes* 1991;40(Suppl 2):115–120.
24. Snoeck A, Remacle C, Reusens B, Hoet JJ. Effect of a low-protein diet during pregnancy on the fetal rat endocrine pancreas. *Biol Neonate* 1990;57:107–118.
25. Holemans K, Verhaeghe J, Dequeker J, Van Assche FA. Insulin sensitivity in adult female offspring of rats subjected to malnutrition during the perinatal period. *J Soc Gynecol Invest* 1996;3:71–77.
26. Sodoyez-Goffaux F, Sodoyez JC, De Vos CJ. Maturation of liver handling of insulin in the rat fetus. *Diabetes* 1982;31:60–69.
27. Mulay S, Philip A, Solomon S. Influence of maternal diabetes on fetal rat development: alteration of insulin receptors in fetal liver and lung. *J Endocrinol* 1983;98:401–410.
28. Philipps AF, Rosenkrantz TS, Clark RM, Knox I, Chaffin DG, Raye JR. Effects of fetal insulin deficiency on growth in fetal lambs. *Diabetes* 1991;40:20–27.
29. Canavan JP, Goldspink DF. Maternal diabetes in rats. II. Effects on fetal growth and protein turnover. *Diabetes* 1988;37:1671–1677.
30. Dalinghaus M, Rudolph CD, Rudolph AM. Effects of maternal fasting on hepatic gluconeogenesis and glucose metabolism in fetal lambs. *J Dev Physiol* 1991;16:267–275.
31. Leturque A, Hauguel S, Revelli JP, Burnol AF, Kande J, Girard J. Fetal glucose utilization in response to maternal starvation and acute hyperketonemia. *Am J Physiol* 1989;256:E699–E703.
32. Simmons RA, Gounis AS, Bangalore SA, Ogata ES. Intrauterine growth retardation: fetal glucose transport is diminished in lung but spared in brain. *Pediatr Res* 1992;31:59–63.
33. Liechty EA, Lemons JA. Changes in ovine fetal hindlimb amino acid metabolism during maternal fasting. *Am J Physiol* 1984;246:E430–E435.
34. Girard J, Ferre P, Gilbert M, Kervran A, Assan R, Marliss EB. Fetal metabolic response to maternal fasting in the rat. *Am J Physiol* 1977;232:E456–E463.
35. Mencher D, Shouval D, Reshef L. Premature appearance of hepatic phosphoenolpyruvate carboxykinase in fetal rats, not mediated by adenosine 3':5'-monophosphate. *Eur J Biochem* 1979;102:489–495.
36. Girard J, Caquet D, Bal D, Guillet I. Control of rat liver phosphorylase, glucose-6-phosphatase and phosphoenolpyruvate carboxykinase activities by insulin and glucagon during the perinatal period. *Enzyme* 1973;15:272–285.

37. Nouspikel T, Iynedjian PB. Insulin signalling and regulation of glucokinase gene expression in cultured hepatocytes. *Eur J Biochem* 1992;210:365–373.
38. Bossard P, Parsa R, Decaux JF, Iynedjian P, Girard J. Glucose administration induces the premature expression of liver glucokinase gene in newborn rats. Relation with DNase-I-hypersensitive sites. *Eur J Biochem* 1993;215:883–892.
39. Yasuda K, Yamada Y, Inagaki N, et al. Expression of GLUT1 and GLUT2 glucose transporter isoforms in rat islets of Langerhans and their regulation by glucose. *Diabetes* 1992;41:76–81.
40. Issad T, Coupe C, Pastor-Anglada M, Ferre P, Girard J. Development of insulin-sensitivity at weaning in the rat. Role of the nutritional transition. *Biochem J* 1988;251:685–690.
41. Leturque A, Postic C, Ferre P, Girard J. Nutritional regulation of glucose transporter in muscle and adipose tissue of weaned rats. *Am J Physiol* 1991;260:E588–E593.
42. Van Assche FA, Aerts L. Long-term effect of diabetes and pregnancy in the rat. *Diabetes* 1985; 34(Suppl 2):116–118.
43. Holemans K, Aerts L, Van Assche FA. Evidence for an insulin resistance in the adult offspring of pregnant streptozotocin-diabetic rats. *Diabetologia* 1991;34:81–85.
44. Aerts L, Sodoyez-Goffaux F, Sodoyez JC, Malaisse WJ, Van Assche FA. The diabetic intrauterine milieu has a long-lasting effect on insulin secretion by B cells and on insulin uptake by target tissues. *Am J Obstet Gynecol* 1988;159:1287–1292.
45. Holemans K, Van Bree R, Verhaeghe J, Aerts L, Van Assche FA. *In vivo* glucose utilization by individual tissues in virgin and pregnant offspring of severely diabetic rats. *Diabetes* 1993;42:530–536.
46. Ferre P, Leturque A, Burnol AF, Penicaud L, Girard J. A method to quantify glucose utilization *in vivo* in skeletal muscle and white adipose tissue of the anaesthetized rat. *Biochem J* 1985;228:103–110.
47. Kahn CR. Insulin resistance, insulin insensitivity, and insulin unresponsiveness: a necessary distinction. *Metabolism* 1978;27:1893–1902.
48. Holemans K, Aerts L, Van Assche FA. Absence of pregnancy-induced alterations in tissue insulin sensitivity in the offspring of diabetic rats. *J Endocrinol* 1991;131:387–393.
49. Ktorza A, Gauguier D, Bihoreau MT, Berthault MF, Picon L. Adult offspring from mildly hyperglycemic rats show impairment of glucose regulation and insulin secretion which is transmissible to the next generation. In: Shafrir E, Renold AE, eds. *Frontiers in Diabetes Research. Lessons from Animal Diabetes.* London: Smith-Gordon; 1990:555–560.
50. Aerts L, Van Assche FA. Islet transplantation in diabetic pregnant rats normalizes glucose homeostasis in their offspring. *J Dev Physiol* 1992;17:283–287.
51. Grill V, Johansson B, Jalkanen P, Eriksson UJ. Influence of severe diabetes mellitus early in pregnancy in the rat: effects on insulin sensitivity and insulin secretion in the offspring. *Diabetologia* 1991;34:373–378.

DISCUSSION

Dr. Stuart Campbell: I would like Professor Battaglia to follow on from the statement he made that glucose restriction does not cause IUGR. I find that slightly difficult to accept for the following reason, which is that Peter Soothill showed very elegantly that the insulin-to-glucose ratio was low in IUGR in prenatal samples of cord blood (in other words, a relatively low insulin in relation to the glucose levels that were already low), and it has also been shown that the β islet cells are reduced in volume and in percentage, and the volume of the endocrine tissue is reduced. So in other words, there is hypoinsulinemia and there are reduced numbers of β cells; surely low glucose would cause hypotrophy because of low insulin levels.

Dr. Battaglia: In animal research, in the sheep models of severe growth retardation you certainly develop a lower glucose and a lower insulin, just as you would if I starved you. Now if I starve you and you lower your insulin and glucose, we don't say the low insulin and glucose cause you to grow poorly; we say that's a perfectly reasonable adaptation of the body to the fact that your food is restricted. We looked at that in our animal model of growth retardation, in which there is a very small placenta. The only way a small fetus with a small placenta will get enough glucose is by resetting a low glucose concentration and increasing the glucose gradient across the placenta. I would not interpret that as a cause, but rather as an adaptation. So we have to make clear here what we are talking about as cause and effect. As far as Barker's work is concerned, he had no gestational age data. Growth rate implies a change with time. If all you have is the weight of a baby but no age, you can't talk about growth retardation. So I think this is still a very confusing field. I think we need to know a lot more about it. I have no doubt that in fetal life any organ, including the pancreas, will change the way it grows and develops if you impose on it a different environment. So if we restrict the supply of nutrients to a fetus because of a small placenta for a long time, I think we could find changes in many fetal organs, including the pancreas.

Dr. Godfrey: In relation to the epidemiologic data, in six of seven populations in which there *are* gestational age data in relation to later diabetes, the effects we see are independent of gestational age; adjusting for gestational age if anything strengthens some of the associations. In the initial population that we studied, we didn't have gestational age data, but in populations in the United States, in other populations in the UK, Sweden, and India, and in Australian aborigines, associations between size at birth and later diabetes have being shown independently of gestational age at birth.

Dr. Talamantes: I am trying to put all this together. Several years ago, my lab showed that if you fasted mice you got an increase in placental lactogen. More recently, we showed that the increase that you see in pancreatic islets in the β cells is a consequence of mouse placental lactogen or rat placental lactogen in the case of the rat. If in your fasted rats you get an increase in placental lactogen and if you keep them fasted for long enough, you are going to get a hypertrophy of those islets. I am trying to see how that in turn will have an effect in terms of diabetes.

Dr. Van Assche: We didn't look at human placental lactogen, but I can follow your suggestion. We are not claiming to know the origin of this hypertrophy or this hyperplasia. I am not saying it is glucose, because in severe diabetes there is high glucose and low insulin. I think the main point, which could be the critical event leading to fetal problems, is a reduced uteroplacental circulation in all these situations. And that is the thing that we would like to figure out, but we have no data. If there is reduced uteroplacental circulation, we can explain a lot of things.

Dr. Talamantes: In the human, if you increase glucose you are going to reduce placental lactogen. The growth of the islets in humans, shown by the work of Sorenson, depends on placental lactogen, so if you raise the glucose you are going to lower placental lactogen and you are going to have a reduction in β cell multiplication and release of insulin.

Dr. Van Assche: I follow your comments. The only thing is that you can have hyperplasia of the islets with high glucose levels when there is a normal uteroplacental circulation. So there are a lot of mechanisms working against each other. I completely agree with your comment about human placental lactogen, but there are a lot of factors acting together and I don't know which is the final determinant.

Dr. Soothill: In the human fetus, you get low levels of glucose in IUGR, and even after adjusting for the level of glucose the insulin is still lower. One of the ideas we had about why that might be was that the redistribution process might lead to the pancreas, with other organs in the abdomen, being relatively ischemic. Have you any comments about that in relation to your models?

Dr. Van Assche: We have no data in the rat concerning the vascular system. I have shown that in the human, when there is macrosomia there is an increased amount of vasculature in the endocrine pancreas. So your postulation could be right. Your suggestion that there could be a redistribution of the vascular system is also possible.

Dr. Ogata: Are your adult former IUGR rats smaller than normal?

Dr. Van Assche: Their weight is relatively reduced until about 20 to 30 days of weaning, and you could propose that maybe the mammary glands are not developed enough, but then they increase in weight and they are overweight in adulthood.

Dr. Ogata: This complicates the mechanism of insulin resistance. We have used the maternal uterine artery ligation model and have found postnatally—and we have grown our rat pups under reasonably well-controlled nutritional conditions—that up to 4 weeks they remain smaller than expected compared with controls. We have also found evidence of insulin resistance in the neonatal period; for example, PEPCK is not induced as quickly as in the normal, and if you look at group 1 modulation and insulin-sensitive glucose transporter in various tissues, they are reduced and not appropriate to the insulin. But we also have seen that beyond a certain point the rats get fat. To my mind, that changes the possible mechanisms of the insulin resistance, because now you have a big rat, not a small one. I think that complicates the mechanism considerably.

Dr. Van Assche: I agree with you.

Dr. Pardi: The weight of the pancreas of growth-retarded fetuses is reduced compared with controls. If you look at the ratio with total body weight, the difference is much less. Have you any data on the weight of other organs in the same fetuses—brain and liver, for example—to give an idea about the degree of weight loss of the fetal pancreas in growth retardation?

Dr. Van Assche: Let me first give you some explanation about the morphometric data. When we say that the volume density of the endocrine tissue is reduced, it means that there is an absolute reduction. So in comparison with the total body weight and in comparison with the pancreatic weight, we have a particular reduction of the endocrine tissue. Second, of course the body weight is reduced and the placental weight is increased in severe diabetes, and all the other organs are reduced. The liver is reduced in weight.

Dr. Stuart Campbell: As a humble clinician, I had always believed that maternal diabetes caused macrosomia, and that if you had an IUGR fetus associated with maternal diabetes, it was caused by vascular disease and impaired perfusion. Now you found in your severely diabetic rat mothers that you had IUGR with a low percentage of β cells. Did they have vascular disease, or are you saying that severe maternal diabetes can cause IUGR irrespective of maternal vascular disease?

Dr. Van Assche: In the human situation, in the majority of cases of maternal diabetes you have macrosomia, except when there is an association with pre-eclampsia or with vascular disease. In the rat, when there is severe diabetes (and severe diabetes means glycemia levels up to 400 mg%), we have shown that in this situation there are endothelial lesions to the kidney. We have also shown that in the mesometric triangle in the placenta of the rat, which may be equivalent to the region of the spiral artery in the human, endothelial lesions are also found. Therefore, we think that in severe diabetes we have a reduction of uteroplacental blood flow.

Dr. Girard: Perhaps I could suggest a possible explanation for the liver insulin resistance. It could be postulated that these mothers are making more glucose by gluconeogenesis than by glycogenolysis to explain why insulin is less active in this group.

Dr. Godfrey: As mentioned before, a maternal low-protein diet during pregnancy alone is associated with a persistent tendency toward increased hepatic gluconeogenesis. In our Southampton studies, we found that studying liver metabolism in free-living adults is very difficult, but we have done studies of skeletal muscle metabolism and have shown by magnetic resonance spectroscopy and other techniques that thin babies with insulin resistance as adults do have persisting abnormalities of muscle metabolic fuel selection, so marrying up the species differences and the model differences may be important.

Dr. Battaglia: When you say that uteroplacental perfusion may be abnormal, remember that if there is one thing that is well established it is that the hormones that control angiogenesis are linked to cell division in an organ. So if you have cancer tissue with rapid cell growth, you get a lot of angiogenesis, and if you slow down cell division, then the vascular bed also doesn't develop as fully. The change is in the cell division rate of the tissue you are studying, and angiogenesis follows that—they are nicely coordinated. When we talk about reduced uteroplacental perfusion, my question is whether we are talking about a reduction per kilogram of uterine tissue supplied, because at least in the model we work with, in which we measure flows, we don't see a reduction per kilogram of tissue. Certainly if you have a small fetus, you are going to have a low flow in absolute terms, but for me that isn't underperfusion. How do you visualize this uteroplacental problem?

Dr. Stuart Campbell: Normally, uterine blood flow from before pregnancy to late pregnancy increases from 60 ml/min to about 700 to 800 ml/min, so there is a huge increase in the amount of blood flow that the intervillous space requires, and there has to be this adaptation of maternal blood vessels, principally in the spiral arteries. If that adaptation doesn't occur, then there is, I suppose, a relative obstruction to this flow getting into the intercotyledonary space. I think it helps us understand why IUGR occurs if you realize that blood is going right into the middle of the cotyledon and filtering through the villi, and it's obstruction at that level that is the source of a lot of problems relating to IUGR. In diabetes, there might not be a vascular adaptation problem, but there are abnormal blood vessels in the placental bed that prevent the increase in blood flow, just as in sickle cell disease you get pre-eclampsia because of obstruction by clumps of sickling cells in the placental bed. Anything that obstructs the normal perfusion of the intercotyledonary space, causing slowing of the blood, platelet aggregation, and fibrin deposition within these cotyledons, will I think cause this problem.

Dr. Battaglia: Suppose you have a 10-kg mother and a 100-kg mother, and the 100-kg mother is the one in whom you define normal flow, and it goes up to 700 ml/min. But if 700 ml/min occurs in a 10-kg mother she is dead, because there is no perfusion of the brain and other organs. So her adaptation might be 300 ml, perfectly normal, but 300 because she is smaller. I'm trying to get at the problem of when a disease should be called a uteroplacental perfusion problem. I accept that a placenta that is half the size of another will have a reduced blood flow, but for me that is not a uteroplacental perfusion problem.

Dr. Stuart Campbell: In the human fetus, you often see early IUGR with a fetus adapting to a situation of relatively low perfusion with a small placenta; the fetus adapts, almost hibernating in the uterus, and can often get to viability because it has constrained its growth and has grown along a particular path, even if suboptimally. However, in late pregnancy, with a fully grown fetus or a fairly normally growing fetus, when the effects of impaired perfusion to the placenta and secondary obliteration to the villous circulation occur, then you see the fetus becoming acidemic and dying very quickly because the blood flow is inappropriate to its size. These are the problems we see very often in clinical practice.

Dr. Meschia: You keep implying that the blood flow is decreased, but you don't know that. I could say it's because the mass of the trophoblast is less. How do you respond to that?

Dr. Stuart Campbell: I suppose it is because we use Doppler to identify abnormal waveforms in the placental bed, which are typical of failure of trophoblast invasion and therefore identify a group that we believe has impaired perfusion. If you do volume flow studies, which I know are not particularly accurate, we definitively see a reduced volume flow into the placenta.

Dr. Meschia: But there is also a reduced trophoblast mass, so the disease could primarily be a reduction in the growth of the trophoblast.

Dr. Van Assche: I completely agree with the explanation of Professor Campbell, but I also understand your critical approach, because you have another view with your experimental models, and what is flow? The only thing I can say is that when we look at the morphology of the spiral arteries, we find that they are blocked, and you see infarctions of the placenta on the side where there is blocking of the uteroplacental circulation. We are speaking about the reduction of the flow to the placenta.

Dr. Stuart Campbell: What we have shown is that in many normal small IUGR fetuses at term in which there are no clinical abnormalities, the placenta is actually smaller than average quite early on, at about 20 weeks. But in most of those cases in which we find abnormal uteroplacental waveforms, the placenta is within the normal range for volume, so there are abnormal waveforms in a placenta of normal volume. That is why I believe the blood flow is inappropriate for the placenta.

Drug Abuse

Doris M. Campbell

Department of Obstetrics and Gynaecology, University of Aberdeen, Foresterhill, Aberdeen, Scotland, United Kingdom

Substance abuse in pregnancy is generally believed to be on the increase in many of the developed countries of the world. Pregnant women who expose themselves to toxic substances are at risk for adverse outcome. However, it is not entirely clear to what degree any one specific substance abused may affect either the mother or the baby during the course of pregnancy. In any one individual noted to be a substance abuser, there may be several "drugs" used at different stages or indeed at the same stage of gestation in pregnancy. The exact adverse outcome related to the toxicity of any substance is unclear, as lifestyle and socioeconomic factors also play an important role. Additionally, the role played by prescribed drugs is seldom considered.

This review considers, in three sections, substances that are known to be abused in pregnancy and for which there is some evidence of a mechanism that could lead to a poor outcome. Specifically, opiates (heroin and methadone), cocaine, amphetamines, marijuana (cannabis), and alcohol are discussed. Tobacco smoking with its known adverse effects, a problem for about 35% of pregnant women who smoke, is considered in a separate chapter. The first section of this chapter examines what is known about the extent of the problem, the numbers of pregnant women abusing "drugs," and the problems of ascertainment of drug abuse in pregnancy. The second section considers the general principles of placental handling of drugs, and how each specific drug affects placental function and transport of nutrients. The final section looks at assessment of fetal nutrition, and in particular the growth of the baby.

THE EXTENT OF "DRUG" ABUSE IN PREGNANCY

Obtaining reliable information about obstetric populations in this field is extremely difficult. Although some substances (e.g., alcohol) are freely available, others (e.g., cocaine) are illegal in the majority of countries, including the European nations and the United States. Underreporting of the use of illicit substances is likely for fear of reprisal, and for drugs that are readily obtained (both legal and illegal), feelings of guilt about potential harmful effects on the unborn child may lead women to deny their use. There are certain methodologic considerations in examining the nature of the prevalence of substance abuse in pregnancy. Ascertainment of abuse can be either by questionnaire accompanied by an interview or by a laboratory assessment of the drug or a metabolite. Difficulties encountered by both of these approaches have been summarized (1). Questionnaires, either self-completed or backed up by interview, tend to have a reporting bias because of memory problems and an unwillingness to report accurately the use of illegal substances. Laboratory measures, although giving a degree of accuracy, do not always provide a broader picture of the history, pattern, dosage, and timing of use. Zuckerman *et al.* (2) reported that just over half of "identified" cocaine or marijuana users would have been picked up by urinalysis. Additionally, an accepted biochemical marker of drug abuse may itself alter in pregnancy because of physiologic adaptation and change with gestation. Screening for alcohol abuse in pregnancy is known to be problematic. Barrison *et al.* (3) showed that in pregnancy neither mean cell volume nor τ-glutamyl transpeptidase were reliable indicators of alcohol abuse.

It has also been suggested that pregnant women attending for antenatal care may alter their pattern of substance abuse before clinic visits, knowing that they will be asked for a sample of urine. In addition, opiates, for example, may be prescribed in pregnancy as antidiarrheal agents or for pain relief.

As a result, few good epidemiologic studies of substance abuse in pregnancy have been published, and many tend to identify the frequency of use in high-risk populations in inner-city areas, where drug abuse is known to be rife. Table 1 summarizes the incidence of drug abuse in pregnancy in several countries of the world for the specific substances included in this review.

PLACENTAL FUNCTION

With respect to the transfer of drugs from mother to fetus, the placenta should be considered as a lipid membrane. Passive diffusion is the mode of transfer for the majority of drugs, as their molecules are small and lipid-soluble. Maternal, placental, and fetal factors may affect placental transfer (4). Maternal factors include drug disposition during pregnancy, which is affected by changes in body weight, body composition (in particular fat content), and alterations in plasma volume, cardiac output, renal function, steroid hormone levels, and plasma protein concentrations. Secondly, blood flow to the uterus and fetoplacental unit influences the transfer of drugs to the fetus. With respect to placental factors, the permeability of the placenta to drugs depends on molecular size and lipid solubility, and on the surface area and thickness of tissue layers between the capillaries and the blood, which are known to change with gestation. The placenta contains enzyme systems that are involved in the metabolism of certain drugs (e.g., barbiturates) (5). However, its capacity may readily be overwhelmed and is likely to be less than that of either the fetal or the maternal liver. It has been suggested that the human fetal liver is capable of metabolizing drugs, with well-developed enzyme systems from early in gestation. The degree of protein binding and the pH of the fetal circulation relative to that of the maternal circulation, which change throughout gestation, should also be considered. Additionally, placental transfer of drugs would be affected by timing and dosage. This information is particularly difficult to obtain from illegal drug abusers (6). The following subsections examine placental handling and how transport of nutrients is affected by specific substances.

Opiates (Heroin and Methadone)

Opiates, in particular heroin, readily cross the placenta, and morphine and its metabolites have been found in neonatal urine and meconium. Animal studies in sheep have confirmed rapid transfer of all opiates, with fetal levels being lower than those of the mother (7). The elimination half-lives of the opiate drugs was similar in maternal and fetal plasma, and the authors concluded that elimination from the fetus was mainly by placental clearance. Recently, work in humans examining maternal and neonatal plasma methadone levels found a significant relationship between them, but neonatal levels were consistently lower (8). Lower levels of opiates in the fetus relative to the mother could also be explained by high fetal tissue (liver and brain) uptake (8) or accumulation of significant amounts of opiates as nontransferable conjugates in amniotic fluid (7). There are no studies of the effects of opiates in other aspects of placental function.

Cocaine

Although many of the reported effects on the fetus of cocaine may be attributable to uterine vasoconstriction (9), a more active role for the placenta has been postulated. Studies in animals (9,10) show enzymes in the placenta capable of metabolizing cocaine and thus limiting the transfer of cocaine to the fetus. With respect to the human placenta (11), perfusion studies of isolated cotyledons confirm that the placenta could serve as a depot for cocaine, offering a degree of fetal protection; that fetal exposure might be prolonged by slow release of cocaine and its metabolites from a placental store; and that one of the major metabolites of cocaine, benzoylecgonine, does not cross the placenta as readily as cocaine. Increasingly, evidence is emerging from animal work that cocaine limits transplacental transfer of other substances to the fetus (9) and that this may not simply be related to flow, but a direct effect of cocaine on cellular uptake of nutrients. Results of work on human placental cells in tissue culture, both from human placental brush border membrane and from choriocarcinoma cells, suggest that the placenta itself is a direct target for cocaine, which affects transporter systems within the placenta, in particular noradrenaline and serotonin transporters (12). Such actions of cocaine may limit the transfer of essential nutrients to the developing fetus.

TABLE 1. Incidence of drug abuse in pregnancy in various countries

Reference	Opiates	Cocaine	Amphetamines	Marijuana	Multiple drug use	Alcohol
39 Amsterdam, Holland a) 1969–79 b) 1980–89	a) 92 b) 184	a) 0 b) 117	—	—	>50% Users	—
20 Amsterdam, Holland 1974–83	168	—	—	—	—	—
38 Amsterdam, Holland 1987–94	—	21	—	—	—	—
6 Sacramento, USA (n = 1643)	1.2%	8.5%	6.5%	—	2.1%	—
37 Cleveland, USA (n = 168, highly selected)	4.7%	0.6%	20%	—	9%	4.2% Heavy
25 Stockholm, Sweden (approx. 30,000 births)	0.05% (15)*	—	0.23% (69)*	—	—	—
40 London, UK (n = 1000, anonymous screening)	1.7%	1.1%	—	8.5%	0.5%	—

1 US Review of studies	—	—	10–30%	—
23 US Multicenter (n = 7470)	1–17%	—	11%	—
28 Ontario, Canada (n = 583)	2.3%	—	Trimester 1st 3rd Irreg. 7.7% 6.3% Mod. 1.7% 0.7% Heavy 4.0% 3.0%	—
41 Glasgow, UK (n = 2765)	—	—	—	Occas. 33% Mod. 2% Heavy 0%
42 Belfast, UK (n = 95)	—	—	—	Occas. 15% Mod. 22% Heavy 35%
34 Dundee, UK (n = 952)	—	—	—	Early Late Mild 47% 33% Mod. 3% 1% Heavy 1% 1% V. Heavy 1% 0%
32 US Review	—	—	—	1–2% Abusers

* Numbers in groups.

Amphetamines

It has generally been accepted that the mechanism underlying the harmful effects of amphetamine overuse in pregnancy is similar to that of cocaine—namely, decreased uterine blood flow as a result of vasoconstriction and thus a limited transfer of oxygen and nutrients to the fetus. Using methodology akin to that of their cocaine studies, the group from Augusta, Georgia, has shown that amphetamines also inhibit serotonin and norepinephrine transport in the human placenta (13). Although both drugs inhibit both transporter systems, amphetamines inhibit the norepinephrine transporter to a relatively greater degree, whereas cocaine preferentially inhibits the serotonin transporter. Such placental mechanisms would affect the concentrations of these vasoconstrictive substances in the intervillous space and could thus potentially limit transfer of many nutrient substances.

Marijuana (Cannabis)

Compounds derived from the hemp plant, known as *cannabinoids*, have been detected in neonatal urine and meconium, although once again levels in umbilical cord blood have been shown to be lower than those in the mother (7). Animal studies have suggested rather slow transfer of tetrahydrocannabinol, perhaps attributable to its extensive binding to maternal plasma proteins. Little is known about whether cannabinoids affect other placental functions, such as nutrient and oxygen transport, other than by the already known effects of tobacco smoking.

Alcohol

Alcohol and its major metabolite, acetaldehyde, both freely cross the placenta, and it is generally agreed alcohol affects fetal development and growth by direct toxicity rather than by any specific effect of either component on placental transport. Although there have been isolated reports in animals of alcohol interfering with active transport of amino acids across the placenta (14) by inhibition of amino acid transporter systems, others have shown that ethanol has significant fetal effects even when nutrition is well controlled (15).

FETAL NUTRITION

The assessment of fetal nutrition in the outcome of pregnancy in substance abusers has been examined only by consideration of the standard indices of fetal growth. Many workers have simply looked at birth weight without any control of confounding variables. Drugs may alter the length of gestation; for example, cocaine may downregulate β-adrenergic receptors in the myometrium (7), thereby increasing the likelihood of early delivery. Other measurements of the newborn (e.g., birth length, head circumference, skin fold thickness, arm circumference) that reflect fetal nutrition should be undertaken in an attempt to identify different patterns of poor growth related to specific drug abuse. Ultrasonic assessment of fetal growth has not been used but could in the future provide more insight into this problematic area. Importantly, several studies are now considering long-term outcome, including the growth of infants born to mothers who abuse drugs in pregnancy.

Before the impact of specific substances on fetal growth and development can be detailed, several general points must be considered. The first is the selection of cases for review. As a result of the difficulties of identifying women who abuse substances during pregnancy, many researchers have studied women attending specialized substance abuse centers. Such women, who are likely to be the subset of heavy or addicted users, may not be representative of population use, and this may therefore lead to a rather biased picture of outcome. Study designs often lack a suitable control or comparison group, and in this regard many other factors that influence fetal growth are often not considered in the selection of controls. Drug abuse is a marker of a different lifestyle, and other adverse factors, such as prostitution and sexually transmitted disease (in particular HIV infection), may be as important for outcome as the abuse of drugs.

Another major problem encountered in many studies is the recognized use of more than one substance during a pregnancy and the compounding effects of tobacco smoking. It has been suggested (16) that after controlling for environmental factors, many of the effects attributable to substance abuse disappear. For example, it has been postulated that dietary intake in women who are abusing drugs in pregnancy may be worse than in those who are not abusers. Evidence cited to support this hypothesis (17) includes serum levels of folate and ferritin, which themselves are poor markers of maternal nutritional status in pregnancy. Well-conducted, prospectively planned research is therefore needed to determine on a sound basis the effect of substance abuse on fetal nutrition and growth.

In the following sections, each drug is reviewed separately for its effects on fetal growth.

Opiates (Heroin and Methadone)

Opiates have in general been associated with fetal growth retardation and preterm delivery. In Liverpool (18), birth weight, head circumference, and body length were all reduced in the babies of heroin users compared with controls selected by taking the link before and after the index one. Similar findings from the United States have been summarized (19), and differences in outcome compared between heroin and methadone use. A decrease in birth weight in opiate abusers on average is ± 80 g. This review also detailed the proportion of infants that were small for dates and of low birth weight, concluding that there is an increased incidence of small-for-dates babies in heroin users (18%) in comparison with methadone users (12%) (compare the 5% incidence of small-for-dates infants in drug-free populations). In Amsterdam (20), an increase in low birth weight, an increase in gestational age of less than 37 weeks, and a higher proportion under the 10th centile of birth weight for gestational age was confirmed in infants of heroin or heroin and methadone users. Further follow-up of these Dutch infants found that the differences in weight, height, and head circumference between the groups of children decreased as they became older. When the children were ages 4 to 12 years, no difference remained in the offspring of opiate users compared with those of nonusers other than in height, which was only marginally significant. Swedish workers have proposed that there may be fetal brain imprinting with heroin use in pregnancy and labor that might lead to altered behavior patterns in later life.

Cocaine

Although there are sound pathophysiologic mechanisms (see above) whereby cocaine might affect intrauterine growth, relatively recent reviews of the topic have come to very different conclusions (9,16,19). The group from Rochester, New York, claims that cocaine use leads to reduced birth weight and birth length, intrauterine growth retardation, and early gestation at delivery (9,19). Early delivery may result from abruption of the placenta, a recognized complication of cocaine use, or from the previously mentioned effects on the myometrium (7), confirmed recently in an intact animal (the baboon). On the other hand, the group from Pittsburgh, Pennsylvania (16), has concluded that when other risk factors correlated with cocaine exposure are considered, few studies show any effect of prenatal cocaine exposure on growth. Zuckerman *et al.* (2) used multiple regression analysis to control for confounding variables and found that many of the differences in neonatal growth indices in the offspring of cocaine users (either confirmed by urine assays or self-reported) either disappeared or became less significant. This group further examined neonatal body proportions (21). They found that after controlling for other potentially confounding variables, cocaine use, as detected by assays of maternal urine, was associated with a decrease in subscapular fat and of arm fat, but not of arm muscle circumference. They found no association between ponderal index or ratio of arm circumference to head circumference and cocaine abuse. They suggested that these findings would be consistent with the hypothesis that cocaine impairs nutrient transfer to the fetus. Prenatal care alone had a significant impact in decreasing the proportion of infants of low birth weight among cocaine users (22), adding to the belief that there is more involved in the impairment of fetal growth than substance abuse itself. A recent prospective multicenter study from the United States (23) has confirmed that cocaine use is relatively uncommon and not related to adverse birth outcome, with no increase in the frequency of preterm babies or babies of low birth weight. It was concluded that tobacco smoking was much more common and more likely to be related to poor fetal growth than either cocaine or marijuana use. Acceleration of fetal lung maturity, suggested as being associated with cocaine use (24), has important implications for the management of obstetric complications if confirmed in further work.

Amphetamines

There are few reports of amphetamine abuse in pregnancy. Although there are theoretical reasons (see above) for amphetamine abuse to affect fetal growth, as for cocaine, few data are available. A Swedish survey (25) identified 69 women who were all known to have abused amphetamine in the course of pregnancy. A greater proportion of early deliveries and of babies of low birth weight was found compared with the Swedish population in general. These children were born in 1976/77 and have subsequently been followed up for 10 years. Mean body weight and length at 1 and 4 years were below those of a comparison group, but differences were statistically significant only for girls. At 8 and 10 years of age, weight and length of girls were similar to those of the comparison group and Swedish standards, whereas weight and length of the boys were above. The follow-up study of the Swedish workers identified behavioral differences in the children of amphetamine users, and they concluded that although social and environmental factors appear to have less influence on a child's growth, exposure to amphetamines seems to be more influential on a child's behavior pattern in later life. The impact of multiple drug use, assessed by intrapartum urine screening in Sacramento, California (6), found only very small differences in birth weight and head circumference, and no effect on neonatal length with amphetamine use. The effects of amphetamine use in this study were less than those of cocaine and multiple drug use. Previous reports from San Diego, California, and Dallas, Texas (26,27), showed decreased birth weight, birth length, and head circumference in association with amphetamine abuse.

Marijuana

In Ottawa, Fried et al. (28) found no reduction in birth weight, either raw or adjusted for confounding variables such as nicotine, alcohol, parity, maternal weight before pregnancy, and sex of the infant, in marijuana users. They did conclude, however, that heavy marijuana use was associated with significantly decreased length of gestation compared with moderate or irregular use or with non-use. Zuckerman et al. (2) found a negative effect on birth weight and length from marijuana use demonstrated by urinalysis, but not from self-reported use. In a review, Richardson et al. (16) concluded that it was unclear whether marijuana use affected intrauterine growth during pregnancy. There are only a few studies of growth in infancy, and no consistent effect of marijuana has been demonstrated. Recently, Shiono et al. (23), in an extensive multicenter study, reported that marijuana use is relatively common and is not related to adverse pregnancy outcome, but they considered only the proportion of preterm infants and infants of low birth weight. In a detailed neonatal assessment of body composition, Frank et al. (21) concluded that like tobacco smoking, marijuana depresses lean body mass by leading to prolonged fetal hypoxia.

Alcohol

Although it is generally recognized that excessive drinking during pregnancy gives rise to the fetal alcohol syndrome, there is debate as to how much social or moderate drinking affects fetal growth. Fetal alcohol syndrome is a combination of growth retardation, mental retardation, facial abnormalities, and other possible systemic anomalies. Although fetal alcohol syndrome may be diagnosed in the neonate, it may not be recognized until there is postnatal growth retardation accompanied by developmental delay (14,29,30). Fetal alcohol syndrome is not as common as was originally suggested, the incidence now being thought to be approximately 0.3 to 0.5/1000 births (31). A spectrum of effects of alcohol abuse in pregnancy, ranging from impaired fertility and early fetal wastage through birth defects and growth retardation to behavioral problems or a "normal" outcome, has been proposed (31). It is likely that there is a gradation of toxic effects depending on the amount and timing of alcohol use. It is widely debated whether there is a safe limit of alcohol consumption in pregnancy. If indeed there is a spectrum of effects of alcohol in pregnancy, it is perhaps not surprising that different levels of "safe" consumption have been defined. An increased risk for fetal alcohol syndrome has been associated with a daily alcohol intake exceeding 80 g (8 units per day), and fetal growth compromise with as little as 4 units per day (32). Earlier work in London (33) indicated increased fetal growth retardation (percent birth weight less than the 10th centile) when women consumed more than 100 g of alcohol per week. In a population-based cohort study from Dundee, Scotland (34), there was no detectable effect on the outcome of pregnancy of alcohol consumption below 100 g/wk, whereas at higher levels of intake there was impairment of fetal growth (birth weight, length and head circumference) and shorter gestational age. After adjustment for the effect of smoking, social class, maternal size, and other confounding factors, only the relationship with shorter duration of pregnancy remained. In Finland, Halmesmaki (35), demonstrated a dose-dependent alcohol effect on ultrasonically assessed fetal growth and suggested there was potential to limit growth retardation by counseling women and helping them reduce or stop their alcohol intake. This strategy is as yet unproven. The fetal alcohol syndrome is characterized by poor growth postnatally. The workers in Dundee followed up the offspring of their population-based study of alcohol consumption in pregnancy (36) at the age of 18 months, and even at levels in excess of 100 g/wk they found no adverse outcome when both mental and physical development was assessed.

CONCLUSIONS

Although it is accepted generally that there is an increase of substance abuse in pregnancy, the exact magnitude of such an increase is poorly defined. Ascertainment of drug use in pregnancy is difficult. A change in attitude toward such problems, coupled with improved laboratory screening, may be the way ahead in this area.

Animal studies can further help to elucidate mechanisms whereby such drugs might affect placental function and thereby fetal nutrition. However, hypotheses generalized from animal work need to be supported by properly conducted studies in the human.

The assessment of fetal nutrition mainly depends on measurements of the neonate. Improved means of assessing fetal nutrition in the infants of drug abusers should be sought. Properly conducted epidemiologic studies of drug abuse and its affect on pregnancy outcome are needed, based on population screening rather than selection of high-risk cases, with all the problems relating to adverse outcome resulting from a poor lifestyle and multiple drug abuse.

REFERENCES

1. Day NL, Cottreau CM, Richardson GA. The epidemiology of alcohol, marijuana and cocaine use among women of childbearing age and pregnant women. *Clin Obstet Gynaecol* 1993;36:232–245.
2. Zuckerman B, Frank MD, Hingson R, et al. Effects of maternal marijuana and cocaine use on fetal growth. *N Eng J Med* 1989;320:762–768.
3. Barrison IG, Wright JT, Sampson B, et al. Screening for alcohol abuse in pregnancy. *Br Med J* 1982;285:1318.
4. Nau H, Mirkin BL. Fetal and maternal clinical pharmacology. In: Speight TM, ed. *Avery's Drug Treatment: Principles and Practice of Clinical Pharmacology and Therapeutics.* 3rd ed. Auckland, N Z: Adis Press; 1987:79–85.
5. Kyegombe D, Franklin C, Turner P. Drug-metabolising enzymes in the human placenta, their induction and repression. *Lancet* 1973;1:405–406.
6. Gillogley KM, Evans AT, Hansen RL, et al. The perinatal impact of cocaine, amphetamine and opiate use detected by universal intrapartum screening. *Am J Obstet Gynecol* 1990;163:1535–1542.
7. Szeto MH. Kinetics of drug transfer to the fetus. *Clin Obstet Gynecol* 1993;36:246–254.
8. Doberczak T, Kandall SP, Friedmann P. Relationships between maternal methadone dosage, maternal-neonatal methadone levels and neonatal withdrawal. *Obstet Gynecol* 1993;81:936–940.
9. Plessinger MA, Woods JR. Maternal, placental and fetal pathophysiology of cocaine exposure during pregnancy. *Clin Obstet Gynecol* 1993;36:267–278.
10. Little BB, Daniel DA, Stettler RW, et al. A new placental enzyme in the metabolism of cocaine: an *in vitro* animal model. *Am J Obstet Gynecol* 1995;172:1441–1445.
11. Simone C, Derewlany LO, Oskamp M, et al. Transfer of cocaine and benzoylecgonine across the perfused human placental cotyledon. *Am J Obstet Gynecol* 1994;170:1404–1410.
12. Ganapathy V, Leibach FH. Current topic: Human placenta: a direct target for cocaine action. *Placenta* 1994;15:785–795.
13. Ramamoorthy JD, Ramamoorthy S, Leibach FH, Ganapathy V. Human placental monoamine transporters as targets for amphetamines. *Am J Obstet Gynecol* 1995;173:1782–1787.
14. Rosett H, Weiner L, Edelin KC. Strategies for prevention of fetal alcohol effects. *Obstet Gynecol* 1981;57:1–7.
15. Ouellette EM, Rosett HL, Rosman P, Weiner L. Adverse effects on offspring of maternal alcohol abuse during pregnancy. *N Engl J Med* 1977;297:528–530.
16. Richardson GA, Day NL, McGauhey PJ. The impact of prenatal marijuana and cocaine use on the infant and child. *Clin Obstet Gynecol* 1993;36:302–318.
17. Knight EM, Hutchison J, Edwards CH, et al. Relationships of serum illicit drug concentrations during pregnancy to maternal nutritional status. *J Nutr* 1994;124:9735–9805.
18. Gregg JEM, Davidson DC, Weindling AM. Inhaling heroin during pregnancy: effects on the baby. *Br Med J* 1988;296:754.
19. Glantz JC, Woods JR. Cocaine, heroin and phencyclidine: obstetric perspectives. *Clin Obstet Gynecol* 1993;36:279–301.

20. Soepatmi S. Developmental outcome of children of mothers dependent on heroin or heroin/methadone during pregnancy. *Acta Paediatr* 1994;404(Suppl 1):36–39.
21. Frank D, Bauchner H, Parker S, et al. Neonatal body proportionality and body composition after *in utero* exposure to cocaine and marijuana. *J Pediatr* 1990;117:622—626.
22. Racine A, Joyce T, Anderson R. The association between prenatal care and birth weight among women exposed to cocaine in New York City. *JAMA* 1993;270:1581–1586.
23. Shiono PH, Klebanoff MA, Nugent RP, et al. The impact of cocaine and marijuana use on low birth weight and preterm birth: a multicenter study. *Am J Obstet Gynecol* 1995;172:19–27.
24. Hanlon-Lindberg KM, Williams M, Rhim T, et al. Accelerated fetal lung maturity profiles and maternal cocaine exposure. *Obstet Gynecol* 1996;87:128–132.
25. Eriksson M, Zetterstrom R. Amphetamine addiction during pregnancy: 10 year follow-up. *Acta Paediatr* 1994;404(Suppl):27–31.
26. Oro AS, Dixon SD. Perinatal cocaine and methylamphetamine exposure: maternal and neonatal correlates. *J Pediatr* 1987;111:571–578.
27. Little BB, Snell LM, Gilstrap LC. Methylamphetamine abuse during pregnancy: outcome and fetal effects. *Obstet Gynecol* 1988;72:541–544.
28. Fried PA, Watkinson B, Willon A. Marijuana use during pregnancy and decreased length of gestation. *Am J Obstet Gynecol* 1984;150:23–27.
29. Leading article. Fetal alcohol syndrome. *Lancet* 1976;1:1335.
30. Hanson JW. Alcohol and the fetus. *Br J Hosp Med* 1977;18:126–130.
31. Coles CD. Impact of prenatal alcohol exposure on the newborn and the child. *Clin Obstet Gynecol* 1993;36:255–266.
32. Shubert P, Savage B. Smoking, alcohol and drug abuse. In: Jones DK, Steer PJ, Weiner CP, Craik BWB, eds. *High-Risk Pregnancy*. London: WB Saunders; 1994:51–66.
33. Wright JT, Waterson EJ, Barrison IG, et al. Alcohol consumption, pregnancy and low birth weight. *Lancet* 1983;1:663–665.
34. Sulaiman ND, Florey C du V, Taylor DJ, Ogston SA. Alcohol consumption in Dundee primigravidas and its effects on outcome of pregnancy. *Br Med J* 1988;296:1500–1503.
35. Halmesmaki E. Alcohol counselling of 85 pregnant problem drinkers: effect on drinking and fetal outcome. *Br J Obstet Gynaecol* 1988;95:243–247.
36. Forrest F, Florey C du V, Taylor D, McPherson F, Young JA. Reported social alcohol consumption during pregnancy and infants' development at 18 months. *Br Med J* 1991;303:22–26.
37. Golden NL, Kuhnert BR, Sokol RJ, et al. Phencyclidine use during pregnancy. *Am J Obstet Gynecol* 1984;148:254–259.
38. Smit BJ, Boer K, van Huis AM, et al. Cocaine use in pregnancy in Amsterdam. *Acta Paediatr* 1994; 404(Suppl):32–35.
39. Boer K, Smit BJ, van Huis AM, Hogerzeil NV. Substance use in pregnancy: do we care? *Acta Paediatr* 1994;404(Suppl):65–71.
40. Farkas AG, Colbert DL, Erskine KJ. Anonymous testing for drug abuse in an antenatal population. *Br J Obstet Gynaecol* 1995;102:563–565.
41. Rubin PC, Craig CF, Gavin K, Sumner D. Prospective survey of the use of therapeutic drugs, alcohol and cigarettes during pregnancy. *Br Med J* 1986;292:81–83.
42. Halliday HL, Murnaghan CA, Livingstone B, Malcolm S. The use of drugs, alcohol and cigarettes during pregnancy. *Br Med J* 1986;292:486–487.

DISCUSSION

Dr. Battaglia: The fetal alcohol syndrome, in the United States at least, is really confined to alcohol abuse as defined by the Diagnostic and Statistical Manual–III of the American Psychiatric Association, and those children with fetal alcohol syndrome are certainly severely developmentally handicapped, but again I don't know of any one who has followed them through to adolescence. Do you know of any long-term follow-up?

Dr. Doris Campbell: No, I don't know of any long-term follow-up directly on fetal alcohol syndrome. Fetal alcohol syndrome is the end of a spectrum ranging from normal growth, and we really don't know whether we are missing something more subtle with people who drink moderate amounts.

Dr. Talamantes: I wonder whether the effect of the fetal alcohol syndrome on development is not really a nutrition deficiency problem.

Dr. Stuart Campbell: I think not, because there are morphologic features in the fetus that wouldn't be caused by undernutrition.

Dr. Doris Campbell: There is animal work to suggest that there are direct effects of alcohol, when you maintain nutrition artificially. But in the human, we just don't know much about dietary intake coupled with heavy alcohol abuse in pregnancy.

Dr. Battaglia: I think there is a distinction between the baby who may have some effects of alcohol, which, I agree, could be nutritional, and the baby with effects that are clearly teratogenic. For example, this description of the hypoplasia of the middle part of the facies is a true teratogenic effect, and I don't think that has much to do with maternal nutrition. Of all the compounds Dr. Campbell reviewed, alcohol is the only one in animal studies that is clearly teratogenic, and it is a very interesting teratogen in that it acts beyond embryogenesis and has clear effects on fetal development in animals. So that makes it very interesting to get good neurologic and developmental studies in children, because you have effects at a time when the brain is moving cells around in late fetal life, and remodeling at that stage could have some important effects. The Institute of Medicine has just published a study reviewing fetal alcohol syndrome (National Academy Press, 1996), and one issue discussed was whether there is a specific behavioral disorder associated with classic fetal alcohol syndrome beyond simply a marked reduction in IQ. Some people believe that there is such a characteristic behavioral pattern; they seem to be children who as they get older can't assess risk, which gets them into a lot of problems in the school setting. But that isn't clear yet.

Dr. Doris Campbell: The Dundee group did not come up with any differential effect that could be ascribed to increasing the amount of alcohol, but they did point out that the numbers taking over 120 g/wk were very small, and the numbers taking over 120 g/wk in the third trimester were different from the numbers drinking over 120 g/wk in the first trimester. So there is not only the amount to take into account, there is also the changing pattern through pregnancy that could have differential effects.

Dr. Talamantes: It would be very interesting to look at the Japanese population, which does not have the enzyme to metabolize alcohol, and to look at what would happen in those children born from women who consume alcohol in Japan. That would be to me a very interesting study.

Dr. Grahnquist: What about twin studies and alcohol fetopathy?

Dr. Doris Campbell: I have not seen anything relating to twins.

Dr. Grahnquist: My reason for asking this is because I came across twins, and one of them had a clear alcohol fetopathy but the other one didn't, and the mother was a heavy drinker.

Dr. Doris Campbell: Abnormalities in twins are usually discordant and not concordant, so the distribution of blood to each twin comes into the picture as well, and even with monozygotic twins it is very uncommon to get concordance for abnormality.

Dr. Haschke: Any limit for daily alcohol consumption is questionable. Are there any data in relation to the drinking behavior of mothers? There are some mothers who drink continuously during the day, which results in a certain alcohol level in the body, and there are mothers who have periods of very heavy drinking, resulting in very high alcohol concentrations in the body, and then they slow down for a certain period. So there are different drinking types.

Dr. Doris Campbell: The only evidence that I saw relating to binge drinking was on teratogenicity in early pregnancy, when alcohol might be having a direct effect on the fetal cells developing at that time (1). I found no data relating to binge drinking later on in pregnancy.

Dr. Battaglia: That has important public health implications. Health education aimed at reducing drinking in pregnancy works very well for casual drinkers, but they are not the women producing babies with the fetal alcohol syndrome. Those are the very heavy drinkers who are often binge drinkers, and our evidence in the United States shows that you are not going to get anywhere with a public health message with that group. You have to have a different approach, but we don't know what. I don't know about Europe, but in the United States we could really criticize government agencies that support research, because there is a huge amount of money spent on men's drinking and how to treat it and there is very little spent on women's drinking and how to treat it.

Dr. Doris Campbell: There is another variable with alcohol use, and that is the type of drink and whether it is spirits, wine, or beer. Many drinks have contaminating substances that might also be involved.

Dr. Stuart Campbell: The relative reduction in the biparietal diameter related to alcohol intake was clearly important in the Finnish study (2). Did they measure other fetal variables? If there is a small head circumference related to the abdominal circumference, then that is of great significance, but if it is just intrauterine growth retardation, it may be of less significance.

Dr. Doris Campbell: No, they didn't measure any other parameters.

Dr. Battaglia: What would you hypothesize you would find on fetal velocimetry in the smoking mother, given the data that were presented on the development of the fetal capillary bed?

Dr. Stuart Campbell: It fits in with the work by John Kingdom, in which they found a decrease in the number of capillaries in the *terminal* villi. I suspect that it is related to impaired perfusion caused by the nicotine in the smoking, and that impaired perfusion eventually causes attrition of the capillaries in the tertiary villi and ultimately causes fetal hypoxia and centralization of flow to the fetal brain.

Dr. Soothill: We have shown a more than doubling of carboxyhemoglobin in the fetus, so I think oxygen delivery to the tissues is probably more relevant than transport across the placenta.

Dr. Doris Campbell: Some of the studies on smoking might explain the differences between smokers and non-smokers, but I wonder how you would explain the difference that has been found in birth weight when people stop smoking part way through the pregnancy?

Dr. Stuart Campbell: That would fit in with the carboxyhemoglobin story.

Dr. Soothill: Carboxyhemoglobin does seem to be trapped in the fetal circulation—it is more than double the maternal—and this has been shown in neonatal studies as well, presumably because of the high affinity of the fetal hemoglobin. It should be washed out over a period of a week or two, and therefore if oxygen delivery to the fetal tissues is reducing the growth, then that is one possibility.

Dr. Godfrey: With regard to alcohol, there are data from rats suggesting paternal effects of alcohol exposure before conception (3). And on the smoking data, there are very well-described differences in diet between smokers and non-smokers (4). Studies are currently in progress to address whether some of the effects of maternal smoking on fetal growth may be mediated through changes in the mothers' dietary intakes.

Dr. Doris Campbell: Studies in pregnancy have not found major differences in dietary intake between smokers and non-smokers (5,6).

REFERENCES

1. Ernhart CB, Sokol RJ, Martier S, et al. Alcohol teratogenicity in the human: a detailed assessment of specificity, critical period and threshold. *Am J Obstet Gynecol* 1987;156:33–39.
2. Halmesmaki E. Alcohol counselling of 85 pregnant drinkers: effect on drinking and fetal outcome. *Br J Obstet Gynaecol* 1988;95:243–247.
3. Abel EL. A surprising effect of paternal alcohol treatment on rat fetuses. *Alcohol* 1995;12:1–6.
4. Margetts BM, Jackson AA. Interactions between people's diet and their smoking habits: the dietary and nutritional survey of British adults. *Br Med J* 1993;307:1381–1384.
5. Thompson B, Skipper D, Fraser C, et al. Dietary intake of Aberdeen primigravidae in 1950/51 and 1984/85. *J Hum Nutr Diet* 1989;2:345–359.
6. Anderson AS, Campbell D, Shepherd R. Nutrition knowledge attitude to healthier eating and dietary intake in pregnant compared to non-pregnant women. *J Hum Nutr Diet* 1993;6:335–353.

Effects of Maternal Smoking on Placental Structure and Function

K. R. Page, P. Bush, D. R. Abramovich, *P. J. Aggett, M. D. Burke, and #T. M. Mayhew

*Departments of Biomedical Sciences and Obstetrics and Gynaecology, University of Aberdeen, Aberdeen; *Institute of Food Research, Norwich; #Department of Human Morphology, Nottingham University, Nottingham, Scotland, United Kingdom*

The adverse effect of maternal smoking on fetal birth weight is a well-established fact, but the role of the placenta in this phenomenon is not fully understood. During the last 4 years, we have determined the effects of smoking on placental structure and function in Aberdeen women. Mothers were interviewed and completed a questionnaire at their first antenatal clinic and again at their clinic at the 34th week of gestation. The questionnaires established smoking habit (including brand of cigarette smoked) and also determining factors that might confound the study, such as intake of alcohol and caffeine and exposure to environmental tobacco smoke. Medical records were kept, and only healthy subjects with normal uncomplicated pregnancies were included. Plasma cotinine was estimated from a blood sample taken at the 34th-week clinic (all procedures on this project had prior approval of the local ethics committee), and this was used as an objective measure of smoking habit. At delivery, maternal and fetal blood samples were taken and randomized samples of placental tissue were obtained for morphometry, enzyme and heavy metal analysis, and transport studies. Data are presented as the mean ± standard error of the mean. Birth weights of the children born to smokers were 3421 ± 59 g (n = 56), and to nonsmokers they were 3534 ± 75 g (n = 37).

EXPOSURE TO SMOKING

Fifty-eight percent of the patients recruited declared themselves to be smokers. Patient-declared smoking rate correlated significantly with plasma cotinine level, assayed by high-performance liquid chromatography (n = 86; $p < .001$, Spearman rank correlation analysis).

Smoking caused a marked induction in the activity of the cytochrome P_{450}-dependent enzyme ethoxyresorufin-O-de-ethylase (EROD). Activity measured as the mean rate of resorufin production from ethoxyresorufin in placental microsomes was 58.9 ± 12.9 pmol/mg/min in smokers (n = 24) and 5.2 ± 2.8 pmol/mg/min in nonsmokers (n = 14; $p < .001$, unpaired t test). We did not observe any correlation between quinone reductase activity and smoking (quinone reductase activity has been shown to be induced *in vitro* in first-trimester placental tissue by benzo[α]pyrene, a major component of cigarette smoke).

Cadmium is present in tobacco and may interfere with zinc metabolism. The cadmium and zinc content of the placental tissue was measured by inductively coupled plasma mass spectrometry. Smokers showed a significantly higher tissue cadmium content than nonsmokers (24 smokers, 24 nonsmokers; $p < .03$, paired Student's t test), and tissue cadmium content correlated with declared smoking rate (n = 48; $p < .01$, Spearman rank correlation analysis). There was, however, no correlation with smoking for tissue content of zinc or for placental metallothionein content (measured by the silver saturation method).

MORPHOMETRY

Systematic random samples of placental tissue were taken and fixed by immersion in 10% vol/vol formaldehyde. Fifteen classes of morphometric measurements, including surface areas, volumes, and thicknesses of placental tissue components, were examined, but only three of these showed changes correlated with smoking. The fractional volume of the chorionic villi occupied by stromal tissue was 48 ± 1.7% in nonsmokers (n = 11) and 52 ± 0.8% in smokers (n = 27; $p < .05$, unpaired Student's t test), and in the same samples stromal arithmetic mean thickness increased from 12 ± 0.4 μm to 13 ± 0.3 μm ($p < .01$, unpaired Student's t test). These two changes partly reflected a reduction in fetal capillary volume associated with smoking. This was 44 ± 6.3 cm^3 in mothers who smoked five cigarettes a day or less (n = 17), and 28 ± 2.6 cm^3 in mothers who smoked more than five cigarettes a day (n = 13; $p < .05$, unpaired Student's t test).

TRANSPORT STUDIES

The surface of the placenta in contact with maternal blood, the microvillous border, may provide the rate-determining step for the maternofetal transport of a number of different nutrients. We examined uptake of zinc and alanine by microvillous border vesicles prepared from our samples of placental tissue. No difference was observed between smokers and nonsmokers regarding zinc uptake, but there was a significant increase in the sodium-dependent component of alanine uptake of smokers (n = 17) compared with nonsmokers (n = 15; $p < .01$, two-way analysis of variance). Analysis using the Michaelis-Menten equation indicated that this increase was primarily the consequence of a change in maximal uptake rather than an increase in affinity. There was no association with smoking regarding sodium-independent uptake of alanine.

CONCLUSION

EROD activity and morphologic studies clearly indicate that smoking has significant effects on the placenta. The consequences of these effects on fetal development are less easily established. Maternal smoking reduces the fetal capillary volume within the placenta, which could have a detrimental effect on transport function, as it increases the diffusion distance between maternal and fetal blood. We have estimated the diffusive conductance of oxygen in the placenta from our morphometric data. Although our results seemed to show a 13% lower conductance in smokers compared with nonsmokers, this difference was too small to reach statistical significance. It is also possible that the placenta has the capacity to compensate for some of the effects of smoking. Our results show that cadmium derived from cigarette smoke is bound by placental tissues. Work on experimental animals has indicated that by binding cadmium, the placenta can act as a barrier protecting the fetus from environmental sources of this element. The induction of sodium-dependent alanine transport could also represent a change in placental function that would compensate for an adverse maternal environment produced by cigarette smoking. There remains a need to establish better the relative importance of these various factors on fetal growth.

ACKNOWLEDGEMENT

This work was supported by the Tobacco Products Research Trust.

Concluding Remarks

Dr. Battaglia: From my point of view, this conference has been very successful. It was timely to bring people together from basic research and clinical research. We covered a variety of new areas in methodology, ranging from molecular biology to clinically applicable techniques, that can be applied to learn much more about placental function and fetal nutrition. We have touched on how are we beginning to tackle the difficult problem of heterogeneity in growth retardation, and we have started to subdivide cases into more clinically homogeneous groups. That encourages me to think that we will be able to begin directing more specific therapy at subgroups, because it is really necessary first to have a homogeneous subgroup before you attempt therapy. If you try to improve fetal growth when retardation stems from 15 different causes, you can almost tell in advance that it will be unsuccessful, even though you have a few outliers who will be helped. So I think we are getting closer to this.

The discussions that followed each presentation were really excellent; that has been a major contribution to the meeting. Perhaps 5 or 6 years ago we wouldn't have been so careful in how we phrased the questions. Language is terribly important in science, and it is clear we have made progress. Only a few years ago, people were very sloppy in talking about placentation and its development, and in defining what they meant by intrauterine growth retardation. We have clearly gone a long way now in making our language more precise, so we are all talking about the same kinds of patients and the same kinds of problems. For me, this conference has been a real help in that regard. I think we were good in saying where our knowledge ends and where we begin to speculate—where we have hypotheses we would like to test, and that is also useful.

I would like to thank everyone involved. I would like to thank Nestlé for putting on this conference. I think I wrote to them about 7 years ago proposing the topic and I thought they had forgotten about it, but they are a very careful company and wrote me about 2 years ago to say that now is time to do this! It so happens the timing is very good. Young people who have come to this conference are, I hope, leaving recognizing that the tools are in place in the field of obstetrics to answer so many questions that we have posed for many years but now can go out and find definitive answers. One of my mentors used to remind me that it wasn't important to have the first word in the field, it was important to have the last word in the field—that your work should be definitive. I think we are getting to the point where we'll see a lot more definitive work around these obstetric problems, and it is very exciting. So I thank you all for participating, both speakers and observers.

Subject Index

A

Activin
  activity of, 66–67
  immunoreactivity of, 66
Adipose tissue
  lipolytic activity of
    fetal benefit from, 171
    maternal benefit from, 170, 171
    maternal metabolism and, 169–171
Alanine, uptake in smokers vs. nonsmokers, 248
Alcohol abuse
  fetal alcohol syndrome from, 240
  placental transport effect on nutrient transport in, 236
  reduction of amino acid transport with, 151
Alkaline phosphatase, role of, 70
Amino acid(s)
  branched-chain
    in intrauterine growth retardation, 150
    placental utilization of, 23–24
  D- and L-amino acid
    placental transfer of, 186–187, 190
  fetal arterial plasma concentrations, disposal, and clearances of, 53, 53t
  in fetal blood
    comparison in intrauterine growth retardation and appropriate-for-gestational-age, 194–195
  fetal hepatic vs. umbilical circulations, 48–49, 49f
  intrauterine growth retardation and, 194–195, 212
  isoleucine
    placental utilization of, 23
    umbilical venous plasma concentration of
      in IUGR fetuses, 194
    uptake of, uterine vs. umbilical, 22
  loss through villi, 17
  metabolism of, 48–49
  placental delivery of, 21–30
  serine
    conversion to glycine, 24–25
    fetal fluxes of, 51, 51f, 52
  uptake of
    comparison of uterine and umbilical, 21–22
    fetal liver-placental interorgan transport, 48–49
  utilization and production of vs. transport, 21–30
Amino acid transport, 47–48, 147–151
  in diabetic pregnancy, 216–217
  fetal liver-placental system exchange in, 47–48
  in intrauterine growth retardation, 149
  in normal pregnancy, 216
  by passive transfer vs. transporter facilitation, 186–187
  systems in, 148t
    basal membrane, 148
    coordination of, 148
    in fetal liver-placenta interaction, 47–48
    microvillus, 148
Amino acid transporter(s)
  classification of, 149
  in fetal growth, 144
  glutamate, 149
  glutamine, 149
  location of, 144
  molecular biology of, 154
  physiologic studies of, 149
  study techniques for
    cordocentesis, 150
    microvillus, 150
Amino acid transport systems, 148, 148t
  system A, 28–29, 148, 148t, 155
  system L, 148, 154
  system N, 148, 148t
Amphetamine abuse
  effect of
    on adult behavior, 239
    on fetal growth, 239

NOTE: *f* following page numbers indicates figures; *t* indicates tables.

Amphetamine abuse (*contd.*)
    placental transport effect on nutrient transport in, 236
Antiphospholipid antibodies syndrome
    intrauterine growth retardation and, 206–207
    preeclampsia in, 206
    treatment of and fetal growth, 206–209
        aspirin in, 208
        heparin in, 208
        intravenous immunoglobulins in, 206–207
        prednisone in, 208
Arachidonic acid
    in brain
        diet and, 165–166
        in fetal growth, 162
        synthesis of, 159
Aspirin, for antiphospholipid antibodies syndrome, 208
Asymptomatic intrauterine growth retardation (aIUGR). *See also* Intrauterine growth retardation (IUGR)
    definition of, 199
    24-hour maternal diastolic blood pressure monitoring in, 202–203
    maternal blood pressure increase and, 199–203, 210f

B

Birth weight, fatty acids relationship with, 162
Brain, fetal, lipid requirements of, 161
Branched-chain amino acid(s)
    alanine relationship with, 138–139
    deamination of, 23
    in intrauterine growth retardation, 150–151
    leucine, 23
    umbilical venous plasma concentration in intrauterine growth retarded fetuses, 194
    valine, 23

C

Cadmium 5
    binding to placenta, 249
    content in nonsmokers, 249
    interface with zinc metabolism, 248
Cannabis. *See* Marijuana (cannabis) abuse

Carcass analysis
    fall in fetal chloride content, 4, 4f
    of placental transfer of chloride, 2t, 4–5
Carnitine palmitoyltransferase-1 (CPT-1)
    gene expression during perinatal period, 109–110
    changes in, 110, 111f
    regulation of, 112f, 112–113
Carnitine palmitoyltransferase-2 (CPT-2)
    gene expression during perinatal period regulation of, 113–114
Carnitine palmitoyltransferase (CPT) system
    activity of, 108–109, 109f
Chloride
    placental transport of, 4–20
    role of, 3
    uptake into microvillous membrane vesicles, 9, 9f
Chloride transport channels, 10, 11t, 18
    carcass analysis of, 2t, 4f, 4–5
    comparison of first trimester and term, 18–19
    cystic fibrosis transmembrane conductance regulator in, 10, 11t, 18
    cytotrophoblast cells, 3t, 10
    driving forces for, 5t
    implications of, 14
    intact individual villi, 2t, 10
    mechanisms of, 10–12, 12f–13f
    molecular studies of, 3t, 10–11, 11t
    paracellular pathway in, 14, 20
    perfused human placenta in, 3t, 11–13, 13f
    research in, 19
    study techniques for, 4–20
        discussion of, 17–20
        utilization of, 14–15
    transplacental *vs.* paracellular, 12–13
    vesicle studies of, 3t, 8–9, 9f
    in vivo unidirectional fluxes in, 2t, 5–7, 7f–8f
Chloride transporters, 10–11, 11t
    DIDS-inhibitable, 9, 13, 20
Cholesterol, in pregnancy, 171–172, 172f
Cholesterol ester transfer protein (CEPT)
    activity of, 172
Choline phosphoglyceride long-chain polyunsaturated fatty acid, in fetal growth, 162
Cigarettes. *See* Tobacco smoking

Cocaine abuse
  effect on intrauterine growth, 151, 238–239
  nutrient transfer and impairment of, 238
  vs. tobacco smoking, 238–239
Conductance, in chloride transport, 10, 11t, 18
Corticotrophin releasing binding protein (CRH-BP), 66
Corticotrophin releasing hormone (CRH), activity of, 66
Cyclic adenosine monophosphate (c-AMP)
  effects of
    on carnitine palmitoyltransferase (CPT) 1 and 2 gene hepatic expression, 113–114
    on HMG-CoA hepatic gene expression, 114
Cysteine-methionine metabolism, 155
Cystic fibrosis, transport defect in placental tissues, 18
Cystic fibrosis transmembrane conductance regulator (CFTR), in chloride transport, 10, 11t, 18
Cystine aminopeptidase, role of, 70
Cytokines, 69, 70f
Cytotrophoblast cells, 70, 71
  chloride currents in, 10, 11t, 12f
  in chloride transport, 3t, 10

D

Diabetic rats
  first-generation offspring of
    insulin resistance in, 219–220
  glucose homeostasis and
    in first generation offspring, 222
    in second generation offspring, 222–223
    in third generation offspring, 223t, 223–224
  second-generation pregnant offspring of
    glucose intolerance in, 222–223
  third-generation offspring of
    hyperglycemia, hyperinsulinemia, macrosomia, hyperplasia in, 223
Docosahexaenoic acid (DHA)
  in brain
    diet and, 165–166
  in fetal membrane formation, 162–163
  synthesis of, 159

Drug abuse
  identification and incidence of, 231–232, 234t–235t
  placental transport effect on nutrient transport in, 233

E

Eicosanoids, in fetal development, 159
Endocrine function
  of cytokines, 69
  of enzymes, 69–70
  of growth factors, 69
  of neuropeptides, 64–69
  of polypeptide hormones, 62–64
  of steroid hormones, 59–62
  trophic peptide-hormone interactions, 59–74
Endothelin
  action of, 68, 68f
  description of, 68
  interactions of, 70f
  in progesterone release, 73
Enzymes
  controlling fatty acid oxidation and ketogenesis
    regulation of expression of, 107–114
  endocrine function of, 69–70
Epidermal growth factor (EGF) receptor, in trophoblast cell regulation, 37
Epidermal growth factors (EGFs), in progesterone release, 73
Essential fatty acids
  availability from maternal circulation
    fetal benefits from, 171
  effect on fetal lipid metabolism, 157
  fetal requirements for, 161
  head circumferences and, 167
  in maternal hypertriglyceridemia, 174
Estrogens
  estradiol, 62
  estriol, 62
  in maternal hyperlipidemia, 173
  production of, 62
  role of, 62
Ethoxyresorufin-*O*, de-ethylase (EROD), activity and smoking exposure, 247–248

F

Fatty acid oxidation
  expression of enzymes controlling, 107–114

Fatty acid oxidation (*contd.*)
  neonatal hepatic
    hormonal and nutrient control of, 111–114
Fatty acids
  accretion of
    in liver, 160
    in spinal column, 160
  effects of
    on carnitine palmitoyltransferase (CPT) 1 and 2 gene hepatic expression, 112f, 112–113
    liver gene expression and, 118–119
    peroxisome proliferator-activator protein and, 119
Fetal alcohol syndrome
  description of, 240
  effects of, 240
Fetal growth retardation. See Intrauterine growth retardation (IUGR)
Fetal liver-placental system interaction, 47–57
  amino acid in
    net uptake or release of, 48–49
    transport and metabolism of, 47–48
  glutamate exchange in, 52–53, 53t, 54, 54f
  glutamine exchange in, 52, 53
  serine-glycine exchange in, 49–52
Fick principle, in placental amino acid metabolism, 21–22
First trimester, chloride transport in, 18–19
Flux(es). See Amino acid(s); Chloride; Glucose
Follistatin (follicle stimulating hormone suppressing protein), activity of, 68
Food restriction, insulin levels and sensitivity with, 220–222, 222f
Free fatty acid, in adipose tissue lipolysis and effects, 170–171

G

GATA factors, in trophoblast cell regulation, 38–39
Gene expression
  regulation by nutrients during perinatal period, 103–121
    carnitine palmitoyltransferase system in, 108–114
    fatty acids in, 118–119
    glucose in, 120–121

Genomic imprinting, trophoblast cell development and, 33–34
Gestation. See First trimester; Pregnancy; Third trimester
Gestational hypertension. See Hypertension
Glucogenesis, premature, with maternal malnutrition, 218
Glucose
  bidirectional flux of, 145, 147
  gene expression activation by, 120–121
  high-carbohydrate diet replacement of in weanling rat, 219
  high-fat diet replacement of in neonatal rat, 218–219
  intrauterine growth retardation and, 212
  maternal-fetal gradient in normal intrauterine growth-restricted pregnancies, 192, 192f, 193f
  plasma concentrations of
    in offspring of diabetic and food-restricted rats, 219t
    in pregnant offspring and third generation fetuses, 233–234
  relationship of transplacental to umbilical glucose/oxygen quotient, 193, 194f
  restriction of
    intrauterine growth retardation and, 226–227
  umbilical venous-maternal arterial concentrations of, 192, 192f
  uptake of
    in fetal rat, 218
    in placenta of diabetic rats, 105, 106f
Glucose metabolic index, in muscle and tissue, 220, 221f
Glucose tolerance tests, in pregnancy, 211, 212
Glucose transport
  animal models of, 145–146
  in diabetic pregnancy, 216
  glucose transporters in, 143–144
  for growth-retarded fetus, 193
  in normal pregnancy, 215–216
  schematic representation of, 143, 144f
Glucose transporter(s) (GLUTs)
  activity of, 143–144
  differences in, 117
  expression of, 146
    impact of maternal diabetes on, 104–107
    regulation of, 103–104, 105f, 146
  GLUT-1, insulin upregulation of, 147

SUBJECT INDEX

GLUT-3, regulation of, hyperglycemia in, 106–107, 107f
  under intrauterine growth retardation conditions, 144–147
  localization in placenta, 117–118, 144
  in nondiabetic rats
    euglycemic-hyperinsulinemia and hyperglycemic-hyperinsulinemia clamp studies, 106–107, 108f
    ontogenesis of, placental, 104, 105f
    in perinatal period, 218, 219
    protein concentration and, 118
Glutamate
  fetal hepatic output of, 56–57
  fetal hepatic-placental exchange of, 52–53, 53t, 54, 54f
  role of, 149
  uptake of, 22
Glutamate transporters, 57
Glutamine
  fetal hepatic-placental exchange of, 52, 53, 54
  parturition and steroidogenesis linkage and, 56
  role of, 149
Glycerol, adipose tissue lipolysis and effects, 170
Glycine
  formation from serine, 24–25
  placental production of, 24–25
Gonadotropin releasing hormone (GnRH)
  activity of, 65–66
  secretion of, 65, 65f
Growth factors, 69, 70f
Growth hormone binding protein (GHBP), messenger RNA encoding of, 90
Growth hormone (GH)
  binding to receptor, 88, 88f
    initiation of signal transduction pathway via, 88, 88f
  in intrauterine growth, sheep fetus, 99–100
  in stimulation of tyrosine phosphorylation, 88, 89
Growth hormone receptors (GHRs), 88
  deficiency of, Laron syndrome, 98–99
  fetal, 89–93
  gene transcription in, 91f, 91–93, 92f
  messenger RNA encoding of, 89–90
  ovine fetal liver, 90–91
Growth hormone releasing hormone (GHRH), activity of, 67

Growth retardation. *See* Intrauterine growth retardation (IUGR)

H

Head circumference
  essential fatty acids and, 167
  neonatal, relationship with fatty acids, 162
Heparin, for antiphospholipid antibodies syndrome, 208
Hepatocyte growth factor/scatter factor (HGF/SF), in trophoblast cell regulation, 37
Heroin abuse
  vs. methadone
    effect on fetal growth and delivery, 237–238
    placental transport effect on nutrient transport in, 233
Hexokinase (HK)
  ontogenesis of, placental, 104, 105f
  regulation of expression of, 103–104
High-density lipoproteins (HDLs), in pregnancy, 171, 172f, 172–173
Hormone receptors, development within fetus, 85–101
Hormone(s)
  neuropeptide, 64–69
  polypeptide, 62–64
  pulsatile release of, 73
  steroid, 59–62
  human chorionic gonadotrophin (hCG)
    biosynthesis of, 63
    function of, 63
    placental weight and levels of, 60, 60f
    role of, 62–63
    secretion of, 63
    synthesis of, 63
Human growth hormone (hGH)
  amino acid sequence of, 77f
  placental, 64, 70f
Human growth hormone variant (hGH-V), amino acid sequence of, 77f
Human placental growth hormone variant (hPGH-V), 75–83
  amino acid sequence of, 77f
  biologic function of, 78–79
  correlation with insulin-like growth factor-1, 82
  description of, 75
  discovery of, 76

Human placental growth hormone variant
(hPGH-V) (contd.)
  future research directions, 79–80
  genes in, 75–76, 76f
  gestational profile of, 78
  localization of, 78
  structure of
    genes in, 76–77
    protein in, 77, 77f
Human placental lactogen (hPL)
    (somatomammotrophin)
  cross-reactivity of, 82
  description of, 63–64
  fetal liver binding sites for, 93
  glucose and, 227
  placental weight and levels of, 60, 60f
  secretion of, 63–64
Hydroxymethylglutaryl-coenzyme A
    (HMG-CoA), in regulation of gene
    expression during perinatal period,
    114
Hydroxymethylglutaryl-coenzyme A
    (HMG-CoA) synthase
  gene expression during perinatal
    period, 109–110
  changes in, 110, 111f
Hypercholesterolemia, preexisting, fetal
    protection against, 175–176, 176f
Hyperglycemia
  effects of
    on glucose-3 transporter, 118, 121
    on postnatal hepatic metabolism,
      119–120
  in regulation of glucose transporter-3,
    106–107, 107f, 108f, 118
Hyperinsulinemia/insulin resistance, in
    intrauterine growth retardation,
    significance of, 206
Hyperinsulinemia with hypertension
    (syndrome X)
  impaired gestational glucose tolerance
    in, 203
  insulin resistance in, 203
  mechanisms in, 205
Hyperlipidemia
  deviations in maternal and fetal growth
    and, 174–176, 175f
  maternal, 171–173
Hyperoxia
  maternal
    adverse effects for fetus, 135
    benefits for fetus, 134–135, 139
Hypertension
  insulinemia-associated
    insulin resistance and, 203
    mechanisms in, 205–206
  with intrauterine growth retardation
    definition of, 200
    results with 24-hour diastolic blood
      pressure evaluation, 201, 201f,
      202, 203
  without asymptomatic intrauterine
    growth retardation, 200, 201f
Hypertriglyceridemia
  maternal
    deviations in and fetal growth,
      174–176, 175f
    fetal benefits from, 174, 177
  in sucrose-rich diet, 175
Hypoaminoacidemia, reduction in fetal
    growth, 132, 133, 135
Hypoglycemia, fetal, from maternal
    hyperinsulinemia, 205–206
Hypoinsulinemia, fetal glucose uptake in,
    218
Hypoxemia. See Hypoxia
Hypoxia
  effects on fetus
    endocrine, 133–134
    for growth, 129, 129f, 130t, 131–132
    for supply of substrates, 132–133
  fetal
    with marijuana use, 239–240
  hyperoxia for, maternal, 134–135, 139
  maternal
    normobaric, endocrine consequences
      of, 133–134
    reduction of fetal branched-chain
      amino acids, 132, 135, 136

I

Illicit drugs, placental transport effect on
    nutrient transport and, 233–234,
    236
Inhibin
  activity of, 66–67, 67f
  immunoreactive and bioactive, 66–67,
    70f
Insulin
  action in perinatal period, 218–219
  levels and sensitivity with food
    restriction, 220–222, 222f
  plasma concentrations
    in offspring of diabetic and food-
      restricted rats, 219t, 219–220
    in pregnant offspring and third
      generation fetuses, 233–234
  upregulation of GLUT-1 by, 147

Insulin-like growth factor-binding protein (IGF-BP), for glucose transport, 154
Insulin-like growth factors (IGFs)
  action through insulin receptors, 101
  as hormonal mediators, 133–134
  IGF-2, in trophoblast cell regulation, 33, 34, 37, 43
  in intrauterine growth, 100–101
Insulin receptors
  in fetal rat, 218
  role of, 101
Insulin resistance
  in adult offspring of diabetic and food-restricted rats
    euglycemic insulinemic clamp studies of, 220
  maternal
    hyperinsulinemia and hypertension with, 203, 204
  in maternal hyperlipidemia, 173
Intrauterine growth retardation (IUGR), 143–155. *See also* Growth retardation
  amino acid transport in, 147–151
  animal models of, 215–230
    adult offspring of diabetic rats and, 219t, 219–224
    fetal endocrine pancreas and, 217
    heat stress in maternal ewe, 145–146, 150
    insulin action in, 218–219
  asymmetric, 145, 165
  asymptomatic, 199–203, 201f
  branched-chain amino acid transport changes in, 150–151
  causes of, 158
  classification of clinical severity in, 191–192
  etiologic factors in, 199, 200t
  fetal blood sampling for, 191
  fetal endocrine pancreas in, 217
  fetomaternal concentration of amino acids and total α-amino nitrogen and, 194–195, 195f
  glucose in, 192f, 192–193, 193f, 194f. *See also* Glucose
    restriction of, 226–227
  glucose transporters in, 144–147
  insulinemia-hypertension association in, 203–206, 204f
  long-term consequence of, 215–230

  mortality and morbidity risk with, 158–159
  nutrient transport and
    in diabetic pregnancy, 216–217
    in normal pregnancy, 215–216
  placental transport in, 143–155
Intrauterine growth-retarded (IUGR) fetuses
  reduced endocrine pancreas tissue in, 223, 228
Intrauterine growth-retarded (IUGR) perinate
  definition of, 157–158
Intravenous immunoglobulins (IVIG)
  for antiphospholipid antibodies syndrome
    effect on fetal growth, 206–207, 207f, 208–209

K
Ketogenesis
  expression of enzymes controlling, 107–114
  neonatal hepatic
    hormonal control and nutrient control of, 111–114
Ketone bodies
  fetal benefits from, 171
  hypertriglyceridemia and, 174, 177

L
Laron syndrome (growth hormone receptor deficiency), 98–99
Leucine
  disposal of, 195, 196f
  fetal oxidation of, 150
  in intrauterine growth retardation, 150
  maternal heat stress effect on, 150, 155
  transplacental transfer of
    in appropriate-for-gestational-age and small-for-gestational-age babies, 187
  transport of
    in intrauterine growth-retarded *vs.* control animals, 23–24, 27
    protein synthesis and, 28, 29
  umbilical flow of
    in appropriate-for-gestational-age and small-for-gestational-age fetuses, 187

Leucine (*contd.*)
   umbilical venous-maternal arterial plasma concentrations of, 195, 196f
   umbilical venous plasma concentration of
      in intrauterine growth-retarded fetuses, 194
   uptake of
      in appropriate-for-gestational-age fetuses, 185–186
   uterine *vs.* umbilical, 22
   utilization of
      fetal, 23–24, 27, 28, 29
      placental, 23
Linoleic acid, in arachidonic acid synthesis, 159
Linolenic acid, in docosahexaenoic acid synthesis, 159
Lipids. *See also specific, e.g. Low-density lipoproteins (LDLs)*
   endogenous synthesis of, fetal, 160
   in fetal growth
      hormonal control of, 163
      requirements for, 161
      role of, 159
   maternal metabolism of
      fetal growth and, 169–182
      during late gestation, 170f, 170–171
   placental transfer, 160, 161
Lipogenesis, maternal adipose tissue and, 169–170
Lipolysis
   of adipose tissue
      free fatty acid and, 170–171
      glycerol and, 170
      products of, circulation, 170f, 170–171
Lipoprotein:cholesterol ratio, in pregnancy, 171–172, 172f
Lipoprotein lipase (LPL), in pregnancy, 173
Lipoprotein:triglyceride-to-cholesterol ratio, in third trimester, 171, 172f
Liver
   fetal
      lipid requirements of, 161
   neonatal rat
      fatty acid oxidation in, 107–108
      ketogenesis and, 108, 109f
Long-chain fatty acids (LCFAs)
   fetal requirements for, 161
   oxidation of
      in neonatal rat liver, 108, 109f
   polyenoic, in fetal growth, 162
   polyunsaturated, in brain, 161
Low-density lipoproteins (LDLs), in pregnancy, 171, 172, 172f
Lung surfactant glycerophospholipid, fetal, hormone regulation of, 163

M

Macrosomia, maternal diabetes and, 223, 228
Malnutrition
   fetal
      hepatic insulin resistance with, 221
   maternal
      fetal endocrine pancreas and, 217
      intrauterine growth retardation from, 212, 217, 222
      small-for-gestational-age fetuses and, 212
Mannitol, transplacental transfer of, in appropriate-for-gestational-age and small-for-gestational-age babies, 187, 189
Marijuana (cannabis) abuse
   effect of
      assessment of neonates, 239–240
      on gestation, 239
      placental transport effect on nutrient transport in, 236
Mash-2, in trophoblast cell regulation, 38, 43–44
Maternal vascular disease and fetal growth, 199–213
Methadone, placental transport effect on nutrient transport and, 233
Methionine, transport of, 155
Microvillous membrane
   in chloride transport studies, 2t, 10
   transporter systems of, 148
   vesicle studies of
      chloride kinetics in, 8–9, 9f
      power of, 9
Molecular mechanisms of placental development, 31–45
   trophoblast cell in
      development of, 33–34
      lineage of, 31–32, 32t
      regulatory genes of, 36–39
Molecular studies, of chloride transport, 3t, 10–11

N

Neuropeptide(s)
  activin, 66–67
  corticotrophin releasing hormone, 66
  endocrine function of, 69–70
  endothelin, 68
  folliculostatin, 68
  gonadotrophin releasing hormone, 65–66
  growth hormone releasing hormone, 67
  inhibin, 66–67
  interactions of, 70f
  placental vs. hypothalamic, 64–65
  somatostatin, 67
Neurotransmitters, placental, 69
Nicotine, plasma level of, 247
Nutrient transport
  in diabetic pregnancy, 216–217
  illicit drug transport effect on, 233–234, 236. See also specific drug, e.g., Cocaine abuse
  in normal pregnancy, 215–216
Nutrition, in fetus of substance abusers, 236–240

O

Opiate abuse
  effect of
    on fetal growth and delivery, 237–238
    on placental and nutrient transport, 233
Oxygen
  allometric relationship, 139–140
  consumption of and protein metabolism, 183–190
    in appropriate-for-gestational-age fetuses, 185–186
  fetal consumption of, 184–185
    body mass in prediction of, 184–185
    at elective cesarean delivery, 183–190
  role in implantation process, 140–141
Oxygenation in utero
  fetal requirements and, 123, 127f, 128–135
  placental determinants of
    factors influencing, 124t, 124–125
    ontogenic changes in oxygen transfer and characteristics, 125–126
    relation between placental growth and delivery to fetus, 126f, 126–127, 128f
  reduction of
    consequences for fetus, 129, 129f, 130t, 131–134
    therapeutic approaches to, 134–135

P

Pancreas, fetal endocrine, intrauterine growth retardation and, 217
Phenylalanine
  fetal
    reduction in maternal hypoxemia, 132, 135, 136
    uptake and disposal in appropriate-for-gestational-age babies, 185–186
  transplacental transfer of
    in appropriate-for-gestational-age and small-for-gestational-age babies, 187
Phospholipids, in pregnancy, 171–172, 172f
Placenta
  in amino acid delivery, 21–30
  development of
    molecular mechanisms of, 31–45
  insufficiency of
    in antiphospholipid antibodies syndrome, 207–208
  perfused
    in chloride transport, 2t, 11–13, 13f
  size of
    correlation with fetal liver size, 48f, 447
Placental lactogen (PL)
  in activation of JAK2/Stat signal transduction pathway, 95–96
  binding sites for
    fetal liver, 93
  function of, 86–87
  in growth hormone-growth hormone receptor binding, 88, 88f, 95–96, 100
  interaction with growth hormone receptors, 94
  modulation of maternal and fetal metabolism by, 87
  sites of action of, 86, 86f
  structure of, 85–86
  study limitations and, 87
Placental lactogen receptor (PLR), 87–88
  fetal, 93–96
  growth hormone receptor and, 88

Placental lactogen (*contd.*)
  as growth hormone receptor variant, 94–95, 95f
  structural identity of, 94–95, 95f
Placental transfer, in appropriate-for-gestation-age and small-for-gestation-age fetuses, 186–187
Placental transport
  analysis of, 1–2
  approaches to
    homeostatic, 3, 3t
    orientation maintained, 2t, 3
    orientation not maintained, 3, 3t
  of chloride
    study of, 4–20
  in fetal growth retardation, 143–155. *See also* Intrauterine growth retardation (IUGR)
  of illicit drugs, 232–233, 236
    effect on nutrient transport, 233–234, 236
  maternofetal *vs.* transplacental, 1
  study techniques for, 1–20
  substance abuse effect on, 151
Polypeptide hormone(s)
  endocrine function of, 62–63
  human chorionic gonadotrophin, 62–64, 70f
  human growth hormone, 64, 70f
  human placental lactogen, 63–64
  interactions with trophic peptides, 70f
Prednisone therapy, for antiphospholipid antibodies syndrome, 208
Preeclampsia
  in antiphospholipid antibodies syndrome, 206
  with intrauterine growth retardation
    24-hour diastolic blood pressure monitoring results, 201, 201f, 202
    identification of, 200, 201, 202
  normotensive, 213
Pregnancy
  drug abuse in
    fetal nutrition in, 236–240
    identification of, 231–232
    incidence of, 234t–235t
  nutrient transport in
    diabetic, 216–217
    normal, 215–216
Pregnenolone
  progesterone and, 61
  in progesterone production, 61
Progesterone
  metabolism of, 61, 61f

pregnenolone and, 61
production of, 60f, 60–61
role of, 59–60
section of
  modulation of, 66–67, 67f
Protein metabolism and oxygen consumption, 183–190
Protein(s)
  for glucose transporters, 117
  placental
    turnover of, 186
    synthesis of
      amino acid delivery rate and, 187, 190
  transporter, 17

R
Renin, role of, 69–70

S
Serine
  fetal
    fluxes of, 51, 51f, 52
    reduction in maternal hypoxemia, 132, 135, 136
  in glycine formation, 24–25, 28
  maternal plasma, 51
  placental
    metabolism of, 24, 26
    uptake of, 50–51
Serine-glycine exchange, fetal hepatic and placental, 49–52, 50f, 51f
Serine-to-glycine transfer, placental, 24–25, 28
Smoking. *See* Tobacco smoking
Somatomammotropin. *See* Human placental lactogen (hPL) (somatomammotropin)
Somatostatin, activity of, 67
Stat proteins, in signal transduction cascade, 88f, 89
Steroid hormone(s)
  biosynthesis of, 61f
  estrogens, 62
  progesterone, 59–61, 60f, 61f
Syncytiotrophoblast cells, in placental development, 32, 32t, 33, 70, 71, 73
Syndrome X (insulin resistance and hypertension in gestational diabetes), 211

T

Thing-1/*Hxt*/*e*-HAND, in trophoblast cell regulation, 38
Third trimester, maternal plasma lipoprotein:triglyceride-to-cholesterol in, 171, 172f
Tobacco smoking *vs.* cocaine use
  effect on intrauterine growth, 238–239
  effects on placental structure and function, 247–249
Tobacco use, intrauterine growth restriction with, 151
Triglycerides
  accumulation in lipoproteins
    hormonal factors in, 173
    during late gestation, 172–173, 173f
  in pregnancy, 171–172, 172f
Trophoblast cell development
  discovery of genes pivotal to, 34–36, 44
  genomic imprinting and, 33–34
  insulin growth factor-2 gene in, 33
  Mash-2 gene in, 33
  nutrition and, 44–45
  strategies for discovery of genes pivotal to
    gene targeting, 35–36
    transgenic, 32
    in vivo, 34–35
Trophoblast cell lineage, 31–33, 32f
  extravillous, 32t, 33
  future research in, 39–40
  human, 32, 32t, 33
  intravillous, 32t, 32–33
  rodent, 32
Trophoblast cell lines
  placenta-derived, 34
  tumor-derived, 35
  virally transformed, 34–35
Trophoblast cells
  cytotrophoblast, 32, 32t
  syncytial, 32, 32t, 33

Trophoblast regulatory genes
  cytoplasmic signaling components, 37–38
  extracellular signal/receptor systems, 36–37
  nuclear signaling factors, 38–39
  putative, 36t, 36–39
Tyrosine
  phosphorylation of, 88, 89
  reduction in fetal
    in maternal hypoxia, 132, 135, 136

U

Uteroplacental perfusion, fetal effects of reduction in, 228, 229

V

Valine
  placental utilization of, 23
  umbilical venous plasma concentration of
    in IUGR fetuses, 194
  uptake of, uterine *vs.* umbilical, 22
Vascular cell adhesion molecule-1 (VCAM-1), in trophoblast cell regulation, 37
Very-low-density lipoprotein (VLDL) triglycerides
  in pregnancy, 171–172, 172f
  production and plasma increase of, 172, 173f

Z

Zinc
  metabolism of cadmium, 248
  uptake in smokers *vs.* nonsmokers, 248